T0177668

Exploiting Hope

Exploiting Hope

*How the Promise of New Medical
Interventions Sustains Us—and Makes
Us Vulnerable*

JEREMY SNYDER

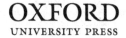

OXFORD
UNIVERSITY PRESS

OXFORD
UNIVERSITY PRESS

Oxford University Press is a department of the University of Oxford. It furthers
the University's objective of excellence in research, scholarship, and education
by publishing worldwide. Oxford is a registered trade mark of Oxford University
Press in the UK and certain other countries.

Published in the United States of America by Oxford University Press
198 Madison Avenue, New York, NY 10016, United States of America.

© Oxford University Press 2021

All rights reserved. No part of this publication may be reproduced, stored in
a retrieval system, or transmitted, in any form or by any means, without the
prior permission in writing of Oxford University Press, or as expressly permitted
by law, by license, or under terms agreed with the appropriate reproduction
rights organization. Inquiries concerning reproduction outside the scope of the
above should be sent to the Rights Department, Oxford University Press, at the
address above.

You must not circulate this work in any other form
and you must impose this same condition on any acquirer.

Library of Congress Cataloging-in-Publication Data
Names: Snyder, Jeremy, author.
Title: Exploiting hope : how the promise of new medical interventions
sustains us—and makes us vulnerable / Jeremy Snyder.
Description: New York, NY : Oxford University Press, [2021] |
Includes bibliographical references and index.
Identifiers: LCCN 2020016482 (print) | LCCN 2020016483 (ebook) |
ISBN 9780197501252 (hardback) | ISBN 9780197501283 (epub) |
ISBN 9780197501269
Subjects: MESH: Therapies, Investigational—ethics | Ethics, Clinical |
Hope | Fraud—ethics | Physician-Patient Relations—ethics | Trust
Classification: LCC R724 (print) | LCC R724 (ebook) | NLM WB 60 |
DDC 174.2/8—dc23
LC record available at https://lccn.loc.gov/2020016482
LC ebook record available at https://lccn.loc.gov/2020016483

This material is not intended to be, and should not be considered, a substitute for medical or other
professional advice. Treatment for the conditions described in this material is highly dependent on
the individual circumstances. And, while this material is designed to offer accurate information
with respect to the subject matter covered and to be current as of the time it was written, research
and knowledge about medical and health issues is constantly evolving and dose schedules for
medications are being revised continually, with new side effects recognized and accounted for
regularly. Readers must therefore always check the product information and clinical procedures with
the most up-to-date published product information and data sheets provided by the manufacturers
and the most recent codes of conduct and safety regulation. The publisher and the authors make no
representations or warranties to readers, express or implied, as to the accuracy or completeness of
this material. Without limiting the foregoing, the publisher and the authors make no representations
or warranties as to the accuracy or efficacy of the drug dosages mentioned in the material. The
authors and the publisher do not accept, and expressly disclaim, any responsibility for any liability,
loss, or risk that may be claimed or incurred as a consequence of the use and/or application of any of
the contents of this material.

1 3 5 7 9 8 6 4 2

Printed by Integrated Books International, United States of America

Contents

Acknowledgments

I would like to thank my family for their support while writing this book and, especially, Leigh Anne Palmer for helping me to refine these ideas over the last 15 years. Anonymous editors provided extremely useful feedback on earlier versions of chapters two and five that were published in *Business Ethics Quarterly* and *Bioethics*, respectively. Thanks to participants in a workshop on "Theoretical Explorations of Exploitation in Practice" for comments on an earlier version of chapter four and members of the New York University Working Group on Compassionate Use and Preapproval Access for comments on chapter seven. Lucy Randall and Hannah Doyle helped guide my manuscript through publication and Audrey McClellan prepared the index. Finally, Iva Cheung did enormous work in improving the clarity and consistency of my ideas throughout the book.

Introduction

"Hope" is the thing with feathers -
That perches in the soul -
And sings the tune without the words -
And never stops—at all -
And sweetest—in the Gale—is heard -
And sore must be the storm -
That could abash the little Bird
That kept so many warm—[1]

BUSHY: Despair not, madam.
QUEEN: Who shall hinder me?
  I will despair, and be at enmity
  With cozening hope: he is a flatterer,
  A parasite, a keeper-back of death,
  Who gently would dissolve the bands of life,
  Which false hope lingers in extremity.[2]

Hope takes many forms. In Emily Dickinson's well-known poem, it sustains and supports people in desperate situations so that they might arrive at a better future. But for Shakespeare's Queen, hope—and false hope in particular—only serves its own ends by prolonging and worsening suffering. In Gustav Klimt's Hope I, which forms the cover for this book, a pregnant woman personifies new life and hope for the future. But this hope creates a vulnerability to loss represented by the skull, diseased faces, and sharp-toothed monster lurking in the background of the painting. Hope protects from despair and defeat but also leads some to deny the limitations of their difficult present, making them vulnerable to exploitation by those who would sell the promise of hope without the reality of its protections.

The power of hope to both give us strength and make us vulnerable to exploitation often appears in popular culture. In John Steinbeck's *The Grapes of Wrath*, the Joad family flees the environmental and economic devastation of Dust Bowl Oklahoma for the promise of a better life in California. As the family prepares to set off, they experience the dual nature of hope. Ma, the matriarch, tells her son Tom that "I hope things is all right in California." She worries that it

seems too nice, kinda. I seen the han'bills fellas pass out, an' how much work they is, an' high wages an' all; an' I seen in the paper how they want folks to come an' pick grapes an' oranges an' peaches. That'd be nice work, Tom, pickin' peaches. Even if they wouldn't let you eat none, you could maybe snitch a little ratty one sometimes. An' it'd be nice under the trees, workin' in the shade. I'm scared of stuff so nice. I ain't got faith. I'm scared somepin ain't so nice about it.[3]

Ma has good reason to be scared of her hope for a better life in California. On the way there, several members of the Joad family leave the group or die. When they finally reach California, they find that many other refugees have arrived before them and that powerful farming interests have worked to make sure that their labor will be exploited and that labor organizing will be disrupted. Even before leaving for California, Ma and Tom are aware of the vulnerability that this hoped-for life creates for them. Ma describes how "it's gonna be, maybe, in California. Never cold. An' fruit ever'place, an' people just bein' in the nicest places, little white houses in among the orange trees." Tom responds, "It done you good jus' thinkin' about it." At the same time, he mentions a friend from California who "says they's too many folks lookin' for work right there now. An' he says the folks that pick the fruit live in dirty ol' camps an' don't hardly get enough to eat. He says wages is low an' hard to get any." In response, a "shadow crossed" Ma's face. She objects, saying that there must be work in California because she's seen advertisements for workers, and it wouldn't make sense to pay for advertisements if there were no need for workers. Tom doesn't have the heart to push back against this hope, responding

> "I don't know, Ma. It's kinda hard to think why they done it.
> Maybe—" He looked out at the hot sun, shining on the red earth.
>   "Maybe what?"
>   "Maybe it's nice, like you says."

Hope for a better life sustains the Joads and gives them purpose. Hope also sets them up for suffering, exploitation, and death. On the one hand, their life in Oklahoma offers no hope and only the promise of unemployment, hunger, and jail. On the other hand, less hope and more realism might have led the Joads to try their luck elsewhere or to be more cautious as they set out for California. This duality of hope—providing sustenance and purpose while making us vulnerable to exploitation and other harms—raises the question of how the value of hope can be taken seriously and even promoted while protecting the hopeful from themselves and from those who see others' hope as an opportunity for their own benefit.

Why an Examination of Exploiting Hope Matters

We often hear stories of people like the Joads who find themselves in terrible and seemingly intractable situations and who are then preyed upon by those offering empty or unrealistic promises of a better life. Frequently these cases are condemned in terms of "exploiting the hope" of another. These accusations are made in a range of contexts, including offers of jobs, safe harbor in another community, and medical interventions. The concept of exploiting hope does heavy lifting in public discourse, identifying a specific form of unethical conduct. However, it is typically unclear why, exactly, "exploiting hope" is considered wrong, what activities can accurately be captured under this concept, and what should be done to protect against this form of wrongdoing. Thus, it is an ethical concept ripe for extended analysis and discussion.

In this book, I offer a close study of the concept of exploiting hope. First, I examine this concept in the abstract. I then apply it to a range of activities in the context of unproven medical interventions. The first half of the book examines how "exploiting hope" is used popularly and then closely analyzes competing understandings of "hope" and "exploitation." This theory-based section culminates in my own account of what it is to exploit hope and when and why doing so is morally problematic. This general account is then used to offer lessons about how to combat such exploitation. In the second half of the book, I examine how hope for improved health from unproven medical interventions can be exploited—by researchers enrolling participants in clinical trials, companies selling unproven stem cell interventions, politicians promising access to experimental medical interventions, and ill individuals and their supporters seeking financial aid for unproven interventions through crowdfunding.

Conceptual Background

While the concept of exploitation is historically associated with Karl Marx, I will generally not focus on his understanding of this concept. Marx's discussion of exploitation is linked to his oft-criticized labor theory of value and the perceived coerciveness of the capitalist economic system. But Marx's argument that justice and rights language is "outdated verbal rubbish" and "ideological nonsense"—as well as his occasional dismissal of the validity of moral claims—casts doubt on whether Marx can be a fruitful source for my account of the moral wrongness of exploiting hope.[4] Nonetheless, some have used Marx's work to inform contemporary accounts of exploitation's ethical dimensions. These interpretations of Marxian exploitation claim that it is morally problematic because it entails (a) taking advantage of an injustice, (b) generating an unfair distribution of resources, or (c) merely using another person.

In the first camp, G. A. Cohen suggests that we can locate the wrongness of exploitation in capitalists' lack of reciprocity—that is, in taking the surplus labor of the worker, capitalists seem to be getting something for nothing.[5] At the very least, Marx's language comparing exploitation to theft indicates that the capitalist economic system is *unjust* when compared with some independent moral standard because capitalism does not ever consider wage labor to be theft. More generally, we can understand exploitation as taking some benefit owed to the worker, thus benefiting from a wrong or injustice. Allen Buchanan notes that comparing exploitation to theft merely pushes the question of what is morally wrong with exploitation on to another, unexplored theory of justice.[6] But whatever this account of justice might be, we can see in Marx an account of exploitation where wrongfully taking advantage of or benefiting from another's vulnerabilities amounts to benefiting from an injustice experienced by another person.

Instead of understanding exploitation as theft, and more generally as a kind of wrong or injustice, we can look instead to the *fairness* of the resource distribution resulting from exploitative relationships. Jon Elster writes that, following Marx's *Critique of the Gotha Programme*, we can understand the appropriation of surplus labor to be wrong unless it is used to meet the needs of those unable to address their own needs. In this case, exploitation is primarily a problem of an unfair distribution of resources. According to Marx, when a society does not live by the slogan "from each according to his ability, to each according to his needs," then its system of resource distribution must rely on exploitation, since the surplus labor of workers is neither returned to them nor given to the neediest. In particular, Elster argues that a person is exploited if "(i) he does not enjoy the fruits of his own labour and (ii) the difference between what he makes and what he gets cannot be justified by redistribution according to need."[7] Locating the wrongness of exploitation in an unfair distribution has the advantage of capturing the notion that the exploiter receives too large a share of the social surplus of an interaction.

Finally, Allen Buchanan suggests that we can locate the wrongness of exploitation within the immorality of treating people as a *mere means* to some end or as an object of mere use. Under this view, the economic relations established by a capitalist economic system contaminate the relationships between individuals outside of labor interactions. The result of these economic relationships is that, "in the labor process, the worker sells the use of his capacities, the control over his mind and body to the capitalist. Thus the labor process accustoms the worker to think of human capacities as saleable. Further, the use of money makes it possible to price and purchase all human capacities—sexual capacities as well as capacities for industrial operations in the labor process."[8] For Buchanan, this process of exploitation is closely connected to Marx's concept of alienation. In the first place, the capitalist economic system alienates the worker from their product by forcing them to sustain a system that provides only for their subsistence while providing the means for their continued subservience. By laboring in the capitalist system, the worker's wage labor "alienates the worker from creative, self-conscious productive activity by robbing him of control over his actions, exhausting his body, and stunting his mind. In this activity, the capitalist utilizes the worker as a mere means, as an alien being, not as a fellow human being with human capacities which must be nurtured if they are to develop."[9] Whether or not this interpretation precisely reflects the original intent of Marx, it does capture another common view of the wrongness of exploitation. By failing to support the uniquely human needs of the worker, exploitative activity demeans that person.

Recent interest in the concept of exploitation was largely sparked by Alan Wertheimer's highly influential book *Exploitation*.[10] Wertheimer focuses on cases of voluntary and mutually beneficial exploitation to develop an account of the wrongness of exploitation distinct from coercion or other forms of involuntariness and outright harms against a baseline of no interaction between the exploiter and exploitee. His general approach to the wrongness of exploitation focuses on how some interactions present an opportunity for exploiters to benefit unfairly from an exchange, to the detriment of the exploitee. Unlike some interpretations of Marx, unfairness in this sense can be tied to a hypothetical fair-market price that sets a baseline for the typical distribution of benefits from an interaction. For example, a market can set a baseline price for the services of a tugboat, and a tugboat captain could exploit passengers of a sinking ship by deviating from that price to derive an unfair benefit from their situation. Wertheimer is clear, however, that a fair-market price is only one means of defining fairness and would not be appropriate across all interactions. More generally, unfairness occurs when one takes special advantage of a situation to receive an unusual gain.

Wertheimer's book led to a reinvigoration of scholarship on the concept of exploitation, applied to a diverse range of topics in ethical and political theory, medicine, business, and elsewhere. Specifically, the focus on voluntary and mutually beneficial interactions, while not denying that exploitation often takes place in a context of coercion and harm, helped to popularize the idea that exploitation is a distinct form of moral wrongdoing. Other authors followed this lead, providing accounts of the distinct moral character of exploitation—some tied to Wertheimer's fairness-based account and others offering alternative understandings of exploitation. Most notably, Ruth Sample's alternative to Wertheimer's account is in line with some interpretations of Marx's understanding of exploitation. Specifically, she argues that exploitation is a form of degradation or failure of respect for others, constituted by neglecting what is necessary for others' well-being, taking advantage of an injustice, or inappropriately commodifying some aspect of another person.[11]

Other authors have followed Sample's lead, offering accounts of exploitation that are not tied to how fairly the interaction's benefits are distributed, but Wertheimer's account of exploitation as unfairness has dominated contemporary discussion of the concept. Frequently in discussions of exploitation in health and business, authors take it for granted that exploitation is taking unfair advantage of another person and use Wertheimer as a default account of exploitation to support this view. Although Wertheimer is clear that a hypothetical fair-market price is only one way to understand fairness in exploitation, these authors frequently adapt this narrow understanding to a wide array of cases. The example of this phenomenon most relevant to this book is found in Adrienne Martin's well-developed account of exploiting hope, in which she treats exploiting hope as synonymous with taking unfair advantage of hope and uses a hypothetical fair market price to create a standard of fairness.[12]

One of my aims in this book, in addition to developing and applying an account of exploiting hope, is to challenge the idea that exploitation should generally be understood as taking unfair advantage of another person. In my previous work on exploitation, I have argued that exploitation should be understood as taking at least three different forms: (1) taking advantage of unfairness within discrete transactions or transactional fairness; (2) taking advantage of unjust structural conditions or structural fairness; (3) and taking advantage of another person as disrespecting them. These include some version of Wertheimer's fairness-based account but also understandings of exploitation more like Sample's, including taking advantage of injustice and failing to meet others' basic needs. Unfairness in discrete transactions, as Wertheimer shows, is effective at explaining the wrongness of exploitation in market exchanges. However, it is more problematic in other respects, including understanding concerns about exploitation against a backdrop of systemic injustice and in more intimate, non-transactional relationships. Not surprisingly, accounts of exploitation as taking unfair advantage of systemic injustice are effective at explaining ongoing, systemic exploitation such as takes place in global manufacturing practices that pay workers less than a living wage. But these accounts are largely limited to the context of transactions against a backdrop of large-scale injustice.

I have previously argued that a respect-based account of exploitation, where individuals fail to act on a specified obligation of beneficence to others, constitutes a third form of exploitation. These three accounts of exploitation are compatible with one another and all are needed to develop a full understanding of the wrongfulness of exploitation across a range of contexts and interactions. However, part of my positive argument in this book is to make the case that this third form of exploitation should be viewed as the most central understanding of exploitation and that the other two forms of exploitation can be understood to flow from this overarching account. Specifically, I will argue that exploitation can be understood as taking advantage of a partial entrustment of another person's well-being. In cases of transactional exploitation that Wertheimer discusses, this entrustment can be seen largely in terms of a duty of rescue that we all share. When we take advantage of unusual deviations from market prices for goods or services necessary to one's well-being, we are taking advantage of a specific vulnerability and failing in this duty of rescue. In the context of systemic injustice, exploitation can be understood as failing in an obligation to promote justice for specific individuals.

Entrustment tells the story of specific, relational obligations. Fairness-based accounts of exploitation are more general. But transactional fairness as in Wertheimer's account is tied to discrete vulnerabilities and contexts that serve, as with a duty of rescue, to entrust certain individuals with others' welfare. And, as I will argue, taking advantage of injustice should be understood as a failure to fulfill specific, political responsibilities that are derived from our relationships to those made vulnerable by these injustices. While these political responsibilities take a different form than partial entrustment with the welfare of certain others, they both involve taking on specified responsibilities for others that are derived from our relationships and context. As I develop and apply my account of exploiting hope, then, I will also make the larger argument that exploitation is best understood as failing to act on the responsibilities in which we are entrusted, choosing instead to benefit unduly from this entrustment.

Outline of the Book

This book is divided into two halves: in the first half I develop a theory-based account of exploiting hope, and in the second half I apply this theory to specific cases where hope was exploited in the development or provision of scientifically unproven or experimental medical interventions. Each half of this book is divided into four chapters.

In the **Chapter 1**, I present and analyze popular uses of "exploiting hope" and its variants, drawn from the press. My aim is to understand how this term is used, to help ensure that my own, theory-driven account is connected to popular use. This is not to say that my own account must mesh fully with the popular use and understanding of exploiting hope. Ideally, my account will help inform popular use of this concept and allow for more consistent use, along with a better understanding of what is objectionable about exploiting hope. This is possible only if my own account draws from the same kinds of interactions and concerns that ground popular use of this concept. My aim of using my account of exploiting hope to illuminate specific cases of exploitation in the second half of this book will succeed only if my account is familiar to those already using this concept.

As one would expect, popular accounts of exploiting hope often focus on cases of desperately poor and sick people struggling to survive or meet their basic needs. But they also include relatively privileged people who are hoping for fame, great wealth, or beauty. These individuals may be forced into exploitative exchanges, but in other cases the exchanges are voluntary. I argue that two factors unite these examples. First, these hopes are *weighty* in the sense of being transformative and having the potential to greatly improve the hopeful person's life. Second, pursuing these hopes involves unusual risk-taking, trust in others, or what I term *leaps of hope* that make the individual especially vulnerable to exploitation. In all these cases, exploiters take advantage of these leaps of hope to benefit themselves with little to no regard for the good of the exploitee. Popular discussion of exploiting hope often takes its wrongness to be self-evident or links it with fraud, use of force, irrationality, or other threats to autonomy, but it is generally unclear on the source of wrongness. These accounts also use the concept of hope interchangeably with "dreams" and frequently pair it with "desperation" and "fear" as motivators for leaps of hope.

Chapter 2 reviews academic accounts of exploitation to see how they fit with and can build on popular uses in the context of hope. I focus on accounts of exploitation in the context of low-wage or sweatshop employment, because the applied literature on exploitation is the most well developed in this area. The dominant understanding of exploitation links it to a form of unfairness, where the exploiter receives an unfair portion of the benefits from a transaction. Following Alan Wertheimer's understanding of this concept, exploitation can be voluntary and mutually beneficial, and thus the wrongness of unfairness is independent of the wrongness of coercion or harm. He argues that a transaction can have features that make it "specially" unfair, as when an employer has a monopoly on employment opportunities in a community. Alternatively, an exchange can be unfair in light of a structural injustice that systematically advantages the exploiter. In these cases, employers may have a political responsibility to address structural injustice to avoid exploiting their employees. In addition to unfairness, contemporary accounts of exploitation also link it to a failure of respect for others. This failure of a duty of respect is linked to a specified duty of beneficence, where our interactions, dependencies, and other entanglements with others serve to specify obligations to aid others in developing and maintaining their distinctive human capacities. I argue that each of these accounts of exploitation is coherent and picks out different kinds of moral wrongs that are useful for understanding exploitation in different contexts. However, exploitation as a failure of respect and structural fairness exploitation are most closely linked to deficits in basic needs and are most useful in understanding concerns around low-wage labor.

Chapter 3 applies academic analyses of the concept of hope to popular usage of "exploiting hope." I largely endorse and adopt Adrienne Martin's account of hope.[13] Martin argues against the orthodox account of hope that understands it as a combination of a desire for some outcome and belief that this outcome is possible. She argues that this account fails to explain the phenomenology of hope and ways it can provide positive, sustaining support. Specifically, the orthodox account does a poor job of explaining hoping for an outcome despite no expectation that it will occur. Rather, she proposes what she calls the *incorporation analysis* of hope, where hoping entails (a) being attracted to an outcome; (b) seeing it as possible; (c) treating this attraction as licensing a reason for certain ways of feeling, thinking, and acting toward that outcome; and (d) treating this attraction as giving sufficient reason for these feelings, thoughts, and actions. This account of hope links it to the concepts of dreaming and fantasizing as well, as hope can involve planning around, acting on, and emotionally engaging with the desired outcome. Hope in this sense can be false, as derived from misinformation or failures in informed and autonomous decision-making, but it need not be so. Fantasizing and planning for the hoped-for outcome is consistent with understanding the actual probabilities of this outcome, including in cases of hoping against all expectation, and active fantasizing about these outcomes can improve health and welfare. At the same time, false hope creates a vulnerability to exploitation, as does persevering in hope at the expense of other, more obtainable options.

The preceding survey of popular accounts of exploiting hope and academic accounts of the concepts of exploitation and hope come together in the **Chapter 4**. I argue that fairness-based accounts of exploitation form a poor basis for understanding the distinctive wrongness of exploiting hope. Transactional fairness misses both that (a) many common examples of exploiting hope are already fair in terms of their market price and (b) exploitees may benefit greatly from these exchanges given the weightiness of the hoped-for outcome. Structural fairness- or justice-based accounts are also problematic in the medical context. A lack of funded access to unproven medical interventions may not be a problem of justice, and thus it is not clear that those lacking access to these interventions are treated unjustly. More generally, structural exploitation can describe some instances of injustices giving rise to the potential for exploitation but not the distinctive character of exploiting hope. Rather, I argue that exploitation understood as a failure of respect gives the best interpretation of what is distinctly wrong with exploiting hope. Specifically, individuals with *weighty hopes* who take risky *leaps of hope* partially entrust their welfare to others. This entrustment creates obligations for others who may exploit their hopes when they use this relationship as an opportunity for gain without duly fulfilling their responsibilities for the hopeful person's welfare. This is true of both genuine hope and false hope, where the hope is based on misinformation, misunderstanding, or fraud.

In the remainder of the book, I apply my account of exploiting hope to cases of hoping against all expectation for better health—specifically those cases involving accessing scientifically unproven medical interventions. **Chapter 5** examines human participation in phase I clinical trials for experimental cancer interventions and phase III clinical trials in low- and middle-income countries. In both cases, people may participate in these trials in the hope of accessing an experimental intervention that will improve their own health or that of their communities. Exploitation of hope is most likely to take place in these contexts when there is confusion about the roles of researchers and the aims of clinical research such that participants misunderstand the likely outcomes of the trial for themselves or their communities. Researchers and their sponsors can contribute to this misunderstanding by not communicating the aims of clinical research clearly or by using the language of hope to encourage trial participation.

While clinical trials are designed to determine the efficacy and safety of new medical interventions, some individuals sell unproven interventions directly to consumers ahead of this evidence. **Chapter 6** examines the case of direct-to-consumer sales of unproven stem cell products to people desperate to solve their perceived health problems. Here, physicians have been willing to misrepresent the evidence supporting such interventions and abuse the trust of their patients to pursue these business opportunities.

In **Chapter 7**, I discuss the promise of early access to unproven interventions through so-called right-to-try legislation. Policymakers and political leaders are frequently accused of exaggerating their achievements, but in this case some of them make specific claims about the promise and achievements of right-to-try legislation to trade on the hope of seriously ill individuals for political gain.

Finally, **Chapter 8** looks at crowdfunding for unproven medical interventions, which typically are not paid for by public or private insurance. This system of fundraising plays a significant role in the exploitation of hope by funneling resources to exploiters and creating a pool of hopeful donors who are often misled about the interventions they are supporting. This case demonstrates the sometimes complex web of the exploitation of hope, where even ill and exploited individuals can be complicit in exploitation, given the need to build hope in others to fund their own hopes.

These cases are intended to add depth to my account of exploitation and give a sense of how it can be operationalized in the context of hope. More generally, my aim is to strengthen my argument that exploitation is best understood as a failure of respect and, more specifically, violating an entrusted vulnerability for one's own benefit. What these cases show is that understanding the exploitation of hope and other entrusted vulnerabilities requires careful consideration of the context of each case, including the roles and responsibilities of putative exploiters. Similarly, responding to these patterns of exploitation requires careful understanding of the character of the exploitative relationship; the social, policy, and regulatory framework in which it takes place; and the range and implications of achievable responses.

1
Talking about Exploiting Hope

What do people mean when they say that someone has "exploited the hope" of another person or that an interaction or situation "exploits hope"? What kinds of activities and interactions give rise to exploiting hope? What, if anything, do people think is unethical about exploiting hope? Is exploiting hope a distinctive kind of unethical activity, or is the term intended more as a rhetorical flourish for condemning bad acts?

This book aims to answer these and other questions about the phrase "exploiting hope." In this chapter, I begin this project by examining how "exploiting hope" and similar phrases are popularly used. That these terms are widely used and are not simply a narrow academic construct is clear. To take one metric, a May 2019 Google search of variations of "exploit," "exploiting," "exploit the," and "exploiting the" combined with "hope" or "hopes" returned over 1.7 million mentions, with "exploit the hope" (1,360,000), "exploit the hopes" (216,000) and "exploiting the hopes" (126,000) by far the most common combinations.

Specifically, I will examine examples of the use of this and similar terms in the popular press to develop a better sense of how non-academics understand and use this term. I do not expect that this exploration will answer the preceding questions or lead to a clear and definitive understanding of the practical and ethical dimensions of this concept. Rather, the aim of this exploration is to better understand the scope of exploiting hope, its distinctiveness in public dialogue, and the features that, according to common use of the term, make it morally problematic. Doing so will help to anchor the more theoretically informed and applied chapters that follow and ensure that the understanding of exploiting hope that I will develop relates to the popular use of the term. That is, I hope to avoid developing an account of exploiting hope that would be unfamiliar to those using this term and disconnected from the more intuitive and less reflective public understanding of what—if anything—is distinctively wrong with acting in this way.

In what follows, I present and analyze uses of the term "exploiting hope" and similar terms from the popular press. These examples are drawn from news publications worldwide, from the past several decades. They include the descriptions of news reporters, press releases from government officials and public agencies, quotes from members of the public, and editorials. They represent not a systematic review of the uses of the term "exploiting hope" and its variations but a cross-section of these uses. This exploration will thus help identify what activities and individuals the term "exploiting hope" is applied to, a sense of what is taken to be wrong with exploiting hope, and what other concepts are used in association with this term.

Hopeful Activities: Seeking a Better Life

To begin, I will consider what kind of activities give rise to concerns about exploiting hope in the popular press. Doing so is useful because it will help to determine the scope of exploiting hope— specifically, if there is a particular form of hope that is taken to be exploitable and specific activities that are more likely to give rise to this concern in popular discourse.

In the popular press, a wide range of activities are criticized as exploiting the hope of individuals. In many cases, these individuals are clearly in a very precarious or vulnerable position—what can be thought of as central or defining cases of exploiting hope where the individual's current situation is desperate in some sense. As should not be surprising, given the central focus of this project on exploiting hope for better health, many of these instances of exploitation are connected to those seeking a treatment for a medical condition, typically where they have been told that no reliable treatment exists. In these situations, sick and desperate people may seek out scientifically unproven or "alternative" interventions that promise improved health. In one typical example of this use of "exploiting hope," Senator and Health Committee Chair Lamar Alexander spoke of balancing scientific progress with "ensuring bad actors do not take advantage of the hope of this exciting field to harm or defraud patients." Responding to the same issue, the commissioner of the US Food and Drug Administration went on to describe a crackdown on two clinics selling unproven and potentially dangerous stem cell interventions to the public:

> Cell-based regenerative medicine holds significant medical opportunity, but we've also seen some bad actors leverage the scientific promise of this field to peddle unapproved treatments that put patients' health at risk. In some instances, patients have suffered serious and permanent harm after receiving these unapproved products. In the two cases filed today, the clinics and their leadership have continued to disregard the law and more importantly, patient safety. We cannot allow unproven products that exploit the hope of patients and their loved ones.[1]

In this example, severe illness can create the potential for the exploitation of hope, especially when those selling medical interventions disregard patient safety and a lack of evidence of efficacy to advance their own interests.

Many cases where exploiting hope is discussed take place outside of health and healthcare. For example, a common concern is human smuggling, understood as transporting individuals across international borders both voluntarily and involuntarily. The crisis of economic migrants risking their lives to gain access to better opportunities in Europe has generated condemnation of the smugglers who take these migrants' money but often subject them to extremely dangerous conditions when crossing the Mediterranean. As one Italian government minister put it:

> We need to rescue those whose boats sink at sea, a task the men of the coastguard have been seeing to for months, but we also need to do everything possible to stop the traffickers of death who exploit the hope of the poor.[2]

Similarly, migration, independent of specific concerns about human smuggling, is a common subject for concerns about exploiting hope. For example, news reports describe a scammer in the US who promised undocumented migrants that she would be able to provide them with legal immigration papers in exchange for a cash fee. When this scam was exposed, the victims not only lost their savings and the opportunity to regularize their immigration status, but also faced deportation. An attorney for these migrants criticized this situation in terms of having their hopes being taken advantage of: "cases in which undocumented immigrants are bilked for promised visas that never appear is an 'overly common' situation. It happens so regularly because people take advantage of the hope for an avenue to apply for immigration benefits."[3]

Other immigration scams are regularly criticized in similar terms. A fraudulent scheme by ethnically Punjabi Canadian men to marry Indian women to allow them to migrate legally to Canada was described as functioning to "exploit the hopes and dreams of Indian families for a better life overseas."[4] In California, a US citizen was arrested for agreeing to adopt adult undocumented immigrants with the promise that doing so would allow them to become legal US citizens. This scheme was condemned by the US Attorney in the case in terms that mixed charges of exploitation with misleading these immigrants: "The indictment returned today alleges a particularly predatory and manipulative type of fraud that takes advantage of the hopes and dreams of undocumented immigrants to extract fees based on false promises."[5]

Another common group of people seen as economically disadvantaged and thus vulnerable to having their hopes exploited are those seeking employment within their home countries. As with many of the preceding cases, these were often linked to scams where desperate individuals were misled and taken advantage of by exploiters. In Australia, for example, scammers posed as a recruiting agency for employers in the natural resources sector. Rather than linking applicants to well-paying jobs, however, scammers stole the victims' identities after asking them to communicate personal information as part of the application process. In this case, "these unethical people are taking advantage of those who are genuinely seeking work in the mining industry. It is callous behaviour that has no other purpose except to exploit the hopes of job hunters as well as their hip pocket."[6] A similar employment scam was described as "particularly cruel as they exploit the hopes of people genuinely looking for work."[7]

In addition to these outright employment scams, people training job seekers for high-paying jobs have been accused of exploiting hope as well. As with the cases described in the preceding, part of the problem in these cases seems to arise from a misunderstanding about the likely outcomes of this training. But whereas employment scams exploit hope by deliberately misleading exploited individuals, misunderstandings and misinformation can lead to charges of exploitation even without a clear intention to defraud. For example, a push to increase employment among newly trained teachers was criticized in terms of the trainees being naive in their expectation of employment. At the same time, the universities and trade schools that trained these teachers were framed as indifferent, profit-seeking institutions that give out academic degrees and other credentials but "do not promise jobs. They run profitable businesses that exploit hope, an expectation for a better future income."[8]

Finally, politicians are often condemned for making empty or false promises to their constituents to gain public office. In some cases, it is the cynicism around these promises and how they are often packaged in aspirational and hopeful language that generates criticism: "Elections are an opportunity for debates about a viable and positive future. As such, election campaigning that exploits the hopes of marginalised populations towards cynical electoral ends, undermines the democratic commitment of the people."[9] Similarly, making empty campaign promises about policy change was seen as "a desperate attempt to exploit the hopes, aspirations and anxieties of Nigerians to wrest the highest political office from the ruling party."[10] While these examples focus more generally on campaign and political rhetoric that affects the decisions of entire communities, these concerns can be directed at how the rhetoric affects specific subgroups as well. Voters who are particularly disadvantaged may thus be more vulnerable to these promises. For example, a political party in Canada was accused of making a series of pre-election promises to help immigrants that was "little more than a political ploy that exploits the hopes of those in search of a better life in Canada."[11] As this accusation demonstrates, worries about politicians exploiting the hopes of voters may be caught up in more general concerns about the welfare of particularly vulnerable groups such as new immigrants.

Hopeful Activities: Reaching for a Life That Is Better than Good

While exploiting hope is often linked to taking advantage of those who are sick, lack decent economic opportunities, or are seeking a safe and stable place to live, the use of this concept is not limited to these cases. In fact, popular use of the idea of exploiting hope is often applied to situations where individuals are not in a clearly desperate situation or in danger of not having their basic needs met.

Rather, they are seeking to greatly improve their lives by achieving some ideal or dreamed-of outcome.

For example, accusations of exploiting hope frequently occur in the context of individuals who are using a lottery or gambling to try to become extremely wealthy rather than to meet their basic needs. As with many of the previous examples, these cases are often connected to fraud or misinformation. In one case, the company American Family Publishers was sued for mailing misleading flyers claiming that the recipient had won or nearly won a large prize as part of a scheme to sell these recipients various products. These flyers motivated the victims to purchase these products in the expectation of winning millions of dollars. The lawyers for these plaintiffs condemned this practice, stating that these "marketing campaigns exploit the hope of the single mother, the recent immigrant and all other Americans striving to reach the American Dream."[12] In a similar case in the UK, police investigated a scam in which victims would receive a call claiming that they had won a large prize but first must pay a tax for that prize. Police in this case stated, "Things like this are money making scams and exploit the hopes and fears of people."[13] Finally, these criticisms are applied in the context of gambling as well, where, again, individuals are seeking a quick path to great wealth. For one critic of casinos in particular, "That human beings have the capacity to feel hopeful is a wonderful thing. It helps people get out of bed in the morning, especially when life gets tough. Casino owners exploit hope as a means to a greedy end."[14]

In other cases, a desire for success or even fame in one's dream job can make people vulnerable to exploitation. In one such example, so-called vanity presses are accused of unreasonably taking advantage of their customers' desire for publishing success and unrealistic views of their own talent to sell them publishing packages that will not actually yield readers or critical respect:

Would-be novelists who believe they are the next Frederick Forsyth but cannot find a conventional publisher pay anything from £2000 to £10,000 to have their manuscripts turned into bound volumes. But promises that the books will actually appear in the shops and be reviewed in the literary pages count for little. The authors for the most part remain obscure, unread and with an attic full of unwanted volumes. The Professional Authors' & Publishers' Association says: "It is a legal racket that allows vanity sharks to exploit the hopes of aspiring writers."[15]

Notably, in this case, the concern is not that these would-be authors need literary success in order to pay their bills and meet their basic needs; rather, vanity presses are accused of taking advantage of a specific kind of hope—described as a vain hope for fame and success where it had not been earned.

As with the desire for professional success and fame, the desire to meet social expectations around appearances and to be seen as fashionable create an opportunity for exploitation. As one commentator put it, the fashion magazine *Vogue* takes advantage of

the hope that a better life lies just around the corner, in the arch of an eyebrow or the rustle of a new silk dress. Cynics might note that, with its inexorable cycles of planned obsolescence, fashion journalism exists purely to exploit this hope. There remains, however, something undeniably and viscerally appealing about a publication that honors our craving for fantasy, glamour and change.[16]

For others, taking advantage of the hope to look fashionable and of social pressure to look a certain way is driven by cynicism in the fashion industry. On this view, we should reject "the fashion industry and the public relations machinery it employs to make people think that clothes matter for reasons other than comfort or style" as this industry takes "advantage of the hopes and fears attendant on the daily act of getting dressed to promote postures of success, importance, prowess or wealth."[17] At its most extreme and dangerous, critics argue that the desire to meet social expectations around appearance can lead to dangerous behaviors such as extreme dieting. This desire to meet social expectations around appearance is described as "a voice that can exploit hopes and dreams and promote blame and guilt."[18]

Hope as a Vulnerability

Thus far, I have presented examples of the range of activities that raise concerns about the exploitation of hope in the popular press. Some cases involved individuals who were in desperate situations, looking for ways to live a decent life. They included persons who are very ill and desperate for a cure or better health, economic migrants willing to risk their safety and lives for better opportunities, unemployed persons seeking stable and better-paying jobs, and marginalized groups looking for politicians and policies that would improve their lives. In other cases, these individuals were seemingly less desperate and had materially better lives but were seen nonetheless as vulnerable to having their hopes exploited. These cases included people hoping for exceptional lives through winning large sums of money, achieving professional success and recognition, and being recognized as fashionable or having a certain desirable appearance. Failing to realize these hopes would still leave them materially secure, particularly from the perspective of the first group of exploitees. However, as with this first group, these individuals had hopes for the future that allowed them to be preyed upon by exploiters.

Despite the many differences between these cases, several factors unite them. First, the victims in these cases are all seeking a better life. That is, the hope that drives these individuals is that the actions they take will allow them to live an adequate, better, or even exceptional life. In the examples discussed in the preceding sections, the hopes underlying each case were generally not small desires for modest life improvements. Rather, they were *weighty* in the sense of being transformative or central to the individual's identity. In some instances, these were hopes key to the individual's survival, as when very ill persons desperately seek medical treatment or others flee violence, political instability, and economic destitution in their homelands. A hope to be seen as fashionable or to achieve professional success and public recognition might seem frivolous by comparison, but even in these cases hopeful individuals are seeking something central to their identity and conception of a good life. This is not to say that hopes in general must be of such import or centrality to one's conception of a good life. However, in the cases where a concern about *exploitation* of hope takes place, these hopes were generally very weighty.

Given the weightiness of the exploitees' hopes in these cases, another common characteristic of these individuals is that their hopes leave them vulnerable to others. More specifically, these hopes led these exploitees to take actions, often accompanied by risk-taking or willingness to trust others, that they otherwise might not have engaged in. For those struggling to live a decent life, these "leaps of hope" include agreeing to dangerous journeys seeking to enter another country without legal documentation, placing their lives in the hands of human smugglers, electing untested politicians, and receiving medical interventions whose safety and efficacy are unproven. Those in the second group generally did not take leaps of hope that threatened their lives and safety; nonetheless, their hopefulness led them to take risky actions that they might not have done otherwise but for the weightiness of their hopes. Many of these risks are financial, as when substantial amounts of money are dedicated to entering a sweepstakes or paying a vanity press to publish one's work. At its most extreme, this risk-taking and willingness to place one's welfare in the hands of others can lead exploitees into financial destitution or compromised health, as when compulsive gamblers hoping for a large payoff go into debt over time, or those seeking a certain fashionable look undertake significant cosmetic surgery or engage in extreme dieting. This common dimension of taking a leap of hope diminishes the differences between the two groups of hopeful people, showing that the weighty hopes that create an opportunity for exploitation leave even the well-off vulnerable to significant and consequential losses.

A further commonality in all exploitative relationships is that exploiters are willing to disregard the truth and even cultivate exploitees' hopes for their own benefit. In many respects, the actions taken by these exploiters are diverse. Often the exploiters are presented as predators, seeking vulnerabilities in others to use for their own advantage. As in the case of exploiters who create fake job ads in order to steal the identities of their victims, they intentionally create traps for their targets, using their targets' hopes to mislead them and allow the fraud to take place. Other exploiters defraud their victims more subtly, as with the sweepstakes companies that knowingly make misleading statements about the likelihood of winning their contests and politicians who are not truthful about the obstacles to their proposed policy changes. In other cases, it is not clear that the exploiter acts to intentionally mislead others— for example, when people in the fashion industry sell an unrealistic image of beauty or unhealthy standards of desirability. In these last cases, it is less clear that these exploiters should be seen as predators of their customers, willfully seeking to mislead them. However, even in these examples, there is a disregard for the likely consequences of their actions and a willingness to take advantage of their customers' hopes for their own benefit.

Why Is Exploiting Hope Wrong?

As seen in the previous section, the cases of exploiting hope I have presented have commonalities in that the hopes involved are weighty and, if realized, have the potential to transform the lives of the exploitees. These exploitees take leaps of hope where they make themselves vulnerable to their exploiters, who do not show sufficient regard for the welfare of the exploitee. Finally, these exploiters in some cases willfully deceive their victims, or at least willfully play into unrealistic conceptions of the likelihood of these hopes being realized.

Discussion of these cases in the popular press often takes it as self-evident that these allegedly exploitative relationships are wrong; in these cases, the reports do not give an explicit accounting of their ethical dimensions. As I will show in the following chapters, it is not in fact obvious what is meant to be ethically problematic about exploiting hope and whether this term picks out a specific form of ethical wrongdoing that can be separated from other forms of unethical behavior. But before trying to develop such an account, I will take a closer look at how this concept is used in the popular press, with the aim of better understanding the range of reasons given for what is wrong with exploiting hope.

The exploiters in many of the cases discussed earlier are criminal predators, creating scams to defraud their victims. In these cases, the wrongness of the exploitation is clearly understood to be caught up in the wrongness of fraud and lying. Typically, in these cases, "hope" is a vulnerability that allows the fraud to take place, creating a desire or need that can be taken advantage of by the fraudster. For example,

> Traffickers are both ruthless and relentless. They know how to exploit the hopes of those desperate to escape poverty or to find shelter from disaster or from strife. Traffickers prey upon the most vulnerable. They target the weak, the despairing, the isolated. And they make false promises and transport their victims across borders to labor without passports or phones in places where the language is unknown and where there are no means of escape.[19]

In this case, would-be immigrants' hope for a better life is a form of desperation that makes them vulnerable to exploitation and more willing to accept the lies of traffickers for lack of better options. This understanding of exploiting hope is seen also in less extreme cases of misleading exploitees, as when women over forty-five seeking to become pregnant via in vitro fertilization (IVF) are led to believe "that IVF can treat any cause of infertility at any age. . . . This can lead to false hope in the individual which can be exploited by unscrupulous practices."[20] By describing the hope here as "false hope," this case makes it clear that the wrongdoing is closely tied to the exploiters' misrepresentations or outright lying.

More subtly, exploiters of hope are sometimes accused not of misrepresenting the truth but of disregarding the fact that their victims are not assessing information rationally. For example, one commentator charges that "revenue from gambling represents the wages of weakness. It preys on foibles, fears and dreams. It exploits hopes against ridiculous odds. It is a cowardly way to fill the public purse, but these days courage seems no match for greed."[21] This kind of accusation can be understood in various ways, but one reading of it is that the consent process is undermined in some way—that is, the hope in this case leads the gambler to act irrationally. They can be said to know that the odds of winning a fortune by gambling are extremely poor but act contrary to this knowledge and their own self-interest. On this view, the exploiter acts wrongly by proceeding with the exchange despite realizing that the victim's reasoning ability is compromised.

Another reading of the charge in the preceding quote is that the exploiter acts wrongly by being motivated by greed, with disregard for the welfare of their victims. This understanding of the wrongness of exploiting hope is consistent with using force or failing to get fully informed consent to the transaction but identifies an additional source of unethical conduct. On this view of the wrongness of exploiting hope, the problem is that the greed of the exploiter leads them to take advantage of or benefit from the exploitee's vulnerability when they ought to refrain from doing so. This greed is also framed as callousness to the victim's desperation, as in the previously discussed case of employment fraudsters.

Connected to this idea that exploiting hope is wrong because it demonstrates greed or callousness on the part of the exploiter is the charge that it is wrong because of the resulting harm to the exploitees. For example, one commentator condemning casino owners as greedy because they exploit the hope of gamblers focuses her concern on less wealthy exploitees:

> If casinos only attracted people with money to burn who could sit at roulette tables and lose their excess wealth to the benefit of casino owners (with a crumb or two deposited in the public trough), it wouldn't matter as much. But studies have shown over and over again that most of the folks who show up will be spending money they need to pay for life's necessities.[22]

On this view, the concern is not simply that the exploitee is misinformed or irrational, or that the exploiter is greedy or callous; rather, exploiting hope can be ethically problematic if it leads the exploitee to lose their savings or to be unable to meet their basic needs. This logic could similarly be applied to differentiate between a wealthy migrant who employs others to help them illicitly gain citizenship to protect their savings from taxation in their home country versus poor and desperate migrants who seek safety and the opportunity to meet their basic needs.

Exploiting Dreams

In the previous section I considered various ways of understanding what the popular press and commentators take to be wrong with exploiting hope. This review presented a range of different possibilities, linked to concerns with lying, undermining autonomy, greed, and harm to others. These examples demonstrate that there is no single, clear explanation in the popular press of what is taken to be wrong with exploiting hope. Moreover, it leaves in question whether exploiting hope is a distinct kind of unethical behavior or whether it is simply shorthand for a range of interactions where one individual wrongfully benefits from another.

In this and the following sections I want to consider as well whether hope is a clear and distinctive concept in the popular use of "exploiting hope." In this section I will examine how exploiting hope and exploiting dreams are often used synonymously. In the next section I will consider contrasting terms that are frequently used in conjunction with exploiting hope.

The term "dreams" is often taken to be closely associated or even interchangeable with "hope(s)" in the context of discussing concerns with exploitation in the popular press. These two terms are often used in conjunction, with no clear indication that they are meaningfully distinct. For example, after a group of Asian women were taken into productive custody as victims of human trafficking, the perpetrators were condemned as a group of criminals that "exploits the hopes and dreams of immigrants."[23] Others offering to facilitate migration by undocumented immigrants are said to "exploit the hopes and dreams of young people."[24] Similarly, those running casinos and other gambling operations engage in a practice that "exploits the hopes and dreams of losers."[25]

In many cases, charges of "exploiting dreams" are made without reference to "hopes" but are applied to cases and in terms that are identical to the previous examples of "exploiting hopes." Discussions of exploiting dreams often focus on actions that intentionally deceive or mislead their victims. Just as worries about exploiting hope were used frequently in the context of human trafficking and undocumented immigration, a scam to defraud would-be migrants with the promise of legal papers to work in the UK was condemned as a practice that "exploits dreams."[26] Human traffickers are, again, condemned in this same way, as when criticizing "people-traffickers who exploit [migrants'] dreams of a new life."[27] Beyond trafficking and migration scams, such accusations of exploiting dreams are brought up against fraudulent providers of supposed medical cures as well. For example, one commentator charged that stem cell clinics selling unproven interventions are "false scientists" who "exploit the dreams of victims of paralysis and other heartbreaking conditions, and their crimes cast a pall all over legitimate efforts as well."[28]

As I demonstrated previously, concerns around fraudsters exploiting hope were not always linked to individuals in desperate situations or lacking basic resources. This is true as well in discussions of exploiting dreams. For example, one case describes a scam in which particularly desirable housing was offered at unusually low rental rates in order to steal renters' deposits. This scam was described in terms of the victims seeing "what we want to see and fraudsters know that—structuring scams to exploit our dreams of romance or wealth."[29] In another case, a fake talent agency took money from would-be models. Despite the low probability of making a career or achieving stardom through modeling, "that is not going to prevent teenagers from dreaming, or unscrupulous operators from trying to exploit those dreams."[30]

As with examples of exploiting hope, "exploiting dreams" was also applied to cases that did not involve outright fraud, such as those where exploitees lacked the basic resources needed for a good or decent life. For example, commentators discussed low-income children's dreams of making a living in professional sports. One commentator on the documentary *Hoop Dreams* wrote, "The movie's message is that basketball is a big business that exploits the dreams of black kids of getting a better life."[31]

Exploitation of dreams for a life of great wealth or success is thought to take place in the absence of fraud as well. Just as commentators expressed concerns that the hopes of would-be authors were exploited by vanity presses, other commentators expressed concern that would-be music stars' dreams were

exploited by reality shows. For example, one former participant in a reality program opined that "when they exploit dreams,
that's heartbreaking."[32] A fan of these shows was quoted elsewhere condemning "the way they exploit the dreams of teenagers
for ratings. It is emotional abuse really."[33] Similarly, one successful
actress spoke of having to navigate sexual abuse and harassment
in the film industry, where there are "unscrupulous film bosses
keen to exploit her dreams of becoming an actress."[34] Outside of
the entertainment industry, unpaid internships that promised
professional success were accused of serving to "exploit dreams
and exclude new talent, undermining the diversity of our profession."[35] Just as lotteries and casinos were charged with exploiting
the hopes of their customers, they are also accused of exploiting
these customers' dreams. Finally, just as the fashion industry was
attacked for exploiting the hopes of those who wanted to meet social expectations about their appearances, similar complaints were
lodged using the language of dreams. For example, tobacco advertising seeking to link smoking with appearing popular or cool to
teenagers was attacked in terms of "the tobacco industry using deceptive advertising to exploit the dreams and the desires of the most
susceptible among us."[36]

What these examples show is that the concept of "exploiting
dreams" is used in much the same ways and for many of the same
cases as "exploiting hope." Both concepts are used in the contexts
of fraudsters deliberately misleading their victims and exploiters
who are willing to benefit from those seeking to improve their
lives. Both are also used to describe interactions where the victims
lack access to basic goods or a decent life, as well as where they
seek fame, wealth, and public affirmation. If there is a difference in
how these two terms are used in the popular press, it is a tendency
to apply the language of "exploiting dreams" more often to those
seeking fame and an exceptional life rather than basic necessities.
Nonetheless, it is clear that, as used popularly, "exploiting hope"
and "exploiting dreams" are largely interchangeable terms used

across the spectrum from consensual, informed relationships to non-consensual, uninformed interactions and from those lacking the means to meet their basic needs to those seeking something exceptional in their lives.

Hope in Contrast

I have shown that, as popularly used, "hopes" and "dreams" are seen as similarly exploitable. These terms are also used frequently in conjunction with contrasting terms that can help to illuminate what is popularly understood to be the scope of exploiting hope and what is objectionable about such interactions. While hopes and dreams conjure up possibilities of a better or even exceptional life for individuals, these contrasting terms have a negative valence and focus on difficulties in the individual's current circumstances or concerns that their life and prospects might worsen.

In many cases, these contrasting terms are used to capture a general sense that the exploited individual's circumstances are very difficult. In this way, statements about exploiting hope are often coupled with descriptions of the "desperation" of the exploitees. For example, unproven medical interventions are said to exploit "the hopes and desperation of those with terminal illness by outlandish promises of miracle cures that there is as yet no evidence to support."[37] This focus on desperation coupled with hope is used in the context of human smuggling and undocumented migration as well. Here, desperation is seen as the motivator for hope, as when a commentator urges that "people smugglers should never be allowed to exploit the hopes of desperate people."[38]

Again, migration schemes are condemned as cases where "criminals seek to take advantage of the hopes and vulnerabilities of families striving to make a home for themselves in this county."[39] This concern is also described in terms of a weakness, as when "they exploit weaknesses in protection and take advantage of the hopes and fears of their victims, preying—for example—on parents' dreams of an education for their children or on an undocumented migrant worker's distrust of law enforcement officers."[40]

Fear, too, is seen as a companion to the exploitation of hope, particularly where individuals are concerned about a worsening of their prospects or some kind of loss. Often, this is a loss of health or even one's life, as when those selling unproven or scam medical interventions take advantage of others: "Advertisements for a variety of pills, tonics, balms, potions and gadgets claim that the products can help halt memory loss and weight gain, ease the effects of menopause, boost energy, and curb arthritis pain. Those claims are mostly false and simply exploit the hopes and fears of older Americans."[41] As with the other contrasting terms, "fear" is not synonymous with hope and dreams but is a characteristic that spurs individuals to seek a better life, as when Hitler's rise to power was fueled by "his ability to exploit the hopes and fears of a crowd simultaneously."[42]

Similar contrasting terms to hopes and dreams are also used for those who are able to meet their basic needs but desire a better or exceptional life. In the case of those who seek to win a fortune though lotteries or gambling, this hope—or even compulsion—can be seen as a vulnerability that can be wrongfully taken advantage of. For example, one commentator takes a negative view toward gambling as a whole and describes the hope of profiting from it as a weakness: "It is only because gambling so profitably exploits the hopes and weaknesses of individuals that our governments insist on monopolizing it"[43] and "revenue from gambling represents the wages of weakness. It preys on foibles, fears and dreams. It exploits hopes against ridiculous odds."[44] Similarly, the self-help and wellness industries are said to "exploit the hopes and fears, if not the hypochondria, of Australians."[45]

In summary, while hopes and dreams are not seen as synonymous with desperation, vulnerability, fear, and weakness, when exploited they are often seen as co-present with these characteristics. Rather than being largely interchangeable, as with hopes and dreams, these latter terms are conditions of need that motivate leaps of hope and dreams that can be exploited by unscrupulous actors.

Lessons Learned and Next Steps

What, then, does this exploration of the uses of "exploiting hope" in the popular press tell us? First, exploiting hope is applied to a wide range of cases. These include instances where the exploited person is hopeful for the means to a minimally decent life, including those who are experiencing very poor health, people risking the dangers of undocumented migration to find safety and economic opportunity, and those seeking employment of any kind. Both desperate individuals and groups can be exploited in these ways, ranging from individuals in employment scams to whole communities exploited by the promises of political parties. Other cases focus on people who are striving for more than a decent minimum—a *great* rather than merely good life. These cases include individuals who reach for fortune through gambling and winning the lottery, fame through literary success and recognition, and desirability and social approval through wearing the latest fashions. What unites these cases is that all these individuals hope for a better life—whether good or great—and, in doing so, become vulnerable to exploitation.

Second, key aspects of these cases are common to all, despite their diversity. While these cases involve individuals who are materially well off and those who lack basic goods needed for survival, in every case the hoped-for benefit was central to the victim's well-being, sense of self, or identity. That is, these hopes were all *weighty* in that they carried great subjective importance to the victim. For this reason, these victims were all willing to take significant risks to their lives, financial well-being, and personal security—what I refer to as *leaps of hope*. This willingness to take leaps of hope created a vulnerability that exploiters could prey upon. In general, these exploiters were predators who knowingly took advantage of their victims' vulnerabilities by misleading them or showing a disregard for the true likelihood of these hopes being realized.

Despite these examples of how "exploiting hope" is commonly used and understood, this exploration also highlights the many areas where the common meaning of this term is unclear or used inconsistently. From these examples, it is not clear what is morally problematic with exploiting hope. Challenges to autonomy and free and informed decision-making are common in these cases. These threats to autonomy can take place when a predatory exploiter intentionally misleads and defrauds an exploitee or simply takes advantage of their irrationality, disregard for the likely outcomes of their actions, or misunderstanding of the likelihood of these outcomes. It is not clear, then, how the wrongness of fraud or other failures of consent relate to and are separable from the wrongness of exploiting hope. Moreover, other cases do not require or emphasize such failures of informed consent. Rather, the wrongness of exploitation can be located in the callousness and greed of the exploiter or in the harm that comes to the exploitee. Taken together, these diverse understandings of the wrongness of exploitation in the popular press leave it unclear what is taken to be wrong with exploiting hope and whether this is a distinct kind of moral wrong.

Another area of confusion created in these cases centers on whether "hope" is meant to pick out a specific concept. As I have shown, in the popular press it is frequently used interchangeably with "dreams." In some cases, it is a kind of irrationality that leads one to take unreasonable risks, and in other cases it is a vulnerability that predators can use to mislead and defraud. It can be a reaction to desperation, fear, and weakness or can stand on its own. In general, it is seen as a vulnerability to be exploited, but it is less clear what that vulnerability is.

Based on this review of the popular uses of "exploiting hope," this is a topic that excites a great deal of public attention and condemnation in specific areas. These popular uses also show that there is little consistency and precision about what is objectionable about exploiting hope. Thus, there is need for a rigorous account of what exploiting hope is, why it is morally problematic, and what should be done about it.

In the following chapters, I will attempt to provide such an account, anchored to the popular understanding and use of exploiting hope reviewed in this chapter. In the next chapter, I examine scholarly accounts of exploitation that can help give sense to the multiple accounts of the wrongness of exploiting hope. Following that, in Chapter 3 I review scholarly accounts of the concept of hope with the aim of identifying a clear sense of hope that is consistent with popular uses of the term in the context of exploitation. I will then present a clear account in the fourth chapter that unites these ideas and that is consistent with popular uses of the idea of exploiting hope while deepening and clarifying our understanding of this concept.

2

What Is Exploitation?

In the previous chapter I reviewed how exploiting hope is discussed in the popular press. This review revealed several common attributes of these cases, including that they typically involve *weighty* needs central to the exploited person's survival or sense of self. The weightiness of these needs typically leads the people in these cases to make *leaps of hope*, understood as risk-taking in the form of trusting or putting one's welfare in the hands of another. Much less clear was what was taken to be morally problematic about exploiting hope in these cases. For the most part, popular discussion of exploiting hope takes it as self-evident that these cases were morally objectionable. This may be due, in part, because these cases often involved fraud, misinformation, and deceit that left the exploited person worse off and, in many cases, dead or badly hurt. The wrongfulness of predators acting to mislead and take advantage of their victims is probably seen to require little explanation. In other cases, exploiters were seen as greedy, overly self-concerned, or insufficiently worried about the needs and sometimes irrationality of exploitees. These concerns can overlap with those around fraud but also stand on their own.

While the wrongness of these cases may seem self-evident, the problem with leaving the wrongness of exploitation unclear or linking it with the wrongness of fraud or other forms of wrongdoing is that doing so makes it unclear whether exploitation is a distinctive moral wrong. If exploitation is not clearly a distinctive form of wrongdoing, then it is also unclear that charging someone with exploiting hope should be taken to mean anything more than stating that they are misleading or mistreating individuals in a vulnerable situation. That is, the charge of exploiting hope might just be a rhetorical flourish rather than a distinctive accusation of wrongdoing.

To determine if exploiting hope picks out a distinctive form of unethical activity, in this chapter I will survey accounts of the wrongness of exploitation before examining the concept of hope in the next chapter. Specifically, I will survey theoretical accounts of exploitation, chiefly through the example of low-wage or sweat-shop labor. I am choosing to focus on the context of low-wage labor rather than the medical context that will be the focus of the ap-plied section of this book because the literature on theories of ex-ploitation applied to labor is especially well developed and diverse. Sweatshop or low-wage labor is associated with wages that fall below a living-wage standard and with long working hours. Like the exploitation of hope, labor of this kind is often described as ex-ploitative and self-evidently immoral.[1] Consider, for example, the charge that "in many of the factories in Mexico, Central America and Asia producing American-brand toys, clothes, sneakers and other goods, exploitation is the norm. The young women who work in them—almost all sweatshop workers are young women— endure starvation wages, forced overtime and dangerous working conditions."[2] In this representative portrayal of sweatshops as ex-ploitative, the poor working conditions are taken as evidence enough that sweatshop employers are acting immorally.

For those who defend sweatshop labor as the first rung on a ladder toward greater economic development, the charge that sweatshop labor is self-evidently exploitative fails adequately to ex-plain the nature of the alleged wrongdoing. While all sides might agree that poor working conditions are unfortunate and unde-sirable, defenders of sweatshop labor argue that they provide the best available alternative for some workers and the best chance at economic development for many low- and middle-income coun-tries (LMICs).[3] Some defenders of sweatshop labor even embrace the label of exploitation.[4] Nicholas Kristof, for example, argues that exploitation is beneficial, and thus, "while it shocks Americans to hear it, the central challenge in the poorest countries is not that sweatshops exploit too many people, but that they don't exploit enough."[5]

Unless there is a clear, widely understood account of why exploitation is a moral wrong, then charging a practice as exploitative will do little to advance debates over whether and why a practice is morally problematic. In 2003, Denis Arnold accurately noted that "the perspectives of moral and political philosophers have been curiously absent from the recent debate over sweatshops in the global economy."[6] Since that time, a considerable body of work has been developed, applying a growing literature on exploitation to sweatshop labor. While many forms of moral wrong are associated with sweatshop labor, I will focus specifically on the worry that low wages allow relatively wealthy employers wrongfully to take advantage of, or gain from, relatively poor workers, especially in LMICs. In particular, I will focus on instances of alleged exploitation in employment relationships that are voluntary and mutually beneficial.

I have two reasons for doing so. First, by restricting this discussion to voluntary and mutually beneficial instances of exploitation, I can isolate the moral wrong of exploitation from other moral wrongs, especially the wrongs of coercion and outright harms to workers. This focus will be particularly important when applying exploitation to hope because the wrongness of exploiting hope is often conflated with the wrongness of fraud or outright harm in popular discussions of this topic. Second, the focus on mutually beneficial and voluntary relationships will allow for arguments that sweatshop labor is not only not exploitative but that it is a morally praiseworthy means of helping to encourage economic growth in poor areas of the world and to provide jobs that pay better and are more stable than any existing alternatives. Similarly, a defender of so-called exploitation of hope in the medical context can argue that giving terminally ill individuals access to unproven interventions is morally praiseworthy because they have nothing left to lose.

In this chapter, I have three goals. First, I will give an overview of the many different uses of the charge of exploitation by examining how the term is used in the literature on sweatshop labor. While it is often not clear what kind of moral wrong is assumed to take place when the charge of exploitation is used, I will demonstrate that many distinct types of exploitation, connected to distinct moral wrongs, are used in the literature on sweatshop labor. Specifically, I will identify two broad categories of exploitation—exploitation as unfairness and exploitation as the mere use of others—with subgroups under each main category. Second, I will discuss which of these senses of exploitation identify clear moral wrongs in the context of sweatshop labor and the exploitation of hope for better health through unproven medical interventions. As I will argue, not all uses of the charge of exploitation persuasively identify clear moral wrongs. Third, I will apply the lessons learned from my exploration of exploitation in sweatshop labor to other relationships. As I will argue, multiple viable models of exploitation in the sweatshop literature can illuminate exploitative practices of relatively well-compensated employees, customers, suppliers, and entire communities. While discussions of theories of exploitation tend to argue for a single, correct account of this moral wrong, my review of the literature on exploitation supports the conclusion that there are multiple reasonable accounts of the moral wrong of exploitation. For this reason, those who would charge that a relationship is exploitative should specify the form of exploitation they believe is taking place. This specification will be particularly important in my discussion of exploiting hope in Chapter 3, where I argue that exploitation as a failure of respect is at the heart of the wrongness of these interactions, especially in the context of unproven medical interventions.

Exploitation as Unfairness

The most common understanding of exploitation generally, and in the literature on sweatshops specifically, interprets exploitation as taking *unfair* advantage of others. In fact, exploitation is often defined as synonymous with taking unfair advantage of others.[7] The link between exploitation and unfairness typically follows from Alan Wertheimer's groundbreaking work on exploitation, where he explicitly describes it in terms of unfairness. As he defines it, "A exploits B when A takes unfair advantage of B."[8] Wertheimer measures the fairness of a transaction according to how the benefits resulting from the transaction are distributed. In many cases, the fairness of this distribution is assessed by comparing it with how these benefits would be distributed under hypothetical fair-market conditions. Other authors develop accounts of exploitation as taking unfair advantage of others but do not use the hypothetical fair-market standard for measuring fairness.[9,10]

The fairness standard marks out a distinct category of exploitation where a transaction is wrongfully exploitative when it results in an unfair distribution of the benefits of a transaction. While there can be endless standards for the fair distribution of the benefits of a transaction, we can divide fairness-based accounts of exploitation into two subgroups: (1) those that emphasize concerns about the fairness of individual transactions without reference to structural justice in the standard of fairness (transactional fairness); and (2) those that do incorporate concerns about structural justice when assessing fairness (structural fairness).

Transactional Fairness

Transactional fairness attempts to limit the scope of the standard of fairness, typically by excluding concerns about the effects of structural justice on the distribution of benefits resulting from an interaction. That is, this standard of fairness limits appeals to background justice or structural reasons as to why one partner to the exchange might be advantaged or disadvantaged relative to other partners. This distinction can be difficult to maintain, but, in the context of sweatshop labor, transactional fairness standards typically appeal to a fair-market exchange between the worker and employer without reference to whether the worker is disadvantaged by institutional structures like unjust global trade laws or the aftereffects of colonialism. Wertheimer's account of exploitation serves as an example of a transactional fairness account or what Robert Mayer calls a neoclassical theory of exploitation.[11]

Under this understanding of exploitation, only when one of a limited set of the exploitee's rights has been violated—or, as Wertheimer puts it, only when "special" unfair advantage is taken of a person—does exploitation take place.[12] As previously noted, Wertheimer argues that in many cases, a hypothetical fair market can be used as a standard for determining whether the terms of an exchange are fair. As he defines it, a hypothetical fair market produces a price that "an informed and unpressured seller would receive from an informed and unpressured buyer."[13] Taking advantage of another person in a pervasive way, as when structural injustice creates systemic, background disadvantages, will not count as exploitation in this view. This act of exploitation may take place through a bilateral or trilateral relationship. That is, the exploiter may be both the rights violator and the individual taking advantage of that violation, or the rights violator and exploiter may be different persons.[14]

The baseline for determining the fairness of a distribution can be altered while still staying within the basic confines of a transactional fairness account of exploitation. Mikhail Valdman argues that Wertheimer's hypothetical fair-market standard should be changed to include only cases that result from an unrefusable offer.[15] An offer can become unrefusable as a result of the high costs of turning down an offer. These high costs, in turn, can be created when the exploiter has a monopoly over a good that the exploitee needs urgently or through other unusual power asymmetries. Under these conditions, the costs of turning down an offer are extremely high, meaning that the exploiter can collect benefits disproportionate to those they could expect if either they did not have monopoly control over some good or the exploitee's need for the good was not urgent, allowing the exploitee to walk away from the offer without an excessive cost. A labor agreement will be exploitative, then, not when it deviates from the terms that would be reached in a hypothetical fair market but when it deviates from a situation where the worker might reasonably turn down the offer, usually by seeking out work from another employer. Importantly, Valdman's account is consistent with many employers offering similarly low wages to potential employees as a result of unjust background conditions. In such a situation, the employer's offer, though very low, will not count as monopoly pricing. Thus, Valdman, like Wertheimer, ties the fairness of an exchange only to the transactional elements of the exchange.[16]

Matt Zwolinski gives a more detailed example of the application of a transactional fairness standard of exploitation to sweatshop labor. He grants the possibility of mutually beneficial exploitation, focusing on Wertheimer's analysis that a relationship can be unfair to the exploitee by insufficiently benefiting them. Thus, to "determine whether a mutually beneficial exchange is exploitative, we must compare the gains made by the parties not (necessarily) to the baseline of no-exchange-at-all, but rather to the baseline in which each party acts within their rights with respect to the other, and ensure that parties are left at least as well off as they would be under *those* circumstances."[17] According to Zwolinski, fair-market exchanges will for the most part ensure that employers do not engage in exploitation. Sweatshop labor will count as exploitative only if employees have a right, claimable on employers, to a living wage.[18]

Zwolinski focuses his account of exploitation in sweatshops on the transformative power of consent and autonomy-exercising choices. He argues that if a choice exhibits even a partial degree of autonomy, then there is a *prima facie* supposition against interfering with that choice. This belief rests on the moral importance of freedom for agents. For Zwolinski, those autonomous choices most central to the identity or core projects of the agent create the strongest claims to noninterference. Because sweatshop workers choose to work the jobs they do to survive and meet their basic needs, these choices are central to the workers' core projects. While we might worry that the workers' rights are being violated through poor working conditions, Zwolinski argues that through their autonomous choices workers can "waive certain claims that we might have had (in the case of workers, the claim not to be told what to do by others, or the claim to certain kinds of freedom of association, for instance)."[19] Rational persuasion and establishing alternative forms of employment to sweatshop labor will not count as cases of external interference.

When choices are made under conditions of limited autonomy, Zwolinski argues, they still signal preferences. Even when an individual faces coercive conditions, ignoring the preferences of the agent under conditions of limited autonomy can be a moral wrong in addition to the coercive act. That is, ignoring a person's preferences shows disregard for that person's welfare, in addition to the disrespect shown by illegitimately limiting their choices in the first place. Therefore, even under conditions of limited autonomy, there is no justification for removing the option of working in a sweatshop if that is the worker's preference from among a limited range of bad options. It is the harm created by removing a preferred option that generates the justification against restricting the worker's choices: "given that many potential sweatshop workers seem to express a *strong* preference for sweatshop labor over the alternatives, acting to remove that option is likely to cause them *great* harm."[20] In short, disregarding an autonomy-exercising choice may harm the agent and is forbidden on that ground.

From these points, Zwolinski generates what he calls "the argument," which maintains that, because sweatshop work is a clear preference of the workers, they are likely to be harmed if this preference is ignored. It is plausible as well that sweatshop work is an autonomous choice. For these reasons, "all else being equal, it is wrong to take away the option of sweatshop labor from workers who would otherwise choose to engage in it."[21] Given that sweatshops are doing something to help their workers, Zwolinski finds it strange that we would condemn these employers as exploitative. While the employer might be able to do more to help their employees, they certainly do more than the vast majority of individuals who do nothing to help the global poor. His analysis of the moral importance of choice supports the notion that providing some benefit in the form of low wages does not violate the workers' rights. That is, each party acts within their rights by making and accepting an offer of wages at market rates. Since Zwolinski argues that exploitation depends on a rights violation, he can conclude that "I do, indeed, believe that claims of sweatshop wages being exploitative are implausible."[22] Here, Zwolinski seems to accept a transactional standard of fairness, where workers do not have a right, claimable on their employers, to a living wage. Because no right is violated within the transaction between employer and worker, exploitation does not take place.

Structural Fairness

One concern with a transactional fairness standard of exploitation like a hypothetical fair-market price is that it fails adequately to consider how structural injustice can disadvantage some parties within a transaction. In the context of sweatshop employment, sweatshop workers may have a weaker bargaining position because they are the victims of socioeconomic injustice, including trade laws that disadvantage citizens of LMICs and histories of colonialism and interventions that have slowed economic development in some parts of the world. This concern persists even in a hypothetical fair market, since transactional fairness does not correct for the disadvantages created by structural injustice. Because sweatshop owners take systemic rather than special advantage of institutional injustice, transactional fairness standards of exploitation are unable to account for the intuition that background injustice can be wrongfully exploited.

An alternative standard for determining the fairness of a transaction—what I will call structural fairness—attempts to correct for the effects of structural injustice. Ruth Sample offers one example of a structural fairness approach to measuring exploitation in sweatshop labor. She gives several accounts of the wrongness of exploitation, including cases where we "fail to respect a person by taking advantage of an injustice done to him."[23] While this account ties the wrongness of exploitation to a failure of respect rather than unfairness, it is the action of taking advantage of the unfairness created by injustice that constitutes a failure of respect. Specifically, she argues that globalization "exploits to the degree to which background injustices experienced by vulnerable nations work to the advantage of their stronger interactors."[24] Persons privileged through the process of globalization, she argues, can unfairly take advantage of the socioeconomic inequality and injustice brought on by trade liberalization.

A weakness of Sample's account is that it is not entirely clear what injustices create the opportunity for exploitation and how one can practically avoid taking advantage of injustice in a thoroughly unjust world. As Matt Zwolinski notes, it would seem strange to accuse someone who enjoys helping—and thus benefits from—victims of injustice of exploiting them, or similarly to condemn someone who sells building supplies to a victim of race-based arson at the normal, fair-market price.[25] This weakness could be addressed by specifying the range of exploitable injustices. For example, structural fairness exploitation can be tied to the failure of international institutions to protect human rights, including the right to a living wage. Exploitation can then be avoided by not taking advantage of this specific injustice. Robert Mayer takes this approach when he uses the price paid for "fair trade" coffee as an example of a structurally just price. This price is fair, he argues, because it is determined through a hypothetical bargain between persons who have a decent minimal standard of living or living wage. This baseline for measuring fairness can be directly contrasted against a transactional fairness standard of a hypothetical fair-market price. In the coffee case, "the initial disadvantage is an insecure standard of living, not a lack of competition. The just price is calculated to be the price which an agent with a secure standard of living would accept, which is greater than the equilibrium price for this good."[26] Both the transactional and structural standards of fairness imagine a hypothetical exchange between parties in order to establish a baseline against which fairness can be measured. Only the structural standard, however, allows broader background factors like a right to a living wage to factor into the calculation.

Transactional vs. Structural Fairness

Given these disagreements about the appropriate standard of fairness for determining when exploitation as a form of unfairness takes place, we should examine the arguments for and against each approach. Wertheimer defends his focus on transactions on the grounds that it would be unfair to ask individuals to make up for the ill effects of long-standing, structural injustice: "even though some fare less well than others by the appropriate principles of social justice, it is unreasonable to expect the better-off party to repair those background conditions by adjusting the terms of a particular transaction."[27] That is, even though unjust socioeconomic structures may create unfair disadvantages for some parties to a transaction, it is not the responsibility of individuals singly to rectify social injustice.

Much of the argument between transactional and structural fairness, then, will turn on the appropriate role, if any, of individuals such as employers in addressing global structural injustice. Those favoring a transactional standard of fairness tend to deny that employers have a special obligation to address the effects of structural injustice as they affect their employees, even if employers gain from this injustice. We have already seen how Wertheimer and Zwolinski deny special obligations for employers. Zwolinski specifically endorses what Wertheimer has called the non-worseness claim. The non-worseness claim maintains that "given that I have a right not to transact with B and that transacting with B is not worse than not transacting with B, it can't be seriously wrong for me to engage in an unfair transaction with B."[28] Zwolinski questions why we would criticize the behavior of an employer in an LMIC that helps the global poor without extending a living wage while ignoring an employer that employs workers only in the US and does nothing to help the global poor.

Chris Meyers, however, takes a more extensive view of the obligations of employers to their employees. Meyers argues that employers in sweatshops exploit their employees when they benefit disproportionately from their labor.[29] He argues that when an individual engages in and benefits from an exploitative relationship, they have an individual responsibility to end the relationship if they can do so without incurring significant hardships.[30] This responsibility exists whether the disproportionate benefit results from transactional or structural asymmetries in bargaining power. Significantly, Meyers uses the discretionary power of CEOs to reduce their own salaries as evidence that they have the discretionary power to increase worker wages. He argues that CEOs "largely determine the strategies and policies that allow or involve sweatshop labor, they benefit enormously from such exploitation in terms of their bloated salaries and other compensations, and they are in a position to do something about it—they have both the power to determine company policy and the means to pay for it with reductions in their own salary."[31] The specific context in which a multinational corporation operates will determine whether Meyers is correct to believe that CEOs of multinational corporations have discretionary power to offer higher wages to their employees.

If they do, Meyers argues that this discretionary power creates an individual responsibility to make up for the disproportionately high wages that they take home. This logic would seemingly apply to other executives within multinational corporations as well. That is, if the discretionary power to create more broadly fair working conditions creates special responsibilities to act on this power, then any employee within a multinational corporation who possesses this power will have the corresponding responsibility. While CEOs will tend to be particularly powerful within corporations, there is good reason to think that a wide range of other executives, particularly in large multinational corporations with widely distributed power structures, will have some discretion over the wages earned by their employees.

But even if CEOs and other executives do have this power, more needs to be said about why the power to set wages creates a special obligation by employers to correct for the transactional and structural unfair working conditions their employees face. If the disproportionately low wages earned by sweatshop workers were the result of unjust institutions rather than a localized vulnerability, then we would still need an argument as to why employers, CEOs, and other executives must individually rectify these injustices lest they exploit their employees.

How, then, might we accommodate Wertheimer's intuition that it would be unfair to hold individual employers responsible for cleaning up the large-scale mess of global injustice while acknowledging the special position of employers in relation to their disadvantaged employees? Iris Young provides one argument for why employers have special, individual responsibilities while remaining sensitive to the worry that structural injustice is created and maintained collectively and is a problem so large that it must be confronted collectively.[32] She differentiates between the backward-looking liability model of responsibility and the forward-looking model of political responsibility. Under the liability model, responsible agents will have voluntarily taken actions that are causally connected to unjust conditions. In the context of sweatshop labor, managers and owners of sweatshops will have the primary responsibility for their workers' low wages, as they are causally responsible for setting these wage levels.

While appropriate in many contexts, the liability model of responsibility faces limitations in that it pays insufficient attention to how social structures constrain the choices available to us. Young notes:

> When confronted with accusations that they wrongly exploit and oppress their workers, however, some of these agents are likely to try to mitigate their responsibility by pointing to factors outside their control. They may claim that they have little choice about the wages they pay and that they cannot afford to give workers time off or invest in better ventilation and equipment. They operate in a highly competitive environment, they may say, where other operators are constantly trying to undercut them. They can stay in business only by selling goods at or below the prices of worldwide competitors, and they can do that only by keeping labor and production costs to a minimum.[33]

In a highly competitive market, wages can only rise so high before the employer will be forced out of business. While these complaints about a lack of options for offering better wages may be overblown in some cases, the liability model of responsibility fails to capture other modes of responsibility when actors face limited options in the context of unjust socioeconomic structures.

Moreover, the liability model of responsibility fails to provide a means for assigning responsibility to other actors who are part of the global structure that promotes and perpetuates low wages for some workers. As a result, the liability model should not be used to explain the full extent of individual responsibility in the face of systemic injustice. What is needed is an account of individual responsibility that acknowledges the role of employers and other powerful parties in perpetuating and benefiting from injustice while being sensitive to the constraints placed on their ability to individually rectify these injustices.

Considering these shortcomings, Young develops an account of what she calls political responsibility. She argues that, though employers are liable for the working conditions in sweatshops, their individual responsibility is better framed as a "political responsibility" to help bring about just social structures. This responsibility is derived from the fact that they "contribute by their actions to the processes that produce unjust outcomes. Our responsibility derives from belonging together with others in a system of interdependent processes of cooperation and competition through which we seek benefits and aim to realize projects. Within these processes, each of us expects justice toward ourselves, and others can legitimately make claims of justice on us."[34] By taking part in these political structures, we all share and have a responsibility to remedy the injustices that derive from these structures.

In practice, actors will face a political responsibility shaped by their position within institutional structures. Young argues that the individual's power to reform institutional structures, privilege accruing from unjust structures, interest in promoting change, and collective ability to initiate change all serve to heighten the individual's political responsibility. Power is understood as the "degree of potential or actual power or influence over processes that produce the [unjust] outcomes."[35] Whereas individuals will not have the resources to respond to all structural injustice, they should focus on those areas where their power to influence change is the greatest. Privilege is understood as benefit received from structural injustice, something that matters to our political responsibility on the understanding that as "beneficiaries of the process, they have responsibilities."[36] Interest speaks to the focus primarily of victims of injustice, where those negatively impacted by unjust structures have a particular interest in changing them. This is distinct from saying that these victims are liable for these injustices or blaming victims for injustice. Finally, collective ability speaks to already existing organizations and resources that can be drawn on to effect change more quickly and efficiently. For example, the existence of labor unions, stakeholder organizations, or other groups will impact the ability to bring about political change. Therefore, even if unjust structures limit the degree of choice that employers have over the wage levels that they may offer while remaining competitive, they may yet have a political responsibility to change these structures. If so, the employer's political responsibility must be fulfilled if the employer is to avoid exploiting their workers. Over the long term, these structural changes can lead to fairer wages for workers, thus mitigating the structural exploitation they face.

Arguments for a political responsibility for multinational corporations have been developed within discussions of corporate citizenship and corporate political responsibility in the context of globalization.[37,38,39,40] These arguments for a political role for corporations are not without their critics.[41,42] By tying structural fairness exploitation to Young's framework, the concern that employers exploit their workers can fit within wider discussions of the ethical obligations of corporations. By appealing to a specific form of exploitation and specific form of potential moral wrongdoing by corporations, general claims of corporate social responsibility can be clarified and strengthened. While the specific wrongdoing of structural fairness exploitation will not describe the totality of corporations' political responsibilities, it can help to detail why corporations and their members may have a political role.

Young's account demonstrates that, rather than choose between the transactional and structural fairness accounts of exploitation, we need both accounts in order to give voice to the full range of exploitation faced by sweatshop workers and other participants in globalized business practices. The mistake is in applying the same duties derived from transactional fairness to structural fairness. While the critics of some accounts of structural fairness exploitation are right to note that it is unreasonable to hold individual employers responsible for rectifying all of the disadvantages created by global injustice for their employees, they are wrong to conclude that global injustice does not give rise to exploitable vulnerabilities. Structural unfairness creates importantly different forms of vulnerability for workers, and, as Young demonstrates, avoiding the exploitation of these vulnerabilities requires a different response than that demanded by market failures and other forms of transactional unfairness. Both transactional and structural fairness exploitation can and must coexist if the full range of exploitation is to be completely explained.

Exploitation as a Failure of Respect

The transactional and structural fairness accounts of exploitation focus on the distribution of the benefits created through an interaction. An alternative view of exploitation associates its wrongness with a failure to treat others with respect or with a loss of dignity for the exploitee. In the context of sweatshop labor, low wage levels can be associated with degrading and disrespectful treatment of the worker.[43] The concern, on this account, is not that the sweatshop workers' wages are unfair or disproportionately small when compared with their employers' profits. Rather, the wage levels amount to a failure of respect by employers for their employees as human persons. This failure of respect may take place in the absence of any unfairness, or it can take place in conjunction with transactional fairness, structural unfairness, or both.

While the requirements of treating others with respect can be understood in many ways, in the context of sweatshop labor, commentators have tended to argue that low wages can serve to treat workers as a mere means to the ends of their employers. This "mere means" language derives from Immanuel Kant's "formula of humanity," which requires that one act so that "you use humanity, whether in your own person or in the person of any other, always at the same time as an end, never merely as a means."[44] For example, Radin and Calkins claim that there is a "strong moral argument against sweatshops, which seemingly exploit people for their labor as a means of profit generation."[45] Treating another person as an end, and not merely as a means, is first typically understood to entail negative duties that proscribe against interfering with others' autonomy. When we coerce, deceive, or manipulate others, we attempt to turn their will to our own ends rather than respecting their self-directing nature as persons. Treating others as ends also requires positive steps to promote their ability to act autonomously. As human persons, we each have physical and psychological needs that, if they are not met, will thwart our ability to act autonomously, just as surely as will coercion, deception, and the use of force. This positive duty of beneficence must also be fulfilled if we are to avoid treating others as a mere means to our own ends.

While this "mere means" language helps to add detail to the claim that low wages can fail to demonstrate adequate respect for workers, we can examine more detailed accounts of exploitation as the mere use of others to determine when and why this form of wrongdoing takes place. The connection of exploitation to a duty not to treat others as a mere means draws heavily on the intuition that treating others as ends requires offering one's employees decent working conditions and a living wage. Norman Bowie argues that respect for persons requires that any employment must be "meaningful." Stemming from both the positive and negative manifestations of the duty to treat others as ends, he argues that a Kantian manager has the obligation to extend to employees a wage that allows them to be somewhat independent and to achieve at least some of their desires. Meaningful work will: (1) give employees the opportunity to exercise their autonomy on the job; (2) support and develop the autonomy and rationality of employees; (3) provide sufficient salary to exercise their independence, provide for their physical well-being, and satisfy some of their desires; (4) enable the development of their rational capacities; (5) not interfere with employees' moral development; and (6) not be paternalistic by interfering with their conception of how to obtain happiness.[46]

Denis Arnold joins Bowie in elaborating the charge that employers exploit their workers by merely using them. They jointly argue that respect for one's employees' autonomy entails the positive step of guaranteeing a living wage for these persons.[47] In doing so, they draw on Onora O'Neill's and Thomas Hill's interpretation of Kantian ethics.[48,49] O'Neill and Hill argue that respect for others' autonomy is not merely a matter of refraining from interfering with others. Noninterference, after all, is compatible with complete indifference toward the needs of others, particularly their physical and psychological needs for maintaining their distinctively human capacities. On this basis, Arnold and Bowie write that

> at a minimum, respect for employees entails that MNEs [multinational enterprises] and their suppliers have a moral obligation to ensure that employees do not live under conditions of overall poverty by providing adequate wages for a 48 hour work week to satisfy both basic food needs and basic non-food needs. . . . Anything less than this means that MNEs, or their suppliers, are not respecting employees as ends in themselves.[50]

Without this support, sweatshop workers may not be able to reason abstractly, maintain their rational and moral capacities, and realize fully their other capacities as autonomous persons.

Arnold and Bowie agree broadly that insufficient wage levels can serve to treat one's employees as a mere means to one's own ends. But their adaptation of the formula of humanity raises the question of how strong the obligation to give one's workers a living wage is, particularly in the face of external pressures on wage levels. Typically, the positive duty of beneficence is understood as an imperfect duty, meaning that one has leeway over when and how it is fulfilled. In the context of sweatshop labor, it is not completely clear how much leeway an employer should have over providing a living wage to her employees. Bowie argues that an employer must honor the self-respect of their employees and that employees maintain self-respect through the independence allowed through a living wage. In an earlier version of his argument, he qualified this position by noting that the requirement to offer a living wage is not absolute to the point that an employer must provide such a wage even if doing so would make them uncompetitive. For an employer, "providing meaningful work is one possible and rather effective way for a firm to honor the requirement that it respect the humanity of its employees and the imperfect obligation of beneficence. However, if the labor market does not permit a firm to honor the obligation of beneficence in this way, it is not required to do so."[51] In this version of the argument, the duty to provide a living wage is imperfect, and employers can fulfill their imperfect duty of beneficence through various means that may include not offering a living wage.

But the duty to offer one's employees a living wage can be understood more strictly. Arnold and Bowie's language stating that employers *must* provide their workers with a living wage or fail in a duty of respect for their workers implies that they understand the requirement to offer a living wage as a perfect duty. By a perfect duty, I mean a duty that does not permit leeway as to when and how it is fulfilled. That is, employers are not given flexibility over when and to whom to provide a living wage but are required to provide this wage to all of their workers. It appears, then, that exploitation as a failure of respect can be understood to give the employer leeway over setting wage levels in the face of external pressures like competition, or it can be interpreted to claim that setting a living wage is a requirement of not exploiting one's employees.

Given these choices, understanding exploitation as a failure of a perfect duty offers the more plausible interpretation of this form of exploitation, though with some important caveats that I will explain in the following. If the duty to offer a living wage to one's workers is based on an imperfect duty of beneficence, then the fact that an employer fails to offer their employees a living wage cannot be taken alone to indicate that they exploit their workers. Other beneficent acts may help the employer fully to fulfill their duty of beneficence. For this reason, tying exploitation to an imperfect duty of beneficence leads to counterintuitive results. It runs contrary to the ordinary use of "exploitation" to think that, because an employer makes an unrelated donation to a charity or engages in other unrelated charitable acts, that they would be excused, morally, for offering their employees wages insufficient to support their distinctly human capacities. That is, these unrelated, beneficent acts would seem to do little to assuage the intuition that the employer is improperly using or taking advantage of *these* workers specifically, especially if they can offer a higher wage.

Given this worry about tying this definition of exploitation as treating others as a mere means to an imperfect duty, we can consider how and why this obligation might take a more fixed or perfect form. Doing so will require a brief departure deeper into Kantian ethics, but this discussion will help us understand the rationale for additional accounts of exploitation as the mere use of others. Depending on our own projects and life plans, we will each have different ends that motivate our actions. Kant maintains, however, that the two obligatory ends that we all should share are our own perfection and the happiness of others.[52] While the end of others' happiness is unspecified in its most general form where it applies to every person, this end can be specified given the circumstances of the actual persons with whom we are connected. Thus, an individual's relationships with other persons, instances where others' basic needs are not being met, and cases where one can render aid to another person at little cost to oneself can all serve to specify the general, imperfect obligation to promote the happiness of others—that is, the duty of beneficence.[53] More generally, when our own happiness becomes determinative of or entwined with the happiness of specific others, this increased capacity to impact these persons' happiness specifies the duty of beneficence.[54] In these cases, to ignore the desperate needs of another person can bring into doubt whether one genuinely takes the happiness of others to be an end for oneself.

Ruth Sample takes advantage of this understanding of a perfect form of the duty of beneficence in her account of exploitation as a failure of respect. On her account, one form of exploitation is tied to a failure of respect for others "by neglecting what is necessary for that person's well-being or flourishing."[55] As with Arnold and Bowie, Sample ties this failure of respect within employment relationships to the failure to provide a living wage. She writes that globalization "exploits to the degree to which the requirements of human flourishing are neglected in the process of gaining advantage."[56] Sample goes on to argue that low wages can be said to violate a perfect form of the duty of beneficence. When we disregard the needs of those with whom we interact, it can bring into question whether we hold a maxim of beneficence at all. She argues that "while imperfect duties allow us some discretion in determining whether to act beneficently in a given case, those situations in which we are confronted by vulnerable others in transactions for advantage could not be, by any reasonable person, *optional* opportunities for beneficent action."[57] Our indifference toward the needs of specific persons within the general pool of the global poor may leave it unclear whether one is committed to the duty of beneficence. But when we transact with a person in need and refuse to alter the terms of the exchange to support their basic needs when we could do so, it may become clear that we do not, in fact, hold such a commitment.

Similarly, in my own work I maintain that "employers do not simply have an imperfect duty to help some of their employees to achieve a decent minimum some of the time; rather, employers are required to cede as much of their benefit from the interaction to their employees as is reasonably possible toward the end of the employees achieving a decent minimum standard of living."[58] I argue that the standard of reasonability for ceding benefits to workers is determined both by the dependence of the worker on the employer for their basic support and a requirement that the employer not retain luxury goods in excess of those used for maintaining a flourishing human life. When the employer violates this perfect form of the duty of beneficence, they exploit their workers. Moreover, through this form of exploitation the exploiter offers what I have called a "demeaning choice" between the status quo and an offer of less than what respect for others requires of the exploiter. When exploitees accept these offers, their "surface endorsement" of the terms of the interaction makes it more difficult to see that they have been exploited.[59]

Assessing Accounts of Exploitation in Sweatshop Labor

I have argued that versions of the transactional fairness, structural fairness, and mere means accounts of exploitation are all defensible. Each of these accounts captures a distinct element of exploitation that can take place in sweatshop labor. But this is not to say that each form of exploitation is equally relevant to the central moral concerns with sweatshop labor. The transactional fairness standard is concerned with a fair distribution of the gains of the interaction. An interaction may be fair by the standards of a hypothetical fair market (or another standard of transactional fairness) but leave workers without sufficient income to meet their basic human needs. Moreover, as the transactional fairness account of exploitation is typically tied to a hypothetical fair-market standard of fairness, it will tend to miss the role of background injustice in creating exploitable vulnerabilities in workers. Insofar as much of the concern with sweatshop labor focuses on the very low wages earned by these workers, the transactional fairness standard will not explain this central concern.

The categories of structural fairness and exploitation as a failure of respect both tend to focus on the most socioeconomically disadvantaged members of society. In the case of sweatshop labor, they both highlight the desperate needs of sweatshop workers—needs that are often not met because of structural injustice. However, the structural fairness account of exploitation, like the transactional fairness account, can become detached from the absolute needs of sweatshop workers. Sample makes this point clear:

> Developing nations are exploited when their basic needs are neglected for the benefit of wealthier trading partners. Many of these needs are not reducible to improvements in income. Such exploitation is often made possible by background injustices. But even when our interactors flourish and perhaps even thrive, they can legitimately complain of exploitation when the distribution of the social surplus of that interaction is tilted in our favor because of injustice.[60]

Structural fairness exploitation, then, can take place even when the basic needs of the exploitees are met. In principle, it is also possible for there to be interactions that do not violate the requirements of structural fairness but fail to meet the basic needs of another person where there is a duty to do so by the standards of a perfect form of the duty of beneficence. In practice, however, structural fairness exploitation will tend to be associated with deficits in the basic needs of the exploitee, though only exploitation as a failure of a perfect form of the duty of beneficence must be tied to such a deficit.

Structural fairness exploitation and exploitation as a violation of a perfect form of the duty of beneficence best reflect the needs and desperation that motivate much of the concern with sweatshop labor. Each of these accounts of exploitation will focus on the absolute needs of exploited sweatshop workers but are tied to different forms of wrongdoing with different remedies if exploitation is to be avoided. This conclusion does nothing to rule out the ability of accounts of transactional fairness exploitation to reveal and explain wrongdoing in other contexts. Rather, the applicability of different accounts of exploitation to different contexts underscores the need for further research into these forms of exploitation and the need for clarity as to the form of exploitation being discussed when this term is applied to specific cases.

Lessons for Accounts of Exploitation in Other Contexts

In my review of exploitation in sweatshop labor, I presented three accounts that identify distinct forms of exploitation tied to different forms of wrongdoing. These forms of exploitation can take place in the same interactions but need not do so. Some forms of exploitation will be more common in certain kinds of interactions than will others, and different forms of exploitation will capture the central moral wrong of different kinds of exploitative relationships. Furthermore, some contexts will require multiple accounts of exploitation to explain fully the range of moral wrongs taking place.

I will now briefly apply these accounts of exploitation to other contexts with the goal of demonstrating how these different forms of exploitation will occur outside of sweatshop labor. I do not claim or intend to discuss every form of exploitation. Instead, I aim to further make the case for the need to understand exploitation as taking different forms and identifying importantly different kinds of moral wrongs. These areas of application will include the exploitation of employees (including, but not limited to, sweatshop labor), the exploitation of customers, the exploitation of suppliers, and the exploitation of governments and communities. In addition, I will discuss the relevance of these accounts of exploitation to wider debates over the limits of corporate social responsibility. This discussion of the different strengths of accounts of exploitation to different contexts will be revisited when I develop an account of exploiting hope in Chapter 4.

Exploitation of Employees

While I have thus far developed my discussion of exploitation in the context of sweatshop labor, exploitation can take place in labor relationships more generally. I have already observed that structural fairness exploitation and exploitation as a failure of respect are best suited to accounting for the most common and morally troubling forms of exploitation in sweatshop labor. But both structural and transactional fairness exploitation are also possible in employment relationships where employees earn more than a living wage.

Structural fairness exploitation may take place if relatively well-paid employees earn less than they would under more just institutional arrangements. For example, back-office workers in India might earn less than they would in the absence of a history of colonial exploitation and unfair trade arrangements. If these unjust actions and structures delayed the economic development of India and reduce the bargaining power of Indian workers in the global marketplace, then the workers would receive a less than fair share of the benefits created through their employment, even if they receive more than enough money to meet their basic needs. Structural fairness exploitation is also possible for relatively highly skilled workers who immigrate to high-income countries, such as skilled health workers. These workers may be vulnerable to structural fairness exploitation if they flee unjust institutional structures such as institutionalized forms of ethnic, religious, or sexual discrimination.[61]

Migrant workers may also face transactional fairness exploitation if the terms of their immigration create an unfair market for their labor. For example, many countries tie these migrants to certain employers or otherwise limit their opportunities for employment, creating an unfair market for their skills. Even if the right of states to limit immigration means that these restrictions on employment are morally permissible, they create an element of unfairness in the market for these migrants' labor, placing a considerable bargaining advantage in the hands of the sole legal employer. If these workers are barred from seeking alternative employment, then they will be unable to gain the higher wages or more favorable terms of employment that they would otherwise be able to command on the open labor market in their new community.[62] Again, the wages and benefits received by these workers may be more than sufficient to meet their basic needs, but the relationship could be exploitative by the standards of transactional fairness given the employer's bargaining advantage.

Exploitation of Customers

Customers may be exploited during business transactions. As with labor exploitation, the type of exploitation taking place will depend in part on the resources of the individual being exploited. All customers, regardless of their resources, are vulnerable to fairness exploitation when a supplier possesses monopoly power over the pricing of some good or service. By definition, a monopoly is a departure from a hypothetical fair market, giving vendors the power to set an unfair price for their goods. Should they choose to take advantage of this power, they can exploit their customers. Monopoly powers may be achieved through a chance concentration of the supply of some good or service in the hands of a single vendor, the collusion of vendors to control the supply of some good or service, or the failure of a government to regulate the market and maintain competition among suppliers. In these cases, transactional fairness exploitation becomes possible. Monopoly powers are also possible as a result of systemic injustice, as when only persons of a certain social group are allowed to sell some good or when systemic injustice has made it impossible for some social groups to participate in the market. In these cases, structural fairness exploitation may take place.

When the customer lacks access to some essential goods, a specific form of exploitation as the mere use of others becomes possible as well. A collapse in the supply of a good or spike in demand, particularly following a disaster, can create a form of exploitation commonly called price gouging.[63] In these cases, a vendor will see an increase in their bargaining advantage if their supplies of some good are not destroyed by the disaster or if they are able to move supplies into the affected area after the disaster. When the goods in question are essential to meeting the customer's basic needs—as in the case of food, water, shelter, and medicines—then the inelasticity of customer demand allows the vendor to raise prices and achieve a windfall profit. These gains for the vendor are unfair, as in typical cases of transactional unfairness exploitation. But in cases of price gouging, the vendor commits the additional moral wrong of failing to modify their actions in response to the needs of their customers. Arguably, these needs, in the context of a disaster, can help specify the vendor's duty of beneficence. If so, they may fail in this duty if they react to the disaster by raising prices on their stocks of essential goods beyond any corresponding increase in their costs or the risks they face.

Exploitation of Suppliers

Suppliers may be exploited when buyers achieve monopsony powers that allow them to control the prices that they will pay for goods and services. As with monopoly pricing by a supplier, monopsony powers allow a buyer to receive an unfair portion of the benefits created by the interaction between buyer and seller. When this unfairness is achieved through a localized market failure, where the buyer can purchase goods at less than a hypothetical fair-market price, then the buyer potentially transactional-fairness exploits their suppliers. Monopsony powers may also be achieved through structural injustice, as when the right to purchase a type of good is restricted to certain social groups or when unjust socioeconomic inequalities have denied members of certain social groups from entering the market. In these cases, structural fairness exploitation becomes possible. Even when the prices paid to the suppliers remain sufficient for the suppliers to meet their basic needs, the price paid in these interactions may be unfair and exploitative.

A form of exploitation as a failure of respect is also possible when the buyer's bargaining power allows them to offer prices to suppliers that are insufficient for them to meet their basic needs. This specific charge has been levied against Walmart in light of that company's ongoing efforts to reduce prices paid to suppliers in China, among other countries.[64] Walmart is accused of using its dominant position as a buyer of a large range of goods to set prices on the market, with annual pressure to reduce prices among its suppliers. These suppliers are forced to continually reduce prices for their goods, leading predictably to pressure on wage levels for their employees, loss of benefits, and a failure to improve working conditions. The pricing pressure exerted by companies like Walmart lead predictably to inadequate wages for the employees of these suppliers, even if the management of the suppliers, with whom the buyer interacts directly, retain a living wage. While the buyer does not directly set the wage levels for the suppliers' workers, the buyer is in a special position of influence over this vulnerable group of workers such that the buyer may have a duty of beneficence toward these workers. By failing to take steps to ensure that cost-cutting pressures do not result in worsening working conditions for its suppliers' employees, the buyer can fail in a duty of beneficence and exploit these workers.

Exploitation of Communities

Entire governments or communities may be exploited during trade and production. A primary instance of this exploitation takes place through unjust international institutions that disadvantage entire communities in their trade relations with other countries. Thomas Pogge has cited such several instances within LMICs.[65] For example, the Agreement on Trade-Related Aspects of Intellectual Property Rights (TRIPS) has been cited as a legal structure that serves to inflate the prices of pharmaceuticals, in many cases beyond the point where they can be afforded in poorer parts of the world. Pharmaceutical companies in the US and other wealthy countries are said to have had a dominant role in shaping and pushing for the passage of TRIPS, and so these companies can rightly be accused of exploiting entire communities, particularly in the developing world.[66] Similar exploitation can take place through other trade pacts, where wealthy interests help to shape these treaties to their own advantage.

These cases are instances of transactional and structural unfairness exploitation and, in some cases, exploitation as the mere use of others as well. Institutional injustice creates the potential for exploitation as the mere use of others when it prevents members of some communities from meeting their basic needs. Insofar as the TRIPS agreement helps to price pharmaceuticals beyond the reach of those in need of these drugs in LMICs, then those responsible for these pricing structures and decisions may fail in a specified duty of beneficence toward entire communities given their power over the health and well-being of the members of those communities.

Powerful groups may also transactional-fairness exploit entire communities. This form of exploitation can take place if individuals take advantage of a global market that gives some parties in certain countries and markets unfair advantages over others. The higher prices for pharmaceuticals paid throughout the world not only exhibit a failure by influential members of the pharmaceutical industry to fulfill a specified duty of beneficence but also arguably allow these companies to shut competitors out of the market, thus creating unfairly high prices for their goods. More generally, a history of aggressive war, colonization, and trade structures that exacerbate inequality between states gives citizens of richer countries the power to shape international structures in a way that secures additional benefits for these already richer countries. When members of the developed world take advantage of these injustices, they participate in a global economic system that is structural fairness exploitative of the less advantaged members of the world.

Conclusion

My aim in outlining some of the forms of exploitation in sweatshop labor and other contexts in this chapter is to make the point that the moral wrong of exploitation can take several different forms. Different kinds of exploitation, with their different kinds of underlying moral wrongs, can take place at different points in interactions, and they can take place simultaneously as well. This point is essential to clarifying the meaning of accusations of exploitation. Merely saying that a relationship is exploitative is insufficient. Without specifying which forms of exploitation are thought to be taking place, charges of exploitation will merely confuse charges of wrongdoing and, over time, may foster skepticism that the charge of exploitation can identify a distinct moral wrong at all.

This lesson is crucial, but it also raises another point about the importance of distinguishing between different forms of exploitation. Different theories of exploitation can define exploitation as either an all-things-considered moral wrong—that is, impermissible in all circumstances—or a reason against an action that can be outweighed by other considerations in some circumstances. In the first case, determining whether a relationship is actually exploitative may turn, in part, on the consequences of preventing the potentially exploitative interaction. That is, a sufficiently beneficial relationship will not count as exploitative if preventing the relationship would lead to hardship for the potential exploitee.[67] Sample, for example, considers a case where mutually advantageous sweatshop employment requires gross inequality. In these cases, she argues, the sweatshop owner "is not degrading the workers but simply doing the best he can. He is not guilty of exploitation."[68]

In the second case, a relationship might be said to be exploitative but morally permissible. This moral permissibility is typically extended in light of sufficient benefits to the exploitee or sufficient hardship if the relationship were prevented. The question of moral permissibility may be limited to whether third parties, such as state regulators, are justified in interfering with an exploitative relationship. While the exploiter may act wrongly in structuring the relationship in a way that exploits another person, this act of exploitation does not necessarily justify restrictions by third parties. As Wertheimer puts it, the question of the moral weight of a relationship (the intensity of the exploitative element) is separable from the moral force of the relationship (whether interfering with the relationship would be permissible).[69]

The question of the moral permissibility of exploitation may also extend to whether exploitation should be counted, all things considered, as an act of wrongdoing by the exploiter. Countervailing considerations, including the potential benefit to the exploitee and lack of other, viable options for the exploiter, will be relevant to this determination. When exploitation is considered a non-conclusive reason against an action, an exploitative but morally permissible relationship may create a form of moral residue, where the exploiter may have a duty to make up for the element of exploitation or to take steps to reduce the structural causes of exploitation. On this view, when sweatshop owners find themselves with no choice but to exploit background injustice—for example, they are "right to do wrong."[70]

On any of these views, a relationship is more likely to be exploitative but morally permissible when it is voluntary and mutually beneficial—the kinds of cases on which I have focused in this chapter. When coercion is used in a relationship or one party is harmed against a baseline of no interaction at all, it is much more likely that the moral force of the relationship will permit interference in the interest of the exploitee. In fact, the exploitee's consent and benefit can be necessary conditions for morally permissible exploitation.

These clarifications are important in light of debates over the consequences of regulations aimed at curbing potentially exploitative relationships. Continuing with the example of sweatshop labor, several of the accounts of exploitation that I considered in this chapter rely on empirical claims about the consequences of wage increases. Some authors argue that wage increases can have undesirable effects on would-be workers in impoverished communities if increased labor costs lead to lower levels of employment.[71,72] In response, other authors cast doubt on the negative impacts of increased wages.[73] Others point to the need to be creative when searching for ways to increase employee welfare while remaining competitive.[74,75,76] The answers to these empirical questions will be essential to determining whether exploitation takes place in specific business relationships, whether an exploitative relationship is permissible, and whether the government is justified in regulating exploitative relationships, depending on one's theory of exploitation. Calls to regulate the development and availability of unproven medical interventions as exploitative will similarly need to be sensitive to contextual details around the impacts of proposed regulations on health and safety, as well as other morally relevant dimensions of each case.

More importantly, the role of the positive consequences in determining whether exploitation takes place becomes more complicated when we realize that multiple forms of exploitation can take place in a single interaction. When exploitation is seen as an all-things-considered moral wrong, determining whether exploitation takes place entails balancing the wrongs of exploitation and the benefits that the interaction would create. Similarly, interpreting exploitation as a non-conclusive reason against an action requires balancing the wrongs of exploitation and the benefits created by the interaction to determine whether the interaction is both exploitative *and* impermissible. While a single element of exploitation may not support the conclusion that a relationship is morally impermissible, the presence of multiple forms of exploitation may support a different conclusion. Should we fail to mark distinctions between different forms of exploitation, then not only will we be left without clarity as to the form of moral wrongdoing alleged by charges of exploitation, but we will also be unable to determine whether an impermissible act of exploitation has taken place at all. The key lesson of this chapter, then, is that a discussion of when practices are exploitative simply cannot get off the ground without first discussing and understanding the different forms that exploitation can take.

In this chapter, I have not described all of the forms of exploitation that can take place. But I have illustrated that exploitation takes at least three distinct forms and that clarity about the forms of exploitation alleged to take place is essential if these charges are to serve as a useful part of the dialogue in applied ethics. While this discussion focused on an example from the context of business, this same point about the need for clarity around what type of exploitation is claimed to be occurring applies elsewhere as well, including the medical context. As I will show throughout this book, concerns with exploitation are common and well justified in a range of contexts within the business of providing healthcare, in medical research and practice, and in the provision of unproven medical interventions.

More specifically, the exploitation of hope is common in these contexts. While we now have a much better understanding of what is morally wrong with exploitation, we now need to explore the nature of hope. Specifically, we need to know more about what kind of vulnerabilities hope can create, such that they can be exploited by others. I will then move on in Chapter 4 to develop an account of exploiting hope by applying the understandings of exploitation developed here to the analysis of hope.

3

What Is Hope?

In the first chapter, I showed that popular use of the term "exploiting hope" and its variants, despite being applied across a wide range of cases, shows some key commonalities. These commonalities include that the sense of "hope" in these cases is generally hope for a substantial improvement in the exploitee's life rather than a marginal change. Whether the exploitee was desperate for this improvement because of poor health or a lack of economic opportunities or was simply seeking fame and fortune, the change hoped for would be transformative or *weighty*. Given the importance of the hoped-for change to their lives, these individuals were willing to take *leaps of hope*, typically taking risky actions that included placing significant control over their welfare in the hands of others. Given the weightiness and riskiness of these actions, hope was seen as an exploitable vulnerability that could be taken advantage of.

The previous chapter toured various accounts of exploitation. I demonstrated that, rather than a single, unified account of exploitation, there are at least three senses of exploitation: transactional fairness, structural fairness, and respect-based accounts. Each of these accounts identified a distinct sense in which taking advantage of another person can be either unethical all things considered or constitute a reason against an action. Moreover, the wrongness at the center of each of these accounts is not merely a failure of consent or outright harm to the exploitee. That is, each of these accounts makes the claim that voluntary and mutually beneficial exploitation is possible and that exploitation is its own, distinct form of wrongdoing.

Yet, the popular use of the charge of exploiting hope tends to focus on concerns with failures of consent and harms to exploitees. The most common type of case from the popular press was an instance of defrauding the exploitee, where the victim's hope for a better life created desperation or credulity that made them vulnerable to believing the lies and misrepresentations of the exploiter. These fraudsters took advantage of their victims' willingness to take a leap of hope in order to gain from them financially while, at best, giving them nothing in return and, at worst, leaving them jailed, destitute, or dead.

Given this focus on fraud and harm in how the concept of exploiting hope is popularly used, it isn't clear that the perceived wrongness in these cases is linked to the wrongness of scholarly accounts of exploitation. While these scholarly accounts of exploitation often overlap with fraud, failures of consent, and harm, the specific wrongness of exploitation is meant to be rooted in profiting from transactional unfairness, taking advantage of structural injustice, or failing in a specified duty of beneficence. If popular use of exploiting hope understands hope as simply a form of credulity that makes hopeful persons vulnerable to fraudsters, then there is a danger that rooting my account of exploiting hope in scholarly accounts of exploitation would result in an understanding of exploiting hope that would be unfamiliar to the public and divorced from common use of this term.

Thus, in this chapter I will examine the concept of hope with an eye toward identifying an understanding of this concept that is consistent with popular uses of exploiting hope and that can be used to develop an account of what is distinctly wrong with such actions. I will review scholarly accounts of the concept of hope to see how these accounts can mesh with the use of hope in the context of exploitation, including seeing hope as being transformative of one's life prospects and creating an exploitable vulnerability. I will also examine how these scholarly accounts apply to other terms used in conjunction with popular usage of hope in the context of exploitation.

Crucially, my aim here is *not* to develop a stand-alone account of the concept of hope. Such accounts have been developed elsewhere and in much greater detail than I will attempt here. Rather, my aim is to use the existing literature on the concept of hope to produce an understanding of hope as it relates to exploitation. Specifically, I seek to explore those aspects of hope that give rise to characteristics or vulnerabilities in individuals that can be exploited.

In what follows, I will borrow heavily from the account of hope developed by Adrienne Martin.[1] Her understanding of hope is particularly fitting for my project for several reasons. First, it aims specifically to give an account of hope in the context of highly leveraged situations, where the outcome is highly valued but not seen as likely. These types of situations, where the hoped-for outcome is central to one's well-being and the individual is willing to take a risky leap of hope, are key to the cases discussed in Chapter 1. Second, Martin's account addresses actions that hope can prompt. These actions are in large part what leads to the opportunity for exploitation, as seen in Chapter 1. Finally, Martin discusses hope in the context of fantasizing, which I will link to the aspect of "dreaming" that is common in popular discussions of exploiting hope.

Theories of Hope

Adrienne Martin summarizes the orthodox contemporary analytic view of hope as "a combination of the desire for an outcome and the belief that the outcome is possible but not certain."[2] This understanding of hope has a long history in the modern period. For example, Hobbes describes hope as an "Appetite with an opinion of attaining," thus combining the standard, key elements of desire or appetite and at least the possibility of the desired outcome to occur.[3] David Hume similarly links hope to uncertainty about a desired or undesirable outcome occurring. Interestingly, he links hope to fear, as "when either good or evil is uncertain, it gives rise to FEAR or HOPE, according to the degrees of uncertainty on the one side or the other."[4] The device of placing hope on one end of a spectrum of uncertainty, with fear on the other end, concurs with the popular uses of exploiting hope that I presented in Chapter 1. In this way, fear that an outcome will not occur accompanies hope that it will.

This traditional account of hope is intended to explain the trivial or thin uses of hope that express a casual desire for an uncertain outcome, as when one expresses hope for nice weather for a picnic. Martin suggests that the best test of these views is in their ability to account for what she calls "hoping against hope" or "hoping for an outcome that one highly values but believes is extremely unlikely."[5] She roots the phrase "hoping against hope" in a passage from Romans 4:18, where St. Paul describes Abraham as he "who against hope believed in hope, that he might become the father of many nations." As Martin acknowledges, this idiom can be confusing and imply irrationality on the part of the hopeful person. That is, hoping against hope can be read to imply that the hoped-for outcome is impossible or that continued hope in the face of extremely difficult odds suggests that they do not understand the degree to which it is unlikely. She notes that this is not her intention in using the phrase, as one can hope despite knowing that the hoped-for outcome is highly unlikely.

The phrase "hope beyond hope" can be clarified by examining the Greek origins of the English translation of Romans 4:18, where the Greek *elpis* can be used to express expectation in addition to hope.[6] Thus, hoping against hope can be understood more specifically as hoping against all expectation of a positive outcome. For the sake of clarity, I will refer to this idea as *hoping against all expectation* for the remainder of this book. This understanding of hope, Martin argues, is the standard against which accounts of hope should be measured. It is also the standard that I will adopt for this project, because it is this form of hope—not a trivial desire, but a

risky leap in the face of odds often understood to be very poor—
that best describes the cases where exploitation is most commonly
at play.

To challenge the standard account of hope, Martin gives the example of two individuals with a terminal cancer diagnosis who have
enrolled in a clinical trial of an experimental cancer drug. Both
desire—and, specifically, hope—that the trial will lead to a cure for
their condition but accept that this outcome is extremely unlikely,
as there is less than a 1 percent chance of this occurring. What
differentiates these two individuals is that the first emphasizes the
long odds against being cured through this trial and focuses on
its potential benefit for others. The second individual, however,
suggests that the trial "keeps her going" and acknowledges that it
has a considerable impact on her emotions and actions.[7] Martin
suggests that the standard understanding of hope can account for
the hope of the first of these two individuals but not the second.

Specifically, Martin notes two ways in which the standard account of hope fails to account for hoping against all expectation.[8]
First, it does not explain the phenomenology or affective content of
hoping against all expectation. Rather than simply a desire for some
positive outcome, hoping against all expectation is a profound and
emotion-laden experience. Moreover, this experience can change
from day to day, even if one's strength of desire and understanding
of the likelihood of that desire being realized does not change. That
is, two individuals can have the same strength of desire and probability estimate of an outcome but very different experiences of
this hope. This criticism meshes with the review of popular uses
of exploiting hope from Chapter 1, where exploitees were typically desperate and emotionally vulnerable individuals taking risky
leaps of hope.

Second, Martin argues that hoping against all expectation
supports these individuals in the face of external challenges. She
writes that understanding hope simply as a desire for a positive
outcome does not capture this idea that hope can have a positive,

sustaining effect on individuals. In the cases of exploitation I've reviewed thus far, hope is seen more as a vulnerability, something to be taken advantage of. This view is biased, of course, as it derives from cases where hope has led to exploitation and harm. For those not exploited, hope can have positive impacts when it is not taken advantage of or otherwise abused by others in whom one's welfare is entrusted.

Increasingly, contemporary accounts of hope have moved beyond the orthodox understanding of hope as a combination of a desire for some outcome and belief that that outcome is possible. For example, Luc Bovens argues that, in addition to desire for an outcome and belief that it is possible, a hopeful person must devote some "mental energy" or "mental imaging" to what the world would be like if that outcome were realized. He justifies this requirement by arguing that it would be incorrect to say that he had hoped that a guest would attend his party unless he had "devoted at least some mental energy to the question whether she would or would not come to the party."[9]

Martin agrees with Bovens that mental imaging of this kind is a necessary condition for hope—specifically that "hope entails at least the disposition to entertain certain kinds of thoughts about the hoped-for outcome."[10] However, she argues that this addition is inadequate to demonstrate why the orthodox definition of hope cannot explain hoping against all expectation. Specifically, in cases of hoping beyond all expectation, she notes that two people could have the same mental images about a desired but very unlikely outcome and expend the same mental energy on this imaging; nonetheless, such imaging is consistent with one person despairing of achieving this outcome or hoping very little for it, while another engages deeply with the outcome, hoping beyond all expectation. Martin concludes from this analysis that understanding how hope engages with our imagination and mental energies is an important element of understanding this concept; however, this element does not fully address the shortcomings of the orthodox account.

Philip Pettit has argued for what he calls "substantial hope" as giving a more robust account of this concept.[11] Substantial hope entails acting as if—or having "cognitive resolve" that—the hoped-for outcome will come about or has a good chance of occurring even if it does not. Such hope is justified, he argues, when it guards against a "loss of heart" or demoralization in the face of long odds or an ebb and flow of evidence of whether the desired outcome will come about. Substantial hope has three specific elements:

1. The agent desires that a certain prospect obtain and believes that it may or may not obtain—these are the conditions for superficial hope—but may do so only at a level of confidence that induces a loss of heart, sapping spirit and effort.
2. The signal danger of this loss of heart prompts the agent to adopt a strategy that consists in acting as if the desired prospect is going to obtain or has a good change of obtaining.
3. This strategy promises to avoid that danger and secure the related, secondary benefit, relevant even for someone relatively optimistic, of ensuring stability across the ups and downs of evidence.[12]

Understood as such, substantial hope has a pragmatic character, acting to protect the individual from loss of hope, and thus steadying the individual and ensuring that they continue to work to realize the hoped-for outcome insofar as it is under their control.

Again, Martin argues that Pettit's view of hope improves on the orthodox definition while still being inadequate. Specifically, the individual acting as if the hoped-for outcome will occur or is likely to occur captures an important element of hoping against all expectation. However, Martin notes that simply acting as if a long-shot desirable outcome will occur without accompanying caution or planning in case it does not occur is more akin to faith than hope. Those who hope against all expectation can also prepare for a negative outcome, as when one "hopes for the best but prepares for the worst." Thus, Martin argues, "precaution is a natural companion of hope" rather than its converse, as Pettit suggests.[13] Pettit's account of hope relies too much on treating the hopeful person as having an incorrect estimation of the likelihood of the desired-for outcome occurring. The key difference, for Martin, is that a hopeful person sees an extremely unlikely but hoped-for outcome as good enough to engage with, whereas Pettit suggests that these individuals simply replace the actual likelihood of this outcome with a fabricated likelihood in their minds. For Martin, "while Pettit is right that hoping means being disposed to act as if the hoped-for outcome is going to occur, or is likely to occur, he is wrong about the hopeful person's *rationale* for acting in this way. The hopeful person doesn't act like this because she has decided to act as if the outcome is indeed more likely to occur than she believes it is; rather, she acts like this because she sees the outcome's probability as good enough to permit it."[14]

Martin's alternative, positive account is termed the *incorporation analysis*. This view holds that hope entails not simply that an individual is attracted to an activity and its consequences. Rather, she incorporates this attraction along with the licensing status of the outcome's probability to create a sufficient justificatory rationale for engaging in the activity. On this incorporation view, to hope for an outcome is to:

1. Be attracted to the outcome in virtue of certain of its features;
2. Assign a probability between and exclusive of 0 and 1 to the outcome;
3. Adopt a stance toward that probability whereby it licenses treating one's attraction to the outcome (and the outcome's attractive features) as a reason for certain ways of thinking, feeling, and/or planning with regard to the hoped-for outcome; and
4. Treat one's attraction and the outcome's attractive features as sufficient reason for those ways of thinking, feeling, and/or planning.[15]

For Martin, these are not necessary and sufficient conditions for hope. Rather, they are present in what she calls hope "*in the fullest sense.*" Thus, we can say that a person who engages in hopeful fantasies about the desired outcome but feels that doing so is inappropriate owing to the unlikeliness of this outcome engages in hopeful activities or something akin to hope even if it is not hope in the fullest sense.

For our purposes, the key element of Martin's incorporation analysis is that hope licenses thinking and fantasizing about, planning for, and engaging emotionally with a desired outcome even if it is unlikely to occur. Martin describes the combination of attitudes toward the desired outcome and attendant feelings as a "syndrome," where distinct elements are incorporated into a unified analysis. This syndrome approach helps to explain the richness of a concept like hope, where engaging emotionally with and planning around a desired outcome can be rationally justified even when one's expectations of that outcome occurring is extremely low.

This view can be criticized as not sufficiently engaging in the emotional aspects of hope. Milona and Stockdale[16] agree with Martin that hope involves a normative assessment—namely, that it justifies engaging in hopeful activities. However, they argue that Martin's incorporation analysis cannot account for cases of "recalcitrant hope," where hope persists despite holding a contradictory judgment that it is inappropriate to engage in hopeful activities. For example, one might engage in hopeful fantasies about becoming romantically involved with an abusive former romantic partner while also feeling ashamed of these fantasies and acknowledging that renewing this relationship would be a bad idea. While Martin could respond that recalcitrant hopes are not hopes in the fullest sense, Milona and Stockdale argue that recalcitrant hopes are common and that such a response would be problematically ad hoc.

Instead, Milona and Stockdale argue that "hope involves a perceptual-like normative assessment." Perceptions, in this sense, involve being presented with things in the world as being a certain way. This contrasts with beliefs, in which the agent takes a stance as to what is true. Perceptions, rather, entail an experience of something as being true, as presented to the person having the experience. From this, Milona and Stockdale argue that hope has a specific phenomenology, an experience of what it is like to have hope. What marks hope beyond a desire for an outcome and belief that the outcome is possible is to be *encouraged* by that possibility. Specifically, they argue that hope is an attitude that involves:

1. The desire for an outcome.
2. The belief that the outcome's obtaining is possible but not certain.
3. Seeing the possible-but-uncertain desired outcome as encouraging to varying degrees.
4. Hopeful feelings.[17]

The virtues of this account, they argue, are that (1) it retains the normative dimension of hope found in Martin's view while allowing for the possibility of recalcitrant hope, (2) explains why hope cannot be unconscious, and (3) takes seriously the idea that hopeful individuals correctly understand the low probability of the hoped-for outcome occurring and nonetheless perceive its possibility as encouraging.

As noted earlier, my aim here is not to develop an independent account of hope. Rather, I am seeking to present an understanding of hope that is consistent with and illuminates the cases of exploitation discussed in Chapter 1 and can serve as the basis of an account of exploiting hope. While Martin and Milona and Stockdale disagree as to whether hope is grounded in beliefs or perceptions, they both offer an understanding of hoping against all expectation where hope is rational or justified and the hopeful person is emotionally engaged and oriented toward taking certain actions in response to this hope. As such, they build on an existing thread of scholarship on hope that rejects the orthodox definition and that I will adopt for the remainder of this project.

Hopes, Dreams, and Leaps

As I demonstrated in Chapter 1 of this project, "hopes" and "dreams" frequently appear together in the popular press in the context of exploitation. Hopes and dreams were used to describe many of the same types of interactions—both consensual and fraudulent—for those seeking basic necessities and those seeking an exceptional life. These terms are treated as largely interchangeable, but it is not clear, as popularly used, if adding "dreams" to the charge of exploiting hope meaningfully deepens our understanding of what is problematic about these interactions or if it is more of a rhetorical flourish.

Recall that Martin endorsed Bovens's claim that hope involves expending mental energy or engaging in mental imaging about the hoped-for outcome. While she argued that this addition to the orthodox account of hope was insufficient as a full account of hope, she agreed that hope entailed such mental imaging or the disposition to engage in certain thoughts about the hoped-for outcome. Specifically, hope is commonly expressed in the form of fantasizing about the realization of this hope. Fantasies, for Martin, are defined by having a narrative structure. Rather than simply taking the form of a static image of the desired outcome, they tell an emotion-laden story about what it will be like for the outcome to take place. Moreover, they have an egoistic function in that they take the form of having one's own desires realized. Furthermore, fantasies have a special role in motivating us to act by solidifying the hoped-for outcome in the individual's mind.[18]

From this, Martin sees the fantasizing aspect of hoping as linked to our common use of "dreaming." Specifically, "when we encourage people to hope, we encourage them to engage in the behaviors expressive of hope—we encourage them to 'dream.' In doing so, we encourage them to engage in an activity whereby they can discover new reasons to pursue the object of hope, as well as new ways of doing so."[19] She grants that dreams and fantasies can sometimes work against taking actions supportive of a hoped-for outcome, as when a fantasy focuses on the obstacles to achieving this outcome. In response, she notes that, while fantasies and dreams may create obstacles to action, "in the modern Western world, we are encouraged toward optimistic dreams, and we are rarely enjoined to fantasize pessimistically. When we encourage people to express their hopes, to 'dream big,' we are therefore encouraging the kinds of fantasies that present reasons in favor of the object of hope."[20] This view of the role of fantasies and dreams as having a largely positive valance and encouraging action matches well with the use of "dreams" in the popular press. There, as with Martin's use, dreams are big goals that motivate people to act and, potentially, leave them vulnerable to exploitation.

This motivating aspect of fantasies and dreams also helps to illuminate a common element I observed in the popular discussions of exploiting hope. As I noted, hope in this context often involves risk-taking and placing oneself in another's hands—or, a leap of hope. While Martin rejects Pettit's account of hope as inadequate, Pettit sees a close relationship between hope and precaution.[21] Specifically, hope entails acting as if the hoped-for outcome will occur in order to provide stability to and firm the resolve of the hopeful individual. For Pettit, hope is the opposite of precaution, where one acts as if the desired outcome will not occur. Pettit gives the example of an individual renovating their house where they wisely budget for cost overruns on the assumption that their carefully planned budget will be stressed and deformed when exposed to the realities of building and builders. This exercise of precaution serves to protect the individual from undesirable but foreseeable outcomes, whereas hope gives them the courage to proceed despite the high risk of failure.

As I have discussed, Martin argues that Pettit misses the mark in viewing precaution and hope as structurally similar concepts with opposing valences. She notes that this view implies that hopeful individuals disregard the actual likelihood of the desired outcome in an act of faith rather than hope. Moreover, she sees hope as consistent with precaution, as when the hopeful individual still prepares a plan for failure. That said, Martin agrees that fantasizing—or dreaming—about a hoped-for outcome has the role of affecting one's agency and actions. She specifically describes "active fantasies," where an individual sees themselves as taking an active role in bringing about the hoped-for outcome. This form of fantasizing or dreaming has a role in two causal mechanisms: "fantasy affecting one's sense of agency and one's sense of agency affecting one's actions."[22] Notably, passive fantasies, where one sees oneself as inactive and not having a role in bringing about the hoped-for outcome, can have a dampening role, diminishing the agency of the individual and making it less likely that they will take action to realize this outcome. What I have identified as leaps of hope in the popular literature, then, coincide specifically with Martin's account of active fantasizing or dreaming.

False and Informed Hope

As I showed in Chapter 1, popular concerns that hope can be exploited are often linked to a failure of consent by the exploitee. Most directly, these are often cases where the exploiter acts deliberately to mislead the exploitee by lying to them about the likely benefits of their interaction. Thus human smugglers, scammers dangling fake job offers, and others take advantage of the exploitee's desperation to improve their circumstances in order to offer them "false" hope—a desired outcome where the probabilities of achieving it are considerably different than the exploiter suggests and, in many cases, zero.

But even in cases that do not involve fraud or other forms of misinformation, those hoping for a better life may also fall victim to deficiencies in their ability to give fully informed consent to participate in the interaction. These deficiencies around informed and autonomous decision-making can also constitute false hope. In the context of clinical trials and medical treatment, several forms of failure of fully formed consent have been conceptualized and documented. These include therapeutic misconception, where clinical research is misunderstood to be a form of personal medical treatment; therapeutic misestimation, where the individual misestimates the likelihood of a benefit or harm from occurring; and therapeutic optimism, where individuals overestimate the likelihood of personal benefit, especially during phase I clinical trials.[23]

In cases of therapeutic misconception, participants in the research mistake the purpose of research. The aim of research is to produce generalizable knowledge about the studied intervention, and direct benefit to the research participant is possible but not the primary goal. When this misconception occurs, the research participant believes the research project is designed to benefit them and other participants. This misconception is ethically concerning in terms of informed consent because it may undermine understanding of the study design specifically. For example, this misconception could lead the research participant to not understand the possibility of receiving a placebo in a randomized trial or to discount the possibility that they could be enrolled in the placebo arm.[24]

When therapeutic misestimation occurs, an individual might not misunderstand the difference between research and clinical care or the purpose of research. However, they may yet fail to understand the risks of a medical procedure or the likely benefits of the procedure, and as a result they may be unable to give fully informed consent to the procedure.[25] Misestimation of this kind has been found in phase I clinical trials, where an intervention is being tested for safety rather than efficacy and may involve subtherapeutic doses of a treatment. In these trials, some trial participants enroll with an unrealistic expectation that the trial will confer direct benefit to them. Horng and Grady suggest that this kind of misestimation may be a threat to informed consent depending on the magnitude of the misestimation and its personal relevance. They argue that the larger the magnitude of the misestimation, the more likely that it will misinform the participant's decision to participate in the trial and thus undermine informed consent. Moreover, if the misestimation of the likelihood of the benefit or risk of harm relates to something of special relevance to the participant—such as hearing loss to a musician—the more likely it is that misestimation will occur.

In cases of therapeutic optimism or unrealistic optimism, an individual believes that their outcome will be "more favorable than that suggested by a relevant, objective standard" or "more favorable than the outcomes of their peers."[26] As with therapeutic misestimation, unrealistic optimism can be understood as a form of bias or cognitive distortion. Unrealistic optimism, as a more general psychological phenomenon, is described as a tendency, when considering the likelihood of future events, to emphasize personal factors that might increase the likelihood of a positive outcome.[27] While this optimism can be linked to medical outcomes, it also applies to other life events like financial success, personal fame, and the success of loved ones. The problem with unrealistic optimism is that other, similarly situated persons will likely have other personal factors that affect their odds of positive outcomes. At a group level, unrealistic optimism takes the form of individuals systematically overestimating the likelihood of positive outcomes.

Therapeutic optimism can be described as a form of situational optimism, where the individual believes that their chances of receiving benefit during clinical research participation or clinical care is greater than other, similarly situated persons. As opposed to persons with an optimistic disposition and who generally emphasize positive aspects of the world as they see it, persons with situational optimism may have an unrealistic understanding of their chances of a positive outcome.[28] This unrealistic understanding will particularly be the case if their understanding of their personal chances of a positive outcome from research or clinical care is not based on a relevant personal attribute or difference from other, similarly situated persons. In these cases, informed consent to participate in research or clinical care will be undermined by an inaccurate understanding of the likely benefits and risks of such participation.

However, hope does not necessarily mean that the person believes they are more likely than the evidence suggests to have a positive outcome or to avoid a negative outcome from receiving medical care. Rather, as Martin shows, a hopeful individual focuses on the potential, positive outcomes of a treatment, justifying attention to and imaginative engagement with this outcome despite, in some cases, its statistical unlikelihood or where its likelihood is unknown. The hopeful person needn't misestimate the likelihood of this outcome or apply the likelihood of this outcome to themselves differently than for others. Knowing the true likelihood of the outcome, the hopeful person turns their attention to this outcome, possibly by fantasizing about and planning around it.[29]

Moreover, hopeful individuals may see advantages in this focus, including to their mental health and personal relationships. Hope, understood in the empirical literature as a psychological disposition toward optimism about the future and goal-directed thinking, has been linked to positive impacts on multiple dimensions of well-being, including subjective, psychological, and social well-being.[30,31] While this understanding of hope is distinct from Martin's conceptualization of hope, there is considerable overlap between these accounts in that hope affects one's ability to face and overcome obstacles to a desired outcome. As with hope understood as goal-directed behavior and planning, Martin's understanding of hope as active fantasizing or dreaming can impact an individual's sense of agency and ability and willingness to try to realize a desired outcome.

Hope, understood in this way, can have a positive effect on health behaviors by helping to support resilience toward achieving healthy goals when obstacles arise and to maintain discipline and motivation in pursuing these goals.[32] Conversely, those with low hope about the future are more likely to engage in negative health behaviors such as binge drinking.[33] Once an individual is ill, hope also has a role in promoting positive and desired outcomes. This effect is generated through multiple pathways, including helping individuals adjust to illness, adhering to recommended medical and rehabilitative practices, and dealing with the stresses and uncertainty of illness.[34] More specifically, hope can help individuals cope with pain in general and chronic pain specifically, in part by ignoring the experience of pain in order to focus on one's goals.[35,36] Hope has been found to help children and adolescents adhere to prescribed medical treatments and to prevent anxiety and depression.[37,38] For individuals diagnosed with cancer, Stanton et al. show that hope is correlated with greater resilience following diagnosis, positive emotional responses after receiving care, and better overall outcomes.[39] They echo Martin's distinction between active and passive fantasizing when accounting for this difference in health outcomes for breast cancer patients. Specifically, they suggest that hopeful individuals engage in more active coping behavior, whereas merely "wishful" individuals did not take on these activities.

These positive outcomes of hoping create independent reasons to hope and plan for positive outcomes, because they can increase their likelihood. That is, insofar as hope alters or sustains our behaviors, there are positive reasons to engage in hoping. In fact, there have been calls for physicians to develop skills in bolstering and maintaining hope in their patients to help them gain these therapeutic benefits, and there is a strong argument that caregivers should encourage hope and optimism in others.[40,41] Given the positive effects of hope and the fact that it can be differentiated from therapeutic misconception, therapeutic misestimation, and situational optimism that mislead the individual about the likely outcome of clinical research or treatment, hoping can represent a rational and fully informed choice. This characterization is true of dispositional optimism, understood as a tendency to see the positive aspects of the world and to take actions to realize these outcomes. It is true also of hope for specific outcomes insofar as this hope does not represent a misunderstanding of one's own situation or unrealistic optimism about the likelihood of that outcome coming about.[42]

Hope as a Vulnerability

As we have seen, hope can involve a fully rational and informed way of seeing the world or a possible outcome. In having hope, individuals can entertain dreams about outcomes and prepare themselves for these outcomes. In some cases, doing so is not only consistent with a full understanding of the likelihood of the desired outcome occurring but can increase that likelihood. But then why is hope seen as an exploitable vulnerability? That is, if hope is a rational response to the world that actually enhances individual well-being, why focus on concerns that hope can be exploited?

One answer to this question is that although hope can involve a rational and fully informed way of seeing the world or a specific outcome, it often does not. In cases of false hope, where one does not have a realistic understanding of the likelihood of an outcome taking place, this misunderstanding creates an exploitable vulnerability. For example, if one's hope for a new life in a new country leads one to misunderstand the likelihood of being smuggled safely to another country and the trustworthiness of hired smugglers and their promises, then this misunderstanding creates a vulnerability that makes it easier for smugglers to take advantage of their victims.

Nonetheless, hope need not always entail a misunderstanding about the probabilities of the hoped-for outcome. So is hope an exploitable vulnerability only when it is based on such a misunderstanding? The cases I reviewed in Chapter 1 suggest, in the popular understanding of exploiting hope at least, that this is not the case. Rather, hope is associated with vulnerability in that individuals are desperate to improve their lives, sometimes driven by fear of death or other serious losses, and are willing to take significant risks to see this improvement. Historically, hope has had a negative connotation frequently not seen in modern, Western discussions of this concept. In one of the earliest discussions of hope, Hesiod tells the myth of Pandora releasing hardships and evils into the world by opening a jar given to her by Zeus. Zeus gave Pandora this jar of evils to punish humankind for accepting Prometheus's gift of fire, which the latter had stolen from the gods. As Hesiod wrote, "Nothing but Hope stayed there in her stout, irrefrangible dwelling. Under the lip of the jar, inside, and she never would venture Outdoors, having the lid of the vessel itself to prevent her."[43] This myth is often interpreted as hope, personified as Elpis, acting to counter the evils released by Pandora on humankind: whereas humans would now face "evils and difficult labour" and "distressing diseases that bring doom closer to each one," hope would help them to persevere against these evils.

However, as Nietzsche points out, hope is actually among the evils in Zeus's jar that are visited on the world. He argues that hope is simply a means to prolong humans' suffering, that the perseverance granted by hope is actually an evil. Thus, hope is "the evil that has remained behind" in Zeus's jar, serving Zeus's purpose "that man, though never so tormented by the other evils, should nonetheless not throw life away but continue to let himself be tormented. To that end he gives men hope: it is in truth the worst of all evils, because it protracts the torment of men."[44] In this view, hope is systematically false, in that any hope for overcoming the evils Pandora released, including difficult labor and disease, is futile. Hope is attached to a failure of rationality—but a systemic one that compels us to persevere in search of an unobtainable end. In this way, hope is contrasted with Promethean forethought or foresight, providing instead impractical and unobtainable fantasies and dreams.[45] As we reach out for these dreamed-of outcomes in the face of current suffering, we create a new vulnerability to having that suffering prolonged or worsened.

While Hesiod, as interpreted by Nietzsche, might be accused of taking an unduly negative view of hope, the concern that hope can protract suffering or steer individuals away from more obtainable goals is legitimate. For example, individuals who hope to have their medical condition cured may struggle to abandon or reassess this goal when faced with a terminal diagnosis.[46] Persevering in hope for a cure in the face of information that their hope is unrealistic or false can have significant negative impacts for the patient, in addition to being based on an incorrect understanding of their medical prognosis. These negative impacts can include unnecessary distress for family members, failure to pursue palliative care options, and neglecting to pursue more realistic and obtainable hopes such as spending more time with loved ones or crossing off items from one's "bucket list."[47]

The weightiness of hope creates additional vulnerabilities for the hopeful individual. While we needn't follow, for example, Aquinas in stipulating that hoped-for outcomes "must be something arduous and difficult to obtain, for we do not speak of any one hoping for trifles, which are in one's power to have at any time,"[48] the hopes discussed in the context of exploitation in Chapter 1 generally focused on outcomes central to the individual's well-being and self-conception. Expressing these weighty hopes creates a new vulnerability in that it leaves one open to loss, disappointment, and depression if that hope is not realized or is otherwise threatened. While friends and family may support this hoped-for outcome, expressing hope to others also creates a vulnerability in that these others may not share or endorse this hope. Deeply felt hopes may also be highly subject to new information, leading the hopeful vulnerable to emotional instability as new information supports or diminishes the likelihood of the hoped-for outcome occurring.[49]

Finally, the weightiness of hope compels some people to take leaps of hope that expose them to exploitation. Hope, in cases of exploitation, is not simply a passive daydreaming of the hoped-for outcome. Rather, both in Martin's conception and in popular cases of exploitation, it often leads to risky action that places oneself to some extent in the hands of others, who may in turn take advantage of that hope—by responding with false promises or by disregarding the vulnerability of the hopeful person in favor of focusing on their own benefit.

In short, the many advantages of hope also give rise to several crucial (and, as I will argue, exploitable) vulnerabilities. Hoping can be a rational and fully informed act. However, it can also be false, leading the hopeful individual to engage in actions based on misinformation. Hope is often accompanied by dreaming or fantasizing that allows the hopeful person to engage with and be sustained by the hoped-for outcome. However, hope can be passive, prompting the hopeful person to avoid attending to more realistic goals or actively leading the person away from these more realistic outcomes. Hope can have important, positive outcomes for one's well-being, in part because it is so often associated with weighty outcomes and needs. But for this same reason, weighty hope leaves us highly vulnerable to great loss and disappointment given that the stakes are often so high in these cases—sometimes matters of life and death. Finally, hope can be a risky undertaking compelled by the great promise of the hoped-for outcome. But at the same time, it leaves the hopeful person exposed to harm, loss, and exploitation.

Taking Stock

The ability of hopeful individuals to understand the likelihood of their hoped-for outcome is relevant to an account of exploiting hope because if they have false hope, they may be too ill-informed or emotional to act autonomously, making them vulnerable to exploiters. False hope is likely present in many or perhaps most cases of exploiting hope. However, I would like to argue that the wrongness of taking advantage of another's ignorance or deficiencies in their rational capacities should be kept conceptually separate from exploitation. Following Wertheimer's argument that exploitation is morally problematic in a distinct way from using fraud or force or harming another, these instances of taking advantage of ignorance or irrationality can be classified as instances of fraud (if the exploiter misrepresents information or knowingly takes advantage of the patients' ignorance) or a failure by the patient to act autonomously.[50]

One reason for keeping exploitation separate from failures of consent or autonomy is that, despite often being in an emotionally vulnerable situation, exploitees may be aware of the costs and likely consequences of their actions and yet choose to take them anyway. For example, patients seeking unproven medical interventions often downplay the possibility that unproven interventions will produce a "miracle" cure or complete recovery from their medical condition; rather, many of them seek small, incremental improvements or a halt or slowing of the degeneration of their health.[51] For many of these patients, the appeal of pursuing unproven interventions was that it allowed them to take an active role in managing their health, even if the hoped-for positive results were modest or nonexistent. This is particularly true for patients with the most severe and often terminal illnesses, for whom their lack of other options and sense of desperation are acute.[52] In these cases, the experience of agency and hope for positive outcomes, rather than the reality of these outcomes, was the most likely benefit—one that they felt was worth the cost of these interventions.[53]

On the one hand, these examples present consenting adults who understand that the medical interventions they are pursuing are unproven—and thus offer little evidence that their health will be improved other than through a placebo effect—but nonetheless find value in acting on this hope for better health. On the other hand, these patients may pay very large sums of money for these interventions without good evidence of health benefits (and indeed some risk of harm). Those providing these interventions can take advantage of this hope despite knowing that they are unable to offer any assurances of benefit and, in fact, have little or no scientific basis supporting the use of the intervention. At first glance, these cases take the form of bad actors exploiting the hope of sick and desperate persons even if the vendor does not act fraudulently and the patient is fully informed. It is not obvious, however, if these specific cases are in fact problematically exploitative (and, if so, why) or whether we are simply conflating these cases with more clearly problematic instances of fraud or failures of autonomy. Thus, in the following chapter I will present my account of why exploiting hope is morally problematic, independent of the moral wrongs of misinformation or even harm to the exploited individual.

4

Exploiting Hope

Queer, rootless families, plucked up by war
To blow along the roads like tumbleweed,
Who fed their wild-haired children God knows how
But always kept a fierce and cringing cur,
Famished for scraps, to run below the cart;
Horsedealers, draft-evaders, gipsymen;
Crooked creatures of a thousand dubious trades
That breed like gnats from the debris of war;
Half-cracked herb-doctor, patent-medicine man
With his accordeon and his inked silk hat;
Sellers of snake-oil balm and lucky rings
And the old, crazy hatless wanderer
Who painted "God is Love" upon the barns
And on the rocks, "Prepare to Meet Thy God"[1]

My aim in this chapter is to identify the distinguishing features and moral wrongness of what is often described as "exploiting hope" or "taking advantage of hope"—insofar as such features exist and such a concept can be isolated from other moral concepts. My purpose in doing so is to determine, first, whether "hope" is the sort of vulnerability that can be meaningfully said to be taken advantage of and, if so, whether there is anything distinctive about the moral wrongness of this form of exploitation.

As I argued in Chapter 2, the concept of exploitation can be broken down into three distinct forms of moral failings: (1)

transactional unfairness, where, within a transaction between two people, one person takes advantage of a situation or vulnerability in the other person to receive an unfair portion of the benefit the transaction creates; (2) structural unfairness, where one person takes advantage of structural injustice to receive an unfair or unjust portion of the benefit created by a transaction with someone disadvantaged by that injustice; and (3) exploitation as a failure of respect, where an individual fails to fulfill a specified duty of beneficence to another person. After considering and putting aside applications of the two fairness-based accounts of exploitation, I will discuss how a respect-based account of exploitation can illuminate what is and is not morally problematic about voluntary and non-fraudulent interactions, focusing on the context of accessing unproven medical interventions.

Transactional Exploitation of Hope

As described in more detail in Chapter 2, Alan Wertheimer[2] develops a transactional account of exploitation, where exploitation can be voluntary and mutually advantageous yet unfair and exploitative. For Wertheimer, exploitation takes place when conditions allow one party to take "special" unfair advantage of another.[3] That is, while everyday transactions may be coerced through the use of force, unjust given historical or structural injustices, harmful, or otherwise morally problematic, the particular moral wrong of exploitation takes place when the exploiter uses special factors that arise to extract unusual advantage from an interaction. For example, it may not be morally problematic for a pharmacist to sell an antidote for a poison at a competitive price under normal conditions, but if a manufacturing error destroys all other supplies of the antidote during a mass poisoning, the pharmacist would act exploitatively by taking advantage of this unusual situation to raise prices in response to the desperation of customers.

Wertheimer typically uses a standard of fairness tied to a hypothetical fair-market price to determine when exploitation has occurred, as can be done in the previous example. However, he is clear that "there is no reason to think that there is a unique principle for fair transactions, given that the contexts in which such transactions occur can vary" and that the appropriate principle of fairness "for distributing educational resources may be different from the best principle for distributing health care."[4] In his later writings applied to the context of clinical testing on human subjects, Wertheimer does not defend a hypothetical fair-market price for use in this medical context and notes the difficulty of producing an account of fair transactions for these cases.[5]

While references to the idea of exploiting hope are made in the academic literature, one of the only, and by far the most well-developed, accounts of this concept is presented by Adrienne Martin. Martin's account of exploiting hope uncritically takes Wertheimer's account of transactional exploitation at face value. She uses the anti-cancer drug Avastin as an example of exploiting hope. She writes that Avastin had been shown in early clinical trials to yield small increases in life expectancy.[6] Because of patent protections and marketing exclusivity for new pharmaceutical products, drug manufacturers such as Genentech, Avastin's maker, can charge extremely high prices for these products. Martin dismisses a common defense of these prices—that they are needed for pharmaceutical companies to recover the costs of drug research and development—and states that "if a hypothetical market price is the correct standard for fair exchange, then the exchange we're concerned about is unfair. There is no competitive market for these drugs, and they would be significantly cheaper if there were."[7] Given this standard of fair exchange, then, the high prices that pharmaceutical patent holders can charge for experimental and unproven interventions can lead to the exploitation of their customers.

Martin does point to a real problem in pharmaceutical pricing generally, where the patent and marketing exclusivity systems in place in much of the world allow for the exploitation of persons desperate for these products. However, linking the wrongness of exploiting hope to the problem of monopoly pricing for pharmaceuticals cannot account for the full range of or even central cases of exploiting hope for better health from unproven medical interventions. That is, this understanding of exploitation as transactional unfairness is far too narrow to serve as a basis of a general account of exploiting hope. Thus, the transactional unfairness of prices for unproven interventions cannot tell the full story of the exploitation of hope stemming from these unproven interventions, migrant smuggling, and other common contexts of exploiting hope, at least if fairness is tied to a hypothetical fair-market price.

One issue is that experimental interventions are often not controlled through a monopoly on the procedure or product. For example, biological materials such as one's own stem cells that are processed and injected back into the patient, surgical procedures such as venoplasty for chronic cerebrospinal venous insufficiency (CCSVI), and other products for which full clinical safety and efficacy testing has not been completed are typically not protected by patents. In these cases, there is the potential for a highly competitive market for these goods and services. While their prices might be high and the hope and desperation of individuals may create considerable demand for them, these prices would not be considered unfair and exploitative on Wertheimer's account as interpreted by Martin.

Competition for unproven interventions can be fierce, especially as regulatory limitations on the ability of vendors to offer these interventions in some jurisdictions has created a global medical tourism market for unproven interventions. For example, venoplasty for CCSVI has been offered as an unproven and potentially unsafe intervention for multiple sclerosis. An online search for clinics offering CCSVI venoplasty quickly yields dozens of results, and clinics offering unproven stem cell interventions for multiple sclerosis and many other medical conditions are even more numerous. While these facilities do not compete solely on price, with their reputations among online communities of patients factoring significantly in their popularity, the global market for many unproven interventions cannot be called uncompetitive. Even when the cost of travel to these clinics is factored in for patients living in jurisdictions that have prohibited access to certain unproven interventions on the grounds of patient safety, many of these facilities are in countries with very low labor costs that likely would make them less expensive than facilities in North America and Europe.[8]

More generally, an account of transactional fairness exploitation where fairness is tied to a hypothetical fair-market price does a poor job of helping us understand charges of exploiting hope as they are popularly used. Recall that I demonstrated in Chapter 1 that smuggling of migrants was a common context in which these charges of exploiting hope are made. In these examples, migrants are seeking a better life—often fleeing war, physical danger, and a near complete lack of economic opportunities. When members of the press, politicians, and the general public call the actions of smugglers exploitative, they are not principally concerned that these individuals are benefiting from monopoly pricing or deviate from the fair-market price for their services. The concern here, and in many other popular discussions of migrant smuggling, is not that the price paid by these migrants is unfair. Rather, it is that these smugglers are benefiting from the migrants' desperation for a better life. Were more smugglers to enter the market for illicit migration to wealthier and safer countries and thus bring the price for their services down, it is not likely that these critics would drop their concerns with exploitation. In fact, there is no clear indication that the existing market for human trafficking is uncompetitive or unfair—that it takes "special" unfair advantage of would-be migrants given the long-standing networks for illicit migration in large parts of the world.

What of other standards of transactional fairness, then—especially those offering a better baseline of fairness for the context of medical care and other non-market interactions? While some other, non-market-based standard of fairness such as a just price may be better suited to these contexts, I am skeptical that it will get to the heart of what people find problematic about selling unproven interventions to persons hoping for improved health. The same is true of migrant smuggling and other common cases of alleged exploitation of hope. For example, even if we drop a fair-market standard for judging fairness in migrant smuggling, it isn't clear that the migrants are treated unfairly in terms of the likely benefits received. Smugglers may receive significant payment for their services, but they do so by risking imprisonment for their services and share some of the physical risks of crossing borders that their customers face. However, if these migrants are sufficiently desperate and face poor prospects for their lives and well-being in their home countries, then in many cases the opportunity to migrate provided by these smugglers presents a potentially massive personal benefit. That is, if these services are potentially life saving and life changing, then the balance of benefit may still fall to the would-be migrants, all things considered.

What this shows is that a focus on transactional fairness is not likely to pinpoint what is distinctively morally problematic with exploiting hope. The concern with these cases is not, at their root, that the exploiter benefits unfairly from the transaction. If that were true, these cases could be resolved by ensuring that the potential exploitee gains more from the transaction or the exploiter gains less. Rather, the source of the moral disquiet with these cases is largely the weightiness of the hoped-for outcome in terms of the exploitees' well-being and the exploitees' willingness to take a leap of hope and make themselves vulnerable to exploiters, not that the resulting distribution of benefits is *unfair* as a result of some special vulnerability within the terms of the transaction.

Structural Exploitation of Hope

If the problem with taking advantage of hope is not a special unfairness tied to the outcome of the transaction, perhaps instead it is structural injustice that leads to unfair results for those purchasing these interventions. This approach to understanding the exploitation of hope is initially promising in that it has the potential to address the major shortcoming of the transactional account. The transactional account does not give voice to concerns that hope itself is being exploited, especially when the hopeful person makes a leap of hope to meet their basic needs. A structural account of exploitation, however, focuses on the injustices that give rise to these needs.

Recall that structural fairness exploitation occurs when an individual takes advantage of structural injustice to gain an unfair share of the benefits of an interaction with someone disadvantaged by this injustice. The concern with this form of exploitation is based on the claim, as Thomas Pogge puts it, that taking advantage of another's needs is particularly morally problematic when this need "is to some extent due not to the poverty of their country but to the injustice of its social institutions and policies."[9] Pogge draws on this point to argue that to avoid taking advantage of structural injustice, one must treat those disadvantaged by injustice as "if this injustice did not exist."[10] Wertheimer rightly criticizes this type of response to structural injustice, noting that it is unreasonable to require individuals singly to address the background injustices from which they benefit.[11] These structural injustices are a collective problem, collectively caused, and they make it epistemically and practically challenging to determine what a fully just world would look like and how to bring it about.

As discussed in Chapter 2, an account of structural exploitation can instead rely on fulfilling collective obligations to address injustices from which one benefits. Iris Young's political conception of justice requires that individuals fulfill their shared responsibility to address structural injustice based on (a) their power to respond to or influence unjust structures, (b) their privilege created through these structures, (c) their interest in reforming these structures, and (d) the collective ability of agents to combine their efforts to reform specific structural injustices.[12] Applied to the context of exploitation, taking advantage of a structural injustice heightens one's privilege created through these structures and may indicate greater power to influence these structures and interest in doing so. Structural exploitation, then, is a failure to fulfill this political responsibility when interacting with those disadvantaged by structural injustices.

While Martin uses Wertheimer's hypothetical fair-market standard of fairness in the context of pharmaceutical pricing, she also argues that a "standard for fair prices" should be developed and enforced for pharmaceuticals. She sets this standard at a rate that would ensure a "decent minimum" of access to necessary medical care as a matter of basic justice but notes that access to cutting-edge treatments may not be required by this standard.[13] While Martin does not explicitly explore a structural version of exploitation, her discussion of the injustice of limited access to medical care opens the door for applying this interpretation of exploitation to the context of unproven medical interventions. If we agree that a failure to provide universal access to a decent minimum of medical care is a structural injustice, then there is reason to think that medical providers who take advantage of this injustice without fulfilling their political responsibility to address this injustice are guilty of exploiting their customers.

Similarly, exploitation of the hopes of would-be migrants can be illuminated by reference to structural exploitation. The injustice in these cases could be linked to highly restrictive migration policies in high-income countries—or even the very presence of migratory limits. If these limits were not in place, would-be migrants would not be legally barred from moving to high-income countries and thus would not be made vulnerable to the dangers of illegal crossings and the actions of human smugglers. Thus, these restrictions could place an unfair burden on would-be migrants that smugglers then exploit. A weakness with this understanding of exploitation in international migration is that the injustice of limits on migration to high-income countries is often challenged within academic discussions of this issue and typically has low public support.[14] This is not to say that defenders of the injustice of closed borders are wrong but that we might look elsewhere for additional support for the concern that would-be migrants to high-income countries are the victims of injustice. Here, we can point to the factors that motivate them to migrate, at great personal risk to themselves and their families, in the first place. These include limited economic opportunities, threats of physical and political violence, oppressive governments, and oppressive cultural practices, among others. The causes of these factors are complex and will be specific to the context in which the would-be migrants live, but in many cases, they can be linked to the historical practices of many of the high-income countries to which they wish to migrate. These factors can include histories of colonialism that have slowed economic development or have drawn international borders in ways that make ethnic strife more likely, international trade laws that systematically disadvantage low-income countries, invasion and war that threaten the safety and opportunities of migrants, and ongoing political and economic interference as part of the struggle for global dominance by high-income countries.[15,16] The details of these contexts will matter, but it is much easier to see that injustice factors into the actions, desperation, and vulnerabilities of many would-be migrants.

How successful is a structural account of exploitation in explaining the exploitation of hope? Returning to Martin's example, while limited access to a decent minimum of medical care does raise concerns about structural exploitation, Martin is right to be cautious in linking exploitation in the sale of unproven medical interventions to a lack of universal access to these interventions.

Given that these interventions are unproven or, in the case of Avastin, of limited proven efficacy, it would be difficult to make the case that justice or a decent minimum of access to healthcare requires access to these interventions. If mandating universal access to these interventions at an affordable rate required public subsidies or other public expenditures, it would be a great *injustice*, given that public resources are finite and expenditures on unproven interventions would reasonably require diverting resources from supporting access to proven treatments. This concern was part of the debate over public financing of the unproven CCSVI intervention in Canada, for example, where critics of such funding noted both the opportunity costs created by this potential diversion of resources and the danger of politicizing public funding of medical care based on interest groups' demands of funding for specific, unproven interventions.[17]

Putting aside arguments that a lack of public funding or private insurance support for unproven interventions is unjust, one could instead look to the vulnerability created by a lack of domestic access to some of these interventions where regulatory bodies have banned their sale. It is not at all clear that these patient protections are unjust, as they follow a long history of public health activities such as the inspection of meat and water for safe consumption, consumer protections around the truthful labeling of food and medicines, and prohibitions on the sale of harmful products. Moreover, the disadvantage to those impacted by these restrictions is reduced greatly by their ability to access these goods and services abroad in many cases. As discussed previously, the financial burden of having to travel abroad for unproven interventions is often little to none, though these customers will face the inconvenience of having to travel for care. Providers of unproven interventions might exploit this alleged structural injustice by providing these services without fulfilling their political responsibility to address this injustice, but, given that their power to do so would be very limited as foreign providers, it is not clear what shape this political responsibility might take.

Similarly, we can consider how well a structural account of exploitation explains the concerns with exploiting the hopes of would-be migrants to high-income countries. As noted earlier, these would-be migrants can be made vulnerable by a range of injustices in their home countries that motivate them to migrate to safer countries with greater social and economic opportunities. Smugglers benefit from these injustices insofar as their livelihood depends on having would-be migrants willing to face great personal danger and cost to cross international borders without permission. Thus, it is fair to say that these smugglers have a political responsibility to address these injustices and that, if they fail to fulfill this responsibility, they structurally exploit their clients.

It is less clear whether this political responsibility can account for exploiting hope as it is commonly understood and in a way that makes it clear that hope, specifically, is being exploited. The smugglers' political responsibility will be determined by their connection to those harmed by unjust structures, power to reform institutional structures, and privilege accruing from unjust structures. The connection to those harmed by unjust political structures seems clear and weighty insofar as the smugglers and would-be migrants enter a business relationship that puts the migrants' safety and future under the control of the smugglers. The other dimensions, however, are much weaker. These smugglers may have considerable power in their immediate context, but their power to reform the global political institutions that compel their clients to migrate abroad is vanishingly small. These are generally globally marginalized individuals who are engaging in criminal activities that are by their nature located away from official power centers and legitimate economic markets. Moreover, while these smugglers directly benefit from or are privileged by these unjust structures in the sense that they provide a business opportunity, their overall position of privilege is less clear. Smugglers may themselves be systematically disadvantaged by the same institutions as their clients. While they are to some extent able to turn this disadvantage into a benefit by making a business of their clients' hopes for a better life, the work of people smuggling is itself physically dangerous and exposes the smugglers to criminal prosecution. Just as the would-be migrants are treated unfairly by the injustices that compel them to seek a better life in high-income countries, some of these smugglers might wish that they could meet their needs through less dangerous and precarious work.[18] This factor, of course, does not excuse the often brutal, misleading, and exploitative actions of these smugglers, but it does bring into question the degree to which they are privileged by the relevant international political structures.

The political responsibilities of these smugglers to address the structural injustices they exploit are likely to be highly contextual and dependent on their position and power within smuggling networks.[19] More powerful agents may have the authority to make their clients' lives more dignified, safer, and easier, but they will have little ability to address the massive structural injustices creating the push to migrate abroad. This disconnect suggests that structural exploitation has *some* potential to explain the wrongness of exploiting hope but less potential to explain what is *distinctive* about this practice. In the case of migrant smuggling, international structural justice creates a drive to migrate abroad despite legal prohibitions against doing so. This drive can be described as a leap of hope, and smugglers take advantage of this leap for their own benefit, seeing these injustices as an opportunity, rather than creating a responsibility to address this injustice. However, this focus on the large-scale drivers of the desperation of migrants and other exploitees does little to illuminate hope as an element of exploitation. Rather, injustice creates a need and exploiters unfairly benefit from this need. On this reading of exploitation, hope largely drops out from the conversation. Structural exploitation may be present in many of these cases of exploiting hope, then, but it isn't clear that it gets at the heart of what is distinctively morally problematic about exploiting hope. Thus, we need take a closer look at a third form of exploitation, where individuals treat others as mere means to their own advantage.

Exploitation, Respect, and Hope

As I discussed in Chapter 2, a third form of exploitation occurs when the exploiter violates some form of the Kantian proscription against treating others as a mere means to one's ends. Applied to exploitation, this failure is typically described in terms of failing to accord others the respect due to them by virtue of their humanity.[20,21] In practical terms, this failure of respect can take the form of failing to fulfill a specified duty of beneficence by disregarding what they need to live a distinctly human life. Applied to the general context of individuals seeking access to unproven medical interventions, those using these interventions want not just better health but also the opportunity to take control over their health and to adopt a more optimistic and hopeful outlook, all of which can be taken advantage of through this understanding of exploitation.

A prominent example of this view is given by Ruth Sample.[22] Sample argues that exploitation takes place when we seek to benefit ourselves while failing to honor the value that all human beings have. In addition to taking advantage of an injustice as in cases of structural exploitation, this failure of respect occurs when we do not give others what they need to flourish and when we treat others as commodifiable. Similarly, I have argued that exploitation takes place when the exploiter fails to fulfill a specified duty of beneficence to another.[23] This specified duty of beneficence requires individuals to help someone who falls below a threshold level of well-being—a duty moderated by their ability to meet their own needs and the extent to which the other person depends on them.

If we understand exploitation to entail a failure of respect or failure to fulfill a specified duty of beneficence toward others, do those selling unproven medical interventions exploit those who are hoping against all expectation that these interventions will improve their health? The answer to this question will depend on the context of these interactions. Of particular concern will be purchases of unproven interventions at very high prices, which potentially conflict with the customer's ability to meet their other needs, including adequate housing and savings. These kinds of interactions appear frequently in news coverage of those seeking unproven interventions, who sell or mortgage their houses,[24] drain their savings or incur large debts,[25] and hold charity fundraisers[26] to cover the costs of these interventions.

In these cases of hoping against all expectation, patients exhaust their own savings and that of others by seeking an intervention that is unlikely to have a lasting, positive health impact. This outcome motivates much of the criticism of those who sell these interventions, including charges of exploiting hope. What they demonstrate is that the concern with "exploiting hope" can be centered on concerns with causing harm. Specifically, exploiting hope can take the form of benefiting from another's desperation in a way that is unlikely to confer any real, lasting health benefits to the customer while costing them significant financial resources that they cannot afford. The customer may well know this, meaning that the concern is not necessarily centered on deception by the exploiter or a failure of consent. Rather, the criticism is that the vendor not only fails to confer much benefit to their customer, but also participates in and facilitates the customer's self-harming action. By participating in and facilitating these hopeful but essentially futile and self-harming activities, the exploiter essentially treats the exploitee as an object of profit rather than an individual deserving respect.

In other cases of customers seeking unproven interventions, however, this concern with harm is not as clearly present because the cost of the intervention is moderate or the customer has enough resources to afford the intervention. Moreover, the advantages of a hopeful attitude can offset moderate costs of pursuing unlikely benefits. As a result, participating in and enabling a hopeful activity it is not inherently morally problematic from the perspective of exploitation. In my own and collaborators' research on persons with multiple sclerosis seeking an unproven intervention for this degenerative disease, the individuals my colleagues and I spoke with generally felt very positively about their decision to spend tens of thousands of dollars for this intervention even when their perceived symptom relief was temporary. These individuals acknowledged that the doctors "didn't make any real promises," but they experienced "positivity," "excitement," and "hope" from this intervention. One person described the advantage gained from this intervention as follows: "I knew what was going to happen to me if I did nothing. And so I was going to do something."[27] As noted in more detail in the previous chapter, the positive effects of accessing unproven interventions has been well documented, rooted in the positive effects of optimism and hope on health independent of the efficacy of the intervention itself.[28,29]

Given the potential benefits of pursuing unproven interventions and other hopeful activities, even for those who will experience significant financial distress as a result, why not simply deny that exploitation takes place in *any* of these cases? We could treat those hoping against all expectation as rational adults, choosing to purchase hope for a better life and using their resources as they see fit. Doing so could be said to be not only consistent with respect for others but required of it insofar as these people are not being defrauded and have been fully informed of the prospects of the hoped-for outcome occurring. In the context of unproven medical interventions, this would mean ensuring that hopeful persons are aware of the lack of scientific basis for any positive effects from the interventions beyond a placebo effect and sustained hope for better health and then allowing them to proceed as they see fit.

Understanding exploitation as a failure of respect gives a general answer to this question: disrespect for others or, more generally, treating them as a mere means to one's own ends can occur even without harming another or assisting a harmful action. Through our relationships with others, the general duty of beneficence becomes specified, creating obligations to promote the good of these others. To see this point in the context of exploiting hope, the concept of partial entrustment is helpful toward understanding why fairness-based accounts of exploitation are inadequate.[30] In the context of researchers' ancillary care obligations—that is, obligations to disclose and treat medical needs outside of the scope of a research project—Richardson and Belsky argue that in some relationships, aspects of an individual's well-being are entrusted to another, creating a responsibility to protect and promote that person's well-being. This partial entrustment arises when the partial trustee is given discretion over how something the other individual cares greatly about will be cared for, making this individual particularly vulnerable to the partial trustee. This kind of entrustment is common in relationships in the medical context. Physicians are entrusted with their patients' overall health, creating a high degree of vulnerability. Researchers are given less discretion over research participants' health.[31] However, aspects of their health related to the research are entrusted, creating limited ancillary care obligations for these researchers.

Richardson clarifies that these obligations can arise whether or not they are intended or consented to. He refers to this phenomenon as moral entanglement, where forming a relationship or other connection can create special obligations to others. These entanglements and their resulting obligations can take many different forms, understood more generally as contexts by which a general duty of beneficence becomes specified—the underlying process by which exploitation as a failure of respect occurs. In the context of partial entrustment, Richardson argues that a waiver of rights can create a moral entanglement related to that right, such that "accepting rights waivers gives one special responsibility for the considerations underlying the relevant rights."[32] As he notes, this interaction can be understood in terms of a transfer of rights and privileges but also of some of the underlying responsibilities that accompany those rights. Thus, "moral rights institute a default division of (forward-looking) moral responsibility: the responsibility to look after one concern or another. Waivers of rights constitute a departure from that default division, shifting responsibilities by shifting rights."[33] In the medical context, it is often specifically a waiver of privacy rights by which one person grants another bodily access and permission to assess their medical needs. These waivers of privacy rights—what Richardson refers to as the creation of intimacies—are typically mutually voluntary, as when a patient grants their physician permission to conduct a medical examination. But even in these mutually voluntary cases, the grant of intimacy can create unintended or non-explicit obligations, as when such an examination yields evidence of sexual abuse.

What is distinctive about partial entrustment in cases of accessing unproven medical interventions is that the customer waives a right of bodily autonomy and thereby authorizes control over a wider range of their overall well-being. This is similar to the waiver of rights that takes place in a typical physician–patient relationship but also more intimate in some respects: if the customer genuinely understands that the intervention is unproven, what the customer is seeking through the interaction is not simply improved health but also (a) a sense of taking control over their well-being, (b) optimism and an improved outlook on life, and (c) a sense of direction and purpose in their lives—that is, *hope* for better health. As the multiple sclerosis patient quoted earlier noted, these patients often want "to do something" even if sustained, improved health is not a likely outcome.

By entering a relationship with their customers, those selling unproven interventions take on discretion over their customers' well-being beyond simply their health. Because these vendors cannot offer a likely chance of improved health without deceiving their patients, they can only promote their customers' well-being if they nurture the benefits of hope in a manner that does not destroy the customers' ability to achieve or protect other elements of well-being. While selling unproven interventions does not necessarily harm customers' well-being, high prices for these goods can do so, particularly because these prices are not offset by likely long-term health gains. For this reason, clinical trials for unproven interventions, where participants are typically not required to pay to participate, are less likely to raise concerns about exploitation than do private sales of these interventions. However, as I will discuss in the next chapter, even these noncommercial clinical research relationships involve partial entrustment that creates the potential for exploitation. Once those providing medical care for profit or for research enter into these relationships, they accept their patients' entrustment of their well-being, and these heightened obligations emerge. Disregarding these obligations solely to promote their own well-being, then, would be a case of exploiting these customers' hopes.

We can look at other alleged cases of exploiting hope to see how the concept of partial entrustment illuminates what is taken to be problematic in these cases. Consider a case where Arthur has a romantic crush on Ben. Arthur spends his free hours thinking of Ben, dreaming of what a relationship with Ben would be like, and, increasingly, coming to believe that his happiness is tied to a future with Ben. Arthur repeatedly asks Ben out on dates and is rebuffed. Realizing that a romantic relationship with Ben is very unlikely, Arthur instead approaches Ben with the following offer: He is willing to do Ben's housework, buy him dinner, and take on any other tasks that he might ask of him in the hope that spending more time together might warm Ben to him. Ben responds that he is not physically attracted to Arthur, finds his personality off-putting, and sees no chance of ever developing romantic feelings toward him. Arthur accepts these statements as fact but reiterates the offer anyway out of a stated interest in keeping his hope for a relationship with Ben alive. Ben accepts Arthur's offer, thinking that he will benefit and that Arthur is a fully informed and consenting adult who seems to find this exchange in his interest.

The exchange between Arthur and Ben is arguably exploitative—to be specific, Ben exploits Arthur's hope beyond all expectation for a romantic relationship with him. As with cases of hope for better health from unproven medical interventions, the concern is that in this case Ben fails to show sufficient concern for Arthur's overall well-being. Arthur is an adult giving fully informed consent to the relationship and determines that the value of extending his hope, however unlikely, for a relationship with Ben is worth the cost of time, financial resources, and the considerable risk to his emotional well-being. By accepting Arthur's proposition, Ben takes on responsibility for many aspects of Arthur's well-being, no matter how clear he has been to Arthur that he should have no hope of establishing a romantic relationship with him. Ben chooses to facilitate an emotional entanglement with Arthur that will foreseeably hurt him over the long term. Through his actions, Ben shows concern only for his own gain from the relationship and fails to act sufficiently to promote the aspects of Arthur's well-being with which he has agreed to be entrusted.[34]

Returning to the issue of exploiting the hopes of would-be migrants, the concept of partial entrustment is illuminating in this context as well. Would-be migrants entrust their well-being and very lives to smugglers as they cross borders without permission, make dangerous passages through deserts and overseas, and enter countries where they might not speak the local language, may not know the local political system and customs, and have little legal protection given their undocumented status. When people smugglers benefit from these hopes for a better life, they do not necessarily do so exploitatively. There is nothing built into the relationship between would-be migrant and smuggler that requires the smuggler to abuse their customers or disregard their needs. They offer a service that requires great risk, vulnerability, and cost but may provide this service with care and caution within the bounds of their practice. Rather, exploitation of hope occurs in these cases when smugglers disregard the needs and vulnerability of their charges, emphasizing their own needs with insufficient regard of those with whose safety they are entrusted. This is represented in the popular discussion of smugglers exploiting hope, where they abandon their charges in leaky boats, traffic them, and show substantial disregard for their well-being. While the entire practice of people smuggling understandably receives criticism, these charges of exploitation are largely reserved for these worst cases of disregard, motivated by the extreme vulnerability of would-be migrants where they have handed over their lives to smugglers who then act with callousness toward this act of entrustment.

These examples show that viewing the exploitation of hope in terms of a failure to protect and promote dimensions of well-being with which one has been entrusted depends on an element of emotional vulnerability and entanglement. By entrusting their well-being to the seller of an unproven intervention, these customers become highly vulnerable to the actions of the seller, both in terms of their physical health and their psychological and emotional well-being as they experience the progress of what is typically a very serious and potentially life-threatening medical condition. These customers are not purchasing what is likely to be a life-saving or even long-term health-promoting intervention. Rather, they seek a means to preserve their optimism about the future, investment in their present care, and positive engagement with those around them. In this way, the entrustment of their well-being in the seller of these unproven interventions encompasses many elements of the customers' well-being, creating significant responsibilities for the seller. In the case of Arthur and Ben, Arthur's hope for a romantic relationship with Ben takes the form of a fantasy relationship despite his being told that a genuine romantic relationship is not a possibility. By accepting the fantasy relationship, Ben sustains Arthur's emotional entanglement with him and allows Arthur to remain highly vulnerable to his actions. Finally, even people smuggling will often include these emotional dimensions. These would-be migrants are again taking great risks and incurring large costs to act on their fantasy of a better life. While relationships with their smugglers will vary and may be brief, these migrants are placed in an exceptionally vulnerable situation that includes the emotional vulnerability of placing their hopes and dreams in the hands of others.

Linking the exploitation of hope primarily to a failure of respect for others fits well with and helps to explain the elements of exploiting hope as this concept is popularly used. First, popular examples of exploiting hope are typically weighty in that they involve very important elements of the hopeful individual's well-being and self-conception. As such, they typically involve leaps of hope such that hopeful individuals are willing to take significant risks to realize their hopes or at least prolong the fantasy of having these hopes realized. This weightiness and willingness to take risks to realize hopes helps explain why interactions with these hopeful individuals are particularly ripe for exploitation: the heightened vulnerability in these relationships creates a heightened element of entrustment for the potential exploiter and therefore a greater degree of responsibility for the potential exploitee's well-being. That is, the hopes that motivate concerns about exploiting hope are typically not trivial. They are central to the hopeful individual's survival and sense of self. When others agree to engage with these hopes, they are thus entrusted with them such that they now have great power over the hopeful person and a concurrent responsibility to show restraint in using this power and respect for their newly vulnerable partial trustee.

Second, this account of exploiting hope fits well with the understanding of hope endorsed in Chapter 3. It recognizes that hoping against all expectation, or as Martin prefers, hoping against all hope, can be justifiable and gives reasons for planning around and emotionally engaging with the hoped-for outcome.

This emotional engagement with hope creates a specific kind of vulnerability that can be abused by others—particularly those entrusted with overseeing the hoped-for outcome. This vulnerability does not simply create a danger that the exploitee will receive an unfair amount of benefit from their interaction with those engaged in their hopes. If so, addressing the exploitation of hope would simply be a matter of adjusting the balance of benefits and risks, of redistributing goods and costs. But this focus seems too material and misplaced given that positive outcomes may be exceedingly unlikely. Rather, linking the exploitation of hope to a failure of respect shows that it is the *relationship* between exploiter and exploitee that is central to the wrongness of these interactions. Certainly, disrespect can be shown through charging excessively for some service or keeping too much of the benefit when a hoped-for outcome is realized. But linking exploiting hope to relationships of partial entrustment helps to explain the other dimensions of exploiting hope that may be common when interacting with individuals hoping against all expectation. These other dimensions include disregard for the emotional vulnerabilities of clients, use of entrustment solely as an opportunity for personal gain, and the non-material aspects of hope, such as planning and emotional engagement, as will be seen in more detail in the following chapters.

Exploiting False Hope

While the account of exploiting hope that I have developed here is distinct from and does not rely on the wrongness of deceiving others or other failures of informed consent, much of the popular discussion of exploiting hope does involve such deceit. While these instances of taking advantage of misinformed hopeful people are often described as exploiting hope, they can also, and more clearly, be described as exploiting false hope insofar as the information on which these individuals base their hopes is not based on a genuine understanding of real probabilities.

False hopes, for these purposes, are created in one of two ways. First, they can be created intentionally by fraudsters who wish to mislead their victims for personal gain. These were the most common forms of false hope in the popular discussions of exploiting hope reviewed in Chapter 1. Intentionally false hopes were created by people smugglers misleading would-be migrants about the safety and conditions of migrating abroad, scammers pretending to offer employment opportunities to those desperate for work, and sweepstakes companies intentionally misleading the public about whether they had already won large sums of money or would be likely to do so.

Other false hopes are more akin to the failures on the part of the individual to fully understand the likelihood of achieving the hoped-for outcome or the terms of an interaction. As discussed in more detail in Chapter 3, in the clinical context false hope can arise from therapeutic misconception, where clinical research is incorrectly understood to be a form of personal medical treatment. Other cases may involve therapeutic misestimation, where the individual misestimates the likelihood of a benefit or harm occurring, or therapeutic optimism, where individuals overestimate the likelihood of personal benefit, especially during phase I clinical trials.[35] Outside of the clinic, false hope can take similar forms, where individuals misunderstand the terms or aims of an interaction, misestimate the likelihood that an interaction will benefit them, or experience other failures of rationality where they are unrealistically optimistic about a positive outcome.

While I have distinguished between cases of false hope based on whether a false understanding of the likelihood of a positive outcome is intentional or not, in practice this distinction may be less clear. In some instances, both forms of false hope may occur in a single case, making it unclear which misunderstandings are intentional and which are not. This can take place, for example, where an individual starts with an unrealistic conception of their likelihood of becoming a successful author, allowing a vanity press to further encourage that unrealistic hope. In others, the intentions of those encouraging false hope may be unclear to others or even to the alleged exploiter themselves. Consider, for example, advertisements for unproven medical interventions that carefully avoid promising successful outcomes but instead subtly encourage the possibility of a positive outcome through imagery, hopeful language, and even patient testimonials that are couched in terms warning the viewer that their results may vary. These advertisers may claim pure intentions, but one can reasonably question whether this is genuinely the case, given their messaging. In other instances, these alleged exploiters are true believers, spreading misinformation that they themselves believe. Here, their intentions may not be to mislead or harm others, but the effects are the same as in cases involving intentional fraudsters.

Regardless of the sources and histories of these false hopes, they create vulnerabilities similar to those in more genuine or better-grounded cases of hope; just as with genuine hope, false hope creates vulnerability and an opportunity for exploitation. Both genuine and false hopes, at least in cases of hoping against all expectation, stem from deep needs and the hopeful individual's sense of self. These needs are the basis of hope and in many cases make individuals vulnerable to rational failures in fully understanding the likelihood of this hope being realized or vulnerable to being intentionally misled about this likelihood. As I have discussed, these weighty needs lead to leaps of hope, a form of risk-taking that may be out of character for the hopeful person and, outside of a situation of great need, not rational. These leaps of hope make hopeful persons vulnerable to harm in general, including by being taken advantage of by those who wish to defraud them through creating a false basis for further hope.

Creating false hope in another—that is, misleading them about the benefits they are likely to receive from an interaction—is a serious form of moral wrongdoing. This wrongdoing, however, is distinct from that of exploiting hope, which can take place without causing or taking advantage of false hope. When a hope is false, whether or not one is responsible for creating that false hope, there are responsibilities not to exploit this hope. These responsibilities take the same general form as with cases of genuine hope in that entering an interaction with a hopeful person creates a relationship with new responsibilities—specifically, a partial entrustment—to exhibit respect toward the vulnerable partner and act with restraint toward their pursuit of their basic needs and self-image. The most relevant difference is that in cases of false hope, the hopeful person is less likely to be able to achieve a positive outcome and their hope may not be justified, thus requiring additional restraint on the part of other parties. This does not necessarily mean that interacting with those engaged in false hopes is always unethical, but it means that the danger of exploitation is heightened.

Conclusion

I have argued that exploiting hope takes place not due to unfair pricing or taking advantage of structural injustice. Rather, the exploitation of hope occurs when one fails to fulfill a duty of respect that is specified by the vulnerability created by the partial entrustment of one's physical and emotional well-being to another. Other forms of exploitation may be co-present with respect-based exploitation of hope. Moreover, exploiting hope may often occur in the context of other bad acts, such as intentionally deceiving others to create exploitable false hopes. Nonetheless, exploiting hope is a distinctive form of bad act distinguishable from these other bad acts.

What is distinctive about exploiting hope as opposed to other forms of respect-based exploitation is the specific kind of vulnerability created by hope. In the kinds of cases that give rise to popular worries about exploiting hope, the hoped-for outcome is weighty and central to the exploitee's well-being and sense of self. This out-come is so central that it spurs potentially risky leaps of hope that create substantial vulnerabilities for the hopeful person. These vulnerabilities and risk-taking combine to create a high degree of entrustment in the actions of potential exploiters. Moreover, especially in instances of hoping against all expectation, the en-trustment is not solely or even primarily focused on the hoped-for outcome occurring. Rather, it is part of a project of planning for and fantasizing about the hoped-for outcome on the part of the hopeful person. As such, entrustment in these cases is not simply about the physical and financial well-being of the hopeful person but also about their emotional well-being as they engage in these hopeful journeys. These hopeful entanglements thus suggest a depth of en-trustment that connotes substantial and distinctive responsibilities for potential exploitees.

Based on this understanding of exploiting hope, those consid-ering interacting with hopeful persons should ask themselves three questions before and during these interactions to prevent exploi-tation. First, *should this interaction happen at all or the partial en-trustment be accepted*? That is, is a respectful, non-exploitative interaction possible in this case? This question is relevant for all cases of supporting hopeful people, but especially so in cases of false hope. Second, if the entrustment is accepted, *how can the hopeful relationship be managed most respectfully*? Respectful interaction with a hopeful person will include restricting one's own demands and, potentially, benefits to ensure that the hopeful person does not harm themselves or others by pursuing the hoped-for outcome. Especially in cases of hoping beyond all expectation, this will in-clude managing the emotional well-being of the hopeful indi-vidual as they pursue emotional sustenance rather than, primarily, material gain. Finally, and primarily in longer-term relationships that develop and change over time, one should ask, *should the hopeful relationship be continued*? This question is essential, as new facts will emerge over time, changing the impacts of pursuing the hoped-for outcome. These facts can include new details about the costs of a medical treatment, likelihood of success for a treatment, or dangers for the hopeful person. In this way, the entrusted person must be wary of when a relationship must be changed or ended to avoid exploitation.

In the following chapters I will put this understanding of exploiting hope and these specific questions to the test by applying them to specific cases of exploitation. Doing so will help to demonstrate the ability of this account of exploitation to illuminate alleged cases of exploiting hope. In the next chapter I look specifically at exploitation of hope in clinical trials and will use these questions and my overall account of exploiting hope to address how to avoid such exploitation in practice.

5

Testing Hope

Exploitation in Clinical Trials

Medical research on humans raises a variety of ethical concerns that have been well documented and have led to increased oversight over time. These concerns derive in part from the fact that participants are generally in a vulnerable position compared with researchers running these clinical trials. This vulnerability stems from several factors. These can include (1) a lack of knowledge relative to researchers, where research participants may struggle to understand terminology and methodology around medical research, limiting the possibility of fully informed consent to research participation; (2) ill health that they believe the trial may address; (3) the inability to give consent to trial participation because of lack of capacity (e.g., where participants are children or adults with dementia) or external pressures (e.g., where participants are prisoners or members of the military); (4) the effects of ill health on decision-making, including pain, fear, and desperation; and (5) a lack of access to medical treatment owing to lack of insurance or savings.

In addition to raising concerns about consent to clinical trial participation, these vulnerabilities have led to a variety of worries about exploitation. While these worries can take many forms, one common concern is that hope for better health, quality of life, or other benefits through trial participation creates an opportunity for researchers and others to exploit potential trial participants. However, charges of exploiting hope in clinical trials are frequently poorly articulated, and the specific type of moral wrong that is charged to have occurred is often unclear. This lack of clarity is problematic. If it is not clear what form of moral wrong is meant by the charge of exploitation, then debates over whether specific practices exploit the hopes of research participants will devolve into different parties talking past one another. Moreover, without a clear understanding of how so-called exploitative relationships in human participant research are exploitative, it will be impossible to respond adequately to those commentators who claim that these practices are *not* morally problematic.[1] Merely reiterating that they are exploitative will at best beg the question against these critics. Therefore, a closer examination of the charge of exploiting hope in the context of research on human participants is needed.

In this chapter, I examine two contexts that create the potential to exploit hope in clinical trials. First, I look at participation in phase I cancer trials, where the trial is designed to test the safety of the highest tolerable dosage of the compound under investigation rather than the efficacy of the compound. In these trials, participants may hope beyond all expectation for better health or other benefits despite the design of the trial, creating the potential for exploitation by researchers who seek to enroll these participants in their trials. Second, I will discuss phase III clinical trials in low- and middle-income countries (LMICs). While these trials are designed to test the efficacy of new treatments and may provide direct benefit to some trial participants, the poverty and lack of medical care experienced by some of these participants raises questions about whether they or other members of their communities will be able to access these treatments should they prove effective. Thus, their hopes for better health for themselves and especially their communities may be misplaced, as other, wealthier individuals will receive the main benefits of any treatments developed through these trials. As I will note, these two examples of exploiting hope in clinical trials illuminate a tension in understanding the roles of researchers conducting these trials. On the one hand, there is a requirement to be clear about the limitations of these trials in providing direct benefits to participants and their communities.

However, these examples show that worries about exploitation of hope are also linked to the failure of researchers and their sponsors to do enough to benefit participants and their communities after these trials have concluded.

Hope in Phase I Cancer Trials

The aim of phase I clinical trials is to collect data about the safety of the medical intervention being studied. In trials of pharmacological compounds, these trials seek specifically to establish what dosage of the compound is safe and tolerable to human research participants. Such testing usually proceeds by initially giving human research participants 10 percent of the dose that has been established to be lethal in rodent testing. The dosage is then increased until human participants experience dangerous toxicity or intolerable side effects from the compound.[2] In this way, the maximum tolerable dose of the compound for humans is established through the trial. These trials are not designed to benefit participants, though benefits may occur. Rather, they set the stage for additional clinical trials, including phase II trials that return preliminary data on the efficacy of the intervention and phase III trials that establish efficacy compared with standard treatment.[3]

By design, participants in phase I trials, including trials for cancer treatments, may receive suboptimal doses of the intervention being tested or may not remain in the trial long enough for the intervention to provide full benefits.[4] Nonetheless, participants can benefit from taking part in these clinical trials. For example, a review of 460 phase I trials for cancer treatments involving 11,935 participants from 1991 to 2002 found that the response rate for trial participants ranged from 4.4 to 17.8 percent, depending on whether anticancer treatments approved by the Food and Drug Administration (FDA) were included in the trial. Other participants were harmed by participation: .49 percent of participants died from toxic events, and

14.3 percent had a serious toxic event.[5] Another review of phase I cancer trials conducted from 2003 to 2006 found partial or complete response in 7 percent of the 180 participants and stable disease in 41 percent.[6] In specific cases, phase I clinical trials for cancer treatments can have very high rates of direct medical benefit, including in a majority of participants.[7]

While these trials are not designed to create direct benefits for participants, and the chances of receiving such benefits are unlikely and variable across trials, hope for better health is a primary reason that participants choose to enter these trials.[8] This hope can motivate participation in several ways. First, it may be a false hope based on a misconception about the purpose of the trial. Because phase I cancer trials are not designed to test the efficacy of a new intervention, the danger of therapeutic misconception in these trials is particularly acute. Importantly, this concern has been borne out in research on these trials. Studies of participants in phase I cancer trials show that they often enroll for the purpose of receiving direct medical benefit.[9] For example, a 1995 survey of twenty-seven phase I cancer trial participants found that 85 percent enrolled in the trial because of possible therapeutic benefit, 11 percent because of trust in their physician, and 4 percent because of family pressures. At the same time, only one-third of participants could state the purpose of the trial.[10] Another study of 396 participants in a phase I cancer trial found that the largest number of respondents (84 percent) stated that the possibility of tumor shrinkage was the most important reason for enrolling in the trial.[11] Finally, interviews with ninety-five phase I cancer trial participants found that 68.4 percent experienced therapeutic misconception and that this misconception was positively correlated with lower formal education and lower family income.[12]

False hopes about the likely outcomes of phase I cancer trial participation may also arise from unrealistic optimism.[13] Recall that this form of false hope comes from incorrectly believing that one's personal attributes or context makes one more likely to receive a benefit than the general population. This form of false hope has been identified specifically in phase I cancer trials. A study of 171 phase I cancer trial participants found that a significant number of these participants felt that they were able to control factors regarding their likelihood of benefiting from participating in the trial, leading to unrealistic optimism about the likely trial results.[14] Other participants felt that optimism about the outcomes of trial participation would increase the likelihood of a positive result for themselves.[15] Another study found that 54.6 percent of participants felt that their chances of benefiting from participating in a phase I cancer trial were greater than those of the general population; however, 37.6 percent of these participants were pessimists, rating their chances of benefit as lower than that of the general population.[16]

Even if the ill person is aware of the purpose of the phase I trial and not under a misconception about the likely benefits of trial participation, their friends and families may have false hopes. These support networks can pressure participants to take part in trials even if the participant understands that doing so is not likely to provide direct medical benefit. That is, these participants may choose to take part in trials to placate others, even if they would prefer not to undergo the rigors of trial participation. In empirical research on participant decision-making, there is evidence that this external pressure impacts participation in at least some cases. For example, in a multisite study of 163 phase I cancer trial participants, 9 percent indicated that they experienced moderate to a great deal of pressure to participate from their families.[17] For one patient, pressure to support their family motivated the continued appearance of optimism for better health as, "I didn't want to be all poopy and down and out for them, 'cause they would just be destroyed."[18]

However, hope for benefit from participating in phase I cancer trials need not be false hope. First, phase I cancer trial participants may experience indirect benefits.[19] These include general improvements to quality of life and specific psychological benefits. Much of this benefit comes from participants' greater sense of agency in taking active steps to address their medical issues, including having a treatment plan defined through their trial participation.[20] Many participants also find benefit in the routine contact with care providers that takes place through trial participation, including regular appointments with specialists and updates on the status of their disease.[21] Participating in these trials can also give participants increased meaning in their lives by contributing to creating generalizable knowledge and potentially new medical treatments, even if they do not directly benefit from these advances.[22] Participation in these trials does not preclude palliative care during the trial and hospice care at the end of the trial, leading to improved quality of life even if the participant's medical prognosis does not improve.[23] In these ways, participation in phase I cancer trials mirrors the more general benefits of hoping beyond all expectation for improved health, discussed in Chapter 3.

In addition to these indirect medical benefits, preserving hope for better health—even while understanding that the likelihood of benefiting from trial participation is low—is itself often seen as valuable. For example, in one study of fifty-eight phase I cancer trial participants in the UK, 85 percent of respondents indicated that they agreed or strongly agreed that joining the trial would give them hope and that this was a reason for participating in the trial.[24] While there are legitimate concerns about how well phase I cancer trial participants understand the low likelihood that they themselves will benefit medically from trial participation, numerous studies show that many participants do understand and choose to participate anyway.[25,26] These findings led Agrawal and Emanuel to argue that they "may reflect a motivation to maintain hope in a difficult situation rather than misunderstanding of the information."[27] More generally, hope can be linked to characteristics such as tenacity and optimism and positively support the participants' overall quality of life.[28] One phase I cancer trial participant described how hope and realism about her chances of better health could be consistent with one another: "You hold on to that tiny glimmer of hope. I know at the back of my mind that I also do it because it might help me in the future. It may also very well be that it doesn't work for me, that's what I more or less expect. But on the other hand, even if it only helps a bit, well. . . . Yes, that's the main reason why I decided to take part in it."[29] While this participant focused on hope for future better health for herself, others discussed hope that participation might help others, including family and friends with a predisposition to the same form of cancer.[30]

While phase I cancer trial participants can choose to participate based on well-informed rather than false hope, certain practices by researchers leading these trials can contribute to false hopes. The need to enroll participants in phase I cancer trials creates incentives for researchers not to emphasize that these trials are not designed to provide treatment or even evaluate the efficacy of new interventions. As Matthew Miller describes his experiences as a cancer researcher, "The direction our conversation took and, it turned out, the likelihood patients would enroll, largely depended on whether and the extent to which we discussed the way the protocol opposed customary medical practice. Yet since terminally ill patients rarely if ever initiate such a discussion, no discussion was easier or more tempting to avoid."[31] Miller also notes that physicians recruiting their patients for participation in phase I cancer trials can conflate the limitations of current medical science with the limits created by the trial methodology. Doing so may be a way of protecting patients' hope, but it also serves the aim of trial recruitment.

Misleading potential trial participants can also serve the interests of researchers who are also physicians and wish to retain the appearance that they continue to serve the interests of their patients. These patients are often desperate to be enrolled even in phase I trials, perhaps in the belief that they might receive therapeutic benefit rather than simply contribute to generalizable knowledge. Miller notes that physician researchers can be tempted to follow the lead of these participants. However, "by accepting their gratitude without exploring the assumptions on which it was based, like so many other custodial acts of acquiescence, I was reinforcing the fiction that we were about to embark on a therapeutic enterprise."[32] In general, there is evidence of a disconnect between the information that physicians and researchers believe they convey to trial participants and the uptake of that information by those participants. Failure by physicians to communicate a participant's medical prognosis or the introduction of any ambiguity around the chances of therapeutic benefit in phase I trials often leads to unrealistic hope by research participants.[33]

Researchers can create even greater potential for conflicts of interest and roles if they are also clinicians and recruit from among their patients for trial participants. Empirical research on patient decision-making shows some evidence of physician pressure impacting the decision to participate in phase I cancer trials. In one case, 7 percent of these participants indicated that they had experienced moderate to a great deal of pressure to participate in a phase I trial.[34] Interviews with trial participants also show that they are often motivated by their perception of their physicians' hopes. One participant noted being told by their physician, "Don't give up hope," while another reported staff sharing a sense of hope with her both when there is reason for hope and even "when there is not hope too."[35]

The language of cancer care also contributes to misunderstanding about the aims of phase I trials. Cancer patients and their families regularly adopt the language of cancer charities and treatment centers, treating cancer care as a battle and using other military metaphors.[36] As an extension of this language, choosing not to pursue every treatment option and clinical trial can be seen as "giving up"—a defeat. Participants in phase I cancer trials regularly use this language when describing their participation, including likening participation to their experience fighting in the Vietnam War and comparing giving up hope to rolling over "on your back, legs in the air, just like a cockroach."[37] When researchers and physicians adopt this language, they contribute to its coercive effect and the potential to misunderstand the aims of cancer research in humans.[38] This language can have important practical impacts, as when having hope is associated with not giving up the "fight" against cancer and thus prompts participants to put off making decisions around end-of-life care.[39]

In practice, because phase I cancer trial design can be complicated and participants' scientific literacy can vary, participants may range in understanding the likelihood that they will benefit from participation in these trials. Rather than a binary of understanding and consenting or operating on a misconception, these participants' hopes for better health will range from false to well-informed. For many of these individuals, hope for better health from phase I trial participation includes fantasizing about and emotional engagement with the hoped-for future that echoes the understanding of hope developed in Chapter 3.

Exploiting Hope in Phase I Cancer Trials

Concerns with exploitation in phase I cancer trials often focus on the design and conduct of trials that enroll healthy individuals. These concerns highlight the worry that, because healthy participants do not stand to receive medical benefits from trial participation, they are likely to be sought out as "cheap labor" by researchers.[40] This concern is associated with more general worries related to consent and vulnerability, where healthy volunteers for phase I medical trials are often seen as poor and relatively uneducated individuals, in some instances working as "professional guinea pigs" who make a living enrolling in phase I trials. Following Wertheimer's transactional fairness account of exploitation, Shamoo and Resnik argue that healthy participants could be exploited in phase I trials if they receive an unfair benefit from the transaction compared with the benefits received by researchers and their sponsors. In this way, participation by healthy individuals in phase I clinical trials is a form of labor, and if the wages or benefits of this labor are sufficiently low, then exploitation can take place, just as with any other form of labor. This possibility of exploitation raises the question of what amount of compensation for labor by healthy participants will be adequate and how to balance against concerns about undue inducement into clinical trial participation. Shamoo and Resnik argue that some amount of compensation is necessary to avoid or at least minimize the exploitation of healthy phase I trial participants.[41]

Rebecca Dresser similarly links concerns with exploitation to the socioeconomic status of healthy participants, worrying that such research "imposes a disproportionate share of exploratory research burdens on low-income people through the use of financial incentives."[42] This focus on socioeconomic disadvantage and an "underclass" of healthy research participants in phase I trials can be read as linked to structural fairness concerns and a structural fairness account of exploitation. In her review of responses to these worries about exploitation, Dresser notes that critics of existing trial recruitment and payment approaches have suggested healthy phase I trial participants should receive access to healthcare generally and possibly access to any treatments developed as a result of their trial participation.[43] These suggestions follow the general track of structural accounts of exploitation, where the unfairness of structural injustice can be addressed by giving individuals the benefits they would have received under just conditions. If access to healthcare is seen as a requirement of justice, then extending this access to healthy trial participants would be a means of addressing structural exploitation.

Whatever the merits of a transactional fairness account of exploitation for addressing concerns about the exploitation of *healthy* phase I trial participants, this type of account is unlikely to be adequate for the concerns raised with regard to ill participants in phase

I cancer trials, because—by virtue of their ill health and in some cases terminal prognosis—any chance of a cure, improved health, improved quality of life, or longer life will be of immense value to them. As such, it is less likely that the distribution of benefits for sick cancer trial participants is unfair by the standards of transactional fairness, even granting that the aim of phase I trials is not to provide effective treatment or test efficacy. That is, the balance of benefits for very ill cancer patients in these trials will often, *ex ante*, fall heavily on the side of trial participants, given their very poor health.

Similarly, focusing on a structural account of exploitation seems to miss the concern around phase I cancer trials involving ill patients. The concern for these individuals is not that they are socioeconomically disadvantaged laborers but that they are desperately ill and driven by hope to participate in these trials. The challenge that they face is not adequate access to healthcare; rather, because of the nature and progression of their disease, there typically is not an effective treatment available to improve their health regardless of their insurance coverage or socioeconomic status. In many cases, these individuals may be relatively privileged members of their communities because they typically have some contact with their health systems before trial participation and are often recruited into trials through their personal physicians or care networks. Thus, for these individuals, granting them access to healthcare following trial participation would not address any deficit in their well-being or worries that their hopes for better health are being exploited.

Concerns specifically about the exploitation of terminally ill participants of phase I cancer trials are often linked to failures of consent and false hope. For example, the *British Medical Journal* described a study that found that many phase I trial participants consented to trial participation because of an expectation of therapeutic benefit. This article noted that consent based on an expectation of therapeutic benefit is leading to fears that "terminally ill patients who take part in phase one trials of chemotherapy are being exploited."[44] George Annas similarly charges that phase I cancer trial participants who hold out hope for better health through trial participation are subject to exploitation:

> Terminally ill AIDS and cancer patients can be harmed, misused, and exploited. It has even been persuasively argued that we as a society have developed a 'cure or kill' attitude that permits us to use the terminally ill as 'volunteers' for our experiments designed to banish death . . . subjects who believe they have 'nothing to lose' and are desperate because of their terminal illness should also be disqualified as potential research subjects because they are unable to provide voluntary, competent, informed or understanding consent to the experimental intervention with such a view.[45]

This charge has been challenged, however, on the grounds that even seriously ill people should be able to make informed choices regarding their health and should not be viewed as so passive and vulnerable as to make consent to trial participation impossible and exploitation inevitable. Seidenfeld et al. make this point by arguing, "Although phase 1 trial participants might be vulnerable in other ways because of their illness, grounds to doubt their capacity as a group to make decisions, understand information, and refuse exploitative offers are largely unsubstantiated when considering their demographic characteristics."[46]

Worries about the exploitation of hope are also expressed when research participants are fully informed about trial participation. Matthew Miller voices concern that the combination of desperate patients entering phase I cancer trials and the fact that these trials are not designed to evaluate the drug's efficacy can result in trials that "trade on patients' hopes."[47] However, he is unclear here about how "trading on" hopes should be understood and why it is morally problematic. Much clearer is the concern raised by Nycum and Reid that terminally ill patients can be exploited in phase I cancer trials when their hopes for better health are treated as part of the benefit of trial participation.[48] They are careful to note that false hope, based on a misconception about the design of the trial or likelihood of experiencing direct medical benefit, could harm the participant because it may lead them to participate in a trial on a false belief about the prospects for benefit. Even for those experiencing hope beyond all expectation that is a well-informed rather than false hope, they caution that such hope should be considered a collateral or indirect benefit that should be treated separately from direct medical benefit. They argue that such collateral hope should not be used to stand in for the objective likelihood of direct medical benefit and used to balance against risks of harm. More specifically, they worry that hope for better health can be exploited by researchers if used to stand in for the reality of likely benefit to trial participants.

Nycum and Reid's concern around the exploitation of hope is based on a transactional fairness view of exploitation, exemplified in the concern that exploitation in these cases results from "an unfair distribution of harms and risks."[49] However, there are at least two reasons to doubt that such an understanding of exploitation is the right way to evaluate exploitation of hope in phase I clinical trials involving ill patients. First, it is not clear that these trials represent a distribution of benefits and harms that is unfair to terminally ill trial participants. Even if the likelihood of direct medical benefit, including increased life expectancy and a cure of the underlying disease, is extremely small, such likelihood might reasonably be viewed as extremely valuable to a terminally ill patient even if coupled with an increased likelihood of pain, suffering, and early death. Moreover, as noted earlier, in practice the likelihood of partial or complete response to the compound being tested is small but not vanishingly so in phase I cancer trials. Thus, worries about unfairness in the distribution of benefits and risks may be misplaced.

Second, by placing the value of hope in a separate, subjective category of benefit, it is not clear that Nycum and Reid have provided an account of exploiting hope. Rather, their worry seems to be that by including the subjective benefits of hope in the calculation of benefits and risks of trial participation, ethics review boards make a category mistake that raises the potential for miscalculation, unfairness, and exploitation. Whatever the merits of their argument for treating the benefits of hope separately from direct medical benefits when evaluating the benefit-to-risk profile of phase I cancer trials, their argument is that hope should not be part of the fairness calculation. Thus, this is less an argument for what is entailed by exploiting hope in clinical trials and more an argument that exploitation can take place when hope is included in the benefit calculation.

Clinical Research in LMICs

As with early-stage clinical trials of cancer therapies, concerns with exploitation are often raised in the context of human participant trials in low-income settings. As I have shown, worries about exploiting hope in phase I cancer trials are driven primarily by how these trials can (often falsely) raise the hopes of desperately ill participants, creating the potential for exploitation. In clinical trials in LMICs, by contrast, worries with exploitation focus on how the benefits of the trials are distributed to participants and their communities. The benefits of these trials are typically more tangible than those in phase I trials because they have already gone through early-stage trials and have shown the potential for efficacy in humans. But whereas the *methodology* of these trials can raise exploitable hopes in phase I cancer trials, *socioeconomic barriers* to accessing care are at the heart of concern regarding clinical trials in LMICs. Limited access to insurance and underfunded public health systems in these settings mean that potential clinical trial participants may not have access to adequate medical coverage, much less cutting-edge treatments like those being tested through clinical trials.

Despite—or potentially because of—these barriers to accessing care, hope for better health does drive participation in phase III clinical trials in LMICs. For many of these participants, their interest in clinical trial participation is driven by hope that their own health will be improved or that they may help to improve the health of those around them. In a meta-analysis of studies of Indian clinical trial participants, 48 percent of participants were motivated by a desire for improved health and 43 percent of participants were motivated by an interest in improving the health of others, including in their own communities and throughout the world.[50] These hoped-for outcomes ranged from protection from HIV infection in HIV vaccination trials to hope for a cure for those facing currently incurable diseases or a terminal diagnosis.[51,52] Similarly, a study of an antiretroviral therapy in HIV-positive individuals from Argentina, Brazil, and Thailand found that the single most important reason for continued participation in the trial was the desire to obtain direct medical benefit (56 percent).[53] This same study gave participants a list of possible reasons for continued participation in the study, and large majorities of participants selected helping patients in their own country (91 percent active arm, 92 percent control arm) and improving their own health (89 percent active arm, 84 percent control arm) as very important to them. More recently, a systematic review of rationales for clinical trial participation in LMICs supported these earlier findings.[54] In this review, an interest in helping others was the most common reason for trial participation, described in terms of doing something good for their own community and feeling solidarity with others suffering from the medical condition being studied. Personal medical benefit was a common motivator as well: the possibility of curing or treating the medical condition being researched or preventing infection was the second most common reason for trial participation, and receiving access to medical treatment and ancillary care was the third most common reason.

Charges of exploitation in relation to clinical trials in LMICs typically focus on the benefits received by trial participants and their communities. A case that appears frequently in the literature on exploitation in research on human participants illustrates these worries: Many premature infants are born with insufficient surfactant in their lungs, leading to respiratory distress syndrome. Surfactant replacement therapy can be used to treat respiratory distress syndrome. Four surfactants were approved by the US Food and Drug Administration (FDA) between 1990 and 2000. In 2000, the US pharmaceutical company Discovery Labs sought approval to conduct a phase III trial of a new surfactant called Surfaxin. Discovery Labs and the FDA agreed that a noninferiority trial comparing Surfaxin with existing treatments would not yield sufficiently high-quality data. Instead, a placebo-controlled trial was proposed for 650 prematurely born infants in Bolivia. All participating infants would receive endotracheal tubes, ventilators, and antibiotics—treatments known to improve the chances of surviving respiratory distress syndrome. Some of these treatments were at the time unavailable to infants in the local community not enrolled in the trial. The hospitals selected for this multicenter trial were chosen because they were not able regularly to provide their patients with surfactant therapy. Therefore, those infants in the placebo arm of the trial would not receive worse treatment than what they would have received otherwise. In fact, insofar as they would not ordinarily have access to endotracheal tubes, ventilators, and antibiotics, their treatment would be better. While Discovery Labs had some discussions about making Surfaxin available to participating hospitals at reduced cost if the therapy was approved, no such agreement was reached.[55]

One element of particular note in this case is that it was arguably beneficial to all parties involved in the trial, and participation was voluntary. While human participant trials in LMICs pose difficulties in obtaining fully informed consent, there is nothing about the case, as it is described, that demonstrates a failure to obtain consent. Moreover, even those participants who were enrolled in the placebo arm of the trial may have received better care and better access to medical resources than they would otherwise have received. Even if these benefits were outweighed by the risks of trial participation, all participants received, *ex ante*, a chance of enrolling in the active arm of the trials and accessing all of its potential benefits. There was a strong chance that this trial would therefore create a favorable balance of costs and benefits for the trial participants.

Putting aside outright harms or a failure of consent, two primary pathways for exploitation have been alleged in this and similar cases. First, the use of a placebo control arm, when proven treatments exist and are the standard of care in wealthier communities, has been said to be exploitative,[56] insofar as researchers take advantage of the poverty of research participants in LMICs to enroll them in trials that would not be permitted in wealthier communities. This lower standard of care works to the advantage of researchers because it gives them the opportunity to conduct their research more cheaply and quickly than might be the case if a higher standard of care—and thus an active rather than placebo control—were used.[57]

Second, the accrual, or lack thereof, of benefits from the trial for trial participants and members of the host community has been cited as a source of potential exploitation. In the Surfaxin case, the expense of this drug, if successful, would have placed it far out of the reach of the communities in which it was being tested, given their limited per-capita expenditures on healthcare. While Discovery Labs did start discussions to provide Surfaxin to the host communities at reduced cost if the drug proved successful, a firm agreement was not reached.[58] Therefore, whereas the researchers and their sponsors would benefit from the trial, the members of the communities participating in the trial would benefit very little by comparison. For some commentators, the disproportionately great benefit received by the researchers serves as clear evidence that exploitation has occurred.[59]

In relation to the exploitation of hope, and specifically hope beyond all expectation of better health, it is this second vector of exploitation that I will focus on. In the Surfaxin trial and many other such trials in LMICs, the compound being tested had gone through laboratory testing and earlier phases of testing in humans to be in a position of clinical equipoise, where it was not yet clear whether the compound being tested was more effective than the existing standard of care. The existence of a placebo arm in these trials and the uncertainty of efficacy for participants in the active arm mean that the estimated *ex ante* chances of improved health are often below 50 percent. Nonetheless, for compounds being tested at this stage of human subject trials, the chances of benefit are not trivial. More unlikely is that the compound, if effective, will be made widely available in the participants' home community, given the structural barriers limiting access to treatment. Individuals in both cases—seeking direct medical benefit and better health for their communities—can reasonably be said to be hoping beyond all expectation for these benefits. However, I will focus on the latter group, given its significantly different focus from the case of phase I cancer trial participants seeking direct medical benefit.

Fairness-Based Exploitation in LMICs

In the context of human participant trials in LMICs, worries about exploitation are typically linked to the fairness of the distribution of trial benefits. In the context of host communities, critics charge that clinical trials can fail to provide fair benefits for the host community, especially when the researchers and their sponsors see significant benefits.[60] If so, clinical researchers and their employers can be said to have exploited the communities that host their studies.

These commentators are often not clear, however, as to what kind of distribution would count as fair in these cases and why.

As discussed in more detail in Chapter 2, one strategy for interpreting the concept of fairness as it applies to exploitation is to focus on the terms of the agreement or transaction between those making an exchange. If the terms of this transaction are unfair—that is, if one party benefits unfairly from the transaction—then that individual has exploited the other. In some cases, the exact standard for measuring fairness in transactional exploitation remains vague. Some commentators couch the fairness standard in the language of inequity with the attitude that, whatever standard of fairness or inequity one endorses, failure to guarantee benefits to the host community marks a clear violation of the requirements of fairness.[61] In other cases, critics worry that benefits received by the researchers and, especially, pharmaceutical companies, can be in some sense "disproportionate" and therefore exploitative.[62]

Other, more detailed accounts of transactional exploitation in clinical trials in LMICs draw on Wertheimer's linkage of unfairness to a deviation from the distribution of benefits that would be achieved under hypothetical fair-market conditions.[63] This adaptation of Wertheimer's approach has the advantage of clarity, where an explicit standard is given for measuring fairness within an interaction. However, it suffers from several shortcomings. First, it is not clear that human participant research should be evaluated by the standards of fairness used in the marketplace. While human subject research does not aim to provide basic healthcare for research participants, it does have an enormous impact on those participants' health and well-being, meaning that market norms of fairness may not be appropriate. Second, critics have charged that a hypothetical fair-market standard—and, more generally, transactional fairness approaches that limit the scope of fairness—fail to take into account forms of unfairness created by the background institutional structures within which these transactions take place.[64]

This understanding of exploitation can lead commentators to miss other elements of exploitation present in clinical trials. Specifically, a transactional fairness approach to understanding worries of exploiting the hopes of participants for their communities can fail to illuminate the link between these two groups. Wertheimer questions any link between individual participation in a clinical trial and community exploitation. He grants that research participants might *feel* disrespected if they believe that their community should benefit from their trial participation. However, this experience of disrespect is contingent on the participant having this feeling and not a general requirement of non-exploitation. More generally, Wertheimer argues that the link between participants and their communities is not best explored through the lens of exploitation but "by principles of beneficence or distributive justice that seek to provide more health care resources to the poorest areas of the world."[65]

The inability of transactional fairness exploitation to account for background fairness motivates the use of a structural fairness account of exploitation as an alternative. Such an account of exploitation will include background, structural inequalities, and injustices when determining whether the distribution of resources resulting from an interaction is fair. As discussed previously, Thomas Pogge offers a problematic interpretation of structural exploitation. He argues that it is morally problematic to take advantage of social injustice, particularly if one has had a role in creating or perpetuating that injustice.[66] He notes that in the Surfaxin case, Discovery Labs could justly be accused of perpetuating poor access to essential medicines in LMICs by being part of a network of pharmaceutical companies that have encouraged a patenting system that reduces access to essential medicines in these countries. But even when the pharmaceutical company or researchers do not directly perpetuate background injustice, this injustice can create a range of vulnerabilities that can unfairly be taken advantage of by placing persons in a worse bargaining position and in a situation of greater desperation than would otherwise have been the case.[67] While many vulnerabilities can be taken advantage of without fault—consider a surgeon benefiting from a patient's blocked artery—the argument is that exploiters are not entitled to benefits accrued by virtue of exploitees being disadvantaged by injustice. By way of comparison, a customer at a pawn shop may not be entitled to retain stolen goods, even if they did not steal them and, at the time of purchase, did not know they were stolen.[68]

Recall that Pogge's general solution to concerns about exploiting structural injustice is to grant victims of this injustice transactional terms akin to what they would receive under more just conditions. Thus, a researcher or their sponsor might also restrict their demands on the victims of injustice to create a hypothetical just exchange price akin to a fair transactional price. This is essentially Pogge's strategy when he argues that Discovery Labs "ought to treat Bolivian infants as if they were citizens of a just country and therefore entitled to some basic health care (presumably including some existing RDS [respiratory distress syndrome] treatment) as a matter of course."[69] This understanding of exploitation, while reproducing the flaws discussed in Chapter 2, is also a poor fit for understanding the exploitation of hope for one's community. Arguably, in a fully just context all community members would have access to at least basic medical services. Thus, it is not clear how researchers and their sponsors should interpret the requirements of just exchanges given that drug makers and researchers do not typically provide free access to their products within wealthier settings.

Structural fairness accounts of exploitation can offer less demanding duties than those implied by Pogge. Instead of requiring that one refrain completely from benefiting from unjust institutions, an account of structural fairness can maintain that one's connection to unjust institutions helps to determine and limit the duty to address injustice.[70] While transactional fairness might demand that all localized unfairness be neutralized, structural fairness can entail a positive obligation by actors to mitigate the effects of injustice and to reform unjust institutions. A swath of global institutions have been claimed to be responsible, in part, for the poor health outcomes of the trial participants. These could include very general institutions like colonialism, a history of neoliberal economic policies, and antidemocratic political interventions in South America.[71] Insofar as this is the case, individuals will have a political responsibility to reform these institutions, in keeping with their connection to them. More to the heart of this discussion, pharmaceutical companies can rightly be held liable for promoting international intellectual property agreements such as the Agreement on Trade-Related Aspects of Intellectual Property Rights (TRIPS) that reduce access to essential medicines in countries like Bolivia.[72] To the degree that these institutions hamper the bargaining position of the parents in the Surfaxin case, researchers can be said to exploit these vulnerabilities through the failure to grant fairer terms of access to the benefits of the trial to the host community.

As I will discuss in the remainder of this chapter, examining the specific relationships of researchers to their participants and other contextual factors such as their power to initiate change is key to understanding exploitation in clinical trials in LMICs and elsewhere. However, even the political responsibility–based understanding of structural fairness exploitation is a poor fit specifically for understanding the exploitation of the hope of LMIC research participants for their communities. As Wertheimer correctly notes, this hope and the exploitation it can engender is a contingent characteristic of specific research participants and not a universal characteristic of research in LMICs. While the political context of researchers, research participants, and their communities is important to diagnosing and responding to exploitation, the specific element of exploiting hope is best understood through the relationship between researcher and participant and the partial entrustment generated through this relationship.

Partial Entrustment and the Roles of Researchers

As an alternative to fairness-based accounts of exploitation in the conduct of phase I cancer trials and phase III clinical trials in LMICs, a respect-based account charges that relatively well-off researchers and sponsors fail to fulfill a specified duty of beneficence to their research participants generated through a relationship of partial entrustment. There is considerable debate over how the roles of researchers should be understood. The primary tension that fuels these debates is between the health needs of human research participants and their communities and the aim of producing generalizable knowledge that can further medical practice. While these two interests do not necessarily conflict, in many cases they make competing claims of researchers in terms of study design and the use of resources.

One interpretation of the researcher's role, called the fiduciary approach, maintains that when conflicts emerge between the aims of creating generalizable knowledge and promoting the good of the research participant, the good of the participant should be given priority because of the researcher's fiduciary responsibility to these individuals.[73] One challenge to this view is that patients typically consent to far fewer benefits than the fiduciary view would require. If patients give free and fully informed consent to less than maximal benefits from the researcher (given that their health and safety are reasonably protected from outright harm), then it is not clear whether the researcher is required to go beyond what is required of these consent documents. However, a range of relationships of full and partial entrustment exist that create duties beyond those contracted to. Moreover, factors such as a lack of other opportunities can motivate individuals to make less than appealing deals. If we simply take all contracts and consensual relationships at face value, these dimensions of and restrictions to choice go missing from consideration.

A more significant concern for the fiduciary view is that research has different goals than clinical care, and the potential individual benefits of research for participants should be balanced against the potential social gains of producing generalizable medical knowledge. This view need not be taken to the extreme that any social good can justify violating patients' rights, including requirements of informed consent; rather, researchers have multiple goods to promote and responsibilities to fulfill, all of which place demands on their conduct.[74]

Thus, the fiduciary view has been challenged by the partial entrustment view, which argues that researchers must balance between the aims of research and the needs of participants, fine-tuned by the degree to which the health of the participant is entrusted to the researcher.[75,76] As discussed in more detail in Chapter 4, Henry Richardson and Leah Belsky's partial entrustment view holds that the degree of responsibility of the researcher for research participants will depend on the depth and character of their relationship. Factors that determine entrustment include the resources available to the researcher, the vulnerabilities of the participant, the intimacy of the relationship, and the terms consented to.[77]

David Resnik worries that this account is flawed in that the partially entrusted party can seek to use consent documents to limit their entrustment and that other factors, such as the expertise of the researcher, should be acknowledged to shape the entrustment.[78] I think that these points are justified but that they can be addressed by Richardson and Belsky's account. Researchers and other parties *can* seek to limit their responsibilities through consent and other legal documents—a worry we will see arise in later chapters of this project. However, part of Richardson and Belsky's argument is that other relational factors, independent of consent documents, shape and expand entrustment. Moreover, Resnik is correct that factors such as the researcher's expertise should be considered when assessing their degree of entrustment of research participants. This factor can be considered along with the resources of the researcher, including not only material goods and financial resources but also human resources.

That said, Resnik correctly emphasizes that researcher roles can vary greatly and that the context of that role is important in understanding the obligations of researchers to research participants. Among the contextual factors are the design of the research project, the benefits and risks of the study, the vulnerability of the participant, the participant's aims or motivations in choosing to participate, the capacity of the researcher to benefit the participant, and the prior relationship of the participant to the researcher. These factors, in the context of a partial entrustment approach to understanding the exploitation of hope, can be used to understand the different responsibilities of researchers to research participants in phase I cancer trials and phase III clinical trials in LMICs.

Exploiting Hope in Clinical Trials

The potential conflict between the interests of participants and the aims of creating generalizable knowledge are present in both cases of exploiting hope in clinical trials that I have discussed in this chapter. In phase I cancer trials, researchers can be conflicted between at least two aims. In the first case, they seek to enroll participants into these trials to proceed to later phases of the trial that will determine the efficacy of the compound being tested. At the same time, they must ensure that participants are fully informed about the design of the trial and are not participating based on false hope about their likely benefits. Resnik notes several factors that will increase the entrustment of the health of sick participants to researchers in these trials, including the small chance of direct medical benefit, the expectation of benefit by trial participants, their vulnerability due to illness, the potential to provide participants with benefits outside of the scope of the trial, and a prior relationship between participant and researcher.[79]

As Resnik notes, part of the difficulty with and confusion about the roles of researchers in clinical trials is connected to the fact that physicians often recruit their own patients into these trials. Thus, they can take on a dual role of physician, entrusted with improving the health and well-being of the patient, and researcher seeking to generate generalizable knowledge without harming participants. Matthew Miller notes that explaining the methodological limitations of phase I cancer trials can be particularly challenging to physicians because they must communicate to their patients that, by design, these trials do not aim to maximize benefits to participants; rather, they seek to establish the largest tolerable dose of the intervention being investigated. These conversations, he notes, redefine the previous physician–patient relationship and distinguish between normal patient care and the aims of research.[80] When researchers in these trials fail to make these terms clear and instead simply take advantage of participants' hope for better health, then they potentially exploit the hope of these participants.

Miller suggests that clarity in communication is key to avoiding playing on the hopes of trial participants. In the case of phase I cancer trials, "unless and until we know whether a given drug is effective, under what conditions, for which malignancies, and at what dose, these trials remain non-therapeutic and ought to be spoken of as such."[81] When hope is extended to these potential trial participants without a good grounding in the methodology of the trial, it serves the interests of the trial recruiters rather than the participants and allows researchers to act as if they were solely serving as the participants' caregivers rather than also in a research role. This clarity is not incompatible with compassion and preserving well-informed hope beyond all expectation of benefit. The purpose of clinical trials should be communicated in a way that acknowledges the value that such research can provide for participants even if it is not designed to provide them with direct medical benefit.

In addition to clarity about the design and aims of phase I cancer trials, researchers and their institutions should avoid using persuasive recruitment language that trades on the rhetoric of hope to persuade cancer patients to join the study. Language that describes a study as "novel" or "promising," especially if coupled with a sense of urgency about deciding on participation, can easily promote false hope and, more problematically, twist a potential participant's self-expressive and measured hope into a more problematic expression detached from reality and encouraged externally.[82] Researchers should not interpret this possibility as a requirement to destroy the hopes of would-be participants but rather as a caution not to hype hope to accomplish their ends of trial recruitment.

Moreover, innovative dosing strategies in phase I cancer trials can increase the likelihood of participants receiving an effective dose of the intervention being evaluated and reduce the potential for false hopes. For example, Kipnis advocates for designing phase I cancer trials to allow individuals whose tumors have progressed to move to cohorts being given higher dosages of the intervention being tested if there are no severe adverse reactions to the intervention generally in the trial thus far. As a result, "the redesigned study effects a fairer distribution of the benefits and burdens of cooperation. It is a less exploitative arrangement."[83] Notably, Kipnis's argument is based on a transactional fairness understanding of exploitation. However, his argument is also based on balancing the aim of research to produce scientifically valid results with the interests of the participant. As such, it also conforms with the duties partially entrusted to researchers designing and managing these trials.

Key to avoiding the exploitation of hope in phase I cancer trials, then, is hewing to the researcher's role as protecting the safety of participants (in conjunction with research ethics boards, regulators, and others) and providing clear information about the aims, design, risks, and likely outcomes of the trial so that participants can balance the value of perpetuating hope and contributing to the creation of generalizable knowledge against personal risks and loss of other opportunities, including spending time with family and pursuing palliative care. Doing so requires a careful balance of competing interests. As Resnik notes, being realistic about the likely benefits of phase I trials is necessary but can reduce the hope of participants. Thus, in order to "not take advantage of participants' hopes that they will be the small group of patients for whom treatment works" while not destroying their hope, researchers "must find a way to help patients understand the risks and benefits of research participation and alternative options (such as palliative care) that does not take away their hope."[84]

In phase III trials in LMICs, researchers face a tension between generating generalizable knowledge about the compound being tested and managing the needs of participants with limited access to healthcare who may be motivated to participate in the trial largely because of the potential for personal benefit or to help their communities. Resnik notes several factors that can make the entrustment of the health of participants to researchers stronger in these trials than in phase I cancer trials. Primary among these is the greater potential for direct medical benefit given the different stage, and thus design, of the trial. Moreover, while participants are often ill in both types of clinical trial, participants in LMICs often have another layer of socioeconomic vulnerability. As with phase I trials, researchers may have the resources and expertise to provide benefits to trial participants and their communities outside of the terms of the trial and may have a previous relationship with both groups.[85]

At the same time, this relationship is primarily between the researcher and the research participant and not the participant's community. As such, worries about exploiting hope for better health for the host community will derive primarily through participants' hopes for their communities. As with the exploitation of hope in the context of phase I cancer trials, avoiding exploiting hope in phase III trials in LMICs will first be focused on clear communication to avoid producing or taking advantage of false hopes for what host communities might receive as a result of the trials. In some regards, the danger of such false hope is greater in phase III trials because these trials are designed to test the efficacy of new treatments. What may be unclear to participants is how likely it is that a successful treatment will be made available to the host community and thus how likely the participant's hope to help others is to be realized.

Outside of taking advantage of research participants' false hopes in phase III trials in LMICs, the primary means of exploiting genuine hopes in this context is when researchers and their sponsors disregard this hopeful motivation for trial participation and treat LMICs as expedient settings for research rather than communities in need of support for better healthcare. A range of arguments have been made for why researchers and their sponsors are responsible for ensuring that host communities benefit from medical research taking place within their boundaries, including potentially having access to any new treatments derived from this research. Researchers and their sponsors may then be in a position to give some of the benefits derived from the research to better provide for the health needs of the host community even above what research participants agree to in consent documents.[86] By failing to ensure access to some of the benefits of the trial for the host community, the researcher or sponsor may fail to fulfill a specified duty of beneficence to help provide for the basic needs of others.

Determining whether one has engaged in exploiting the hopes of research participants in LMICs can depend on the resources available to the researcher and their sponsors, the outcome of the trial, and agreements made before the trial. These factors help determine whether the hopes of trial participants for their communities are being used as a means of encouraging trial participation or if the researchers are acting in good faith, within the limits of their resources and the parameters of the trial, to ensure that their obligations to all parties are fulfilled. Thus, it will not be possible to give a single answer to the question of when the exploitation of hope takes place in these contexts—only to outline the general contours that make such exploitation possible.

Conclusion

Hope beyond all expectation can focus on better health for oneself, on other persons, or both. Thus, exploitable hope can have a variety of targets and is not exclusive to self-directed hope. Phase I cancer trials and phase III clinical trials in LMICs can both give rise to the exploitation of hope in similar ways. These hopes are typically weighty in that they can entail better quality of life, improved health, and longer life expectancy for trial participants and their communities. As a result, trial participants are motivated to participate in clinical trials despite personal risks to their health, loss of other opportunities such as palliative care, and large commitments of time and other resources—what I have referred to as leaps of hope. This hope for better health for oneself or one's community can be built on misinformation about the design and terms of the trial, thus leading to false hopes. In phase I cancer trials, false hope develops primarily through misinformation and misunderstanding about trial design and the genuine likelihood of better health. In phase III trials in LMICs, false hope is less a matter of misinformation about trial design and drug efficacy and is more driven by misunderstanding the intentions of researchers, mechanics of drug purchasing and provision, and even international trade forces such as patenting regimes. Thus, false hopes can be generated both through misunderstanding of the nature of research and medicine and through the power dynamics and economic forces that drive medical innovation. If researchers are not clear on the likely outcomes of these trials and especially if they allow or even encourage misunderstanding in the interest or encouraging trial participation, then they simply take advantage of these false hopes. In both of these cases, then, clarity as to the aims and likely outcomes of these trials is key to avoiding exploitation.

When the hopes of trial participants are not founded on mis-information but represent hope beyond all expectation, they can be exploited. Clinicians in phase I cancer trials are limited in the benefits that they can extend to trial participants because of the na-ture of these trials, but they can take specific actions to protect the interests of participants to whom they are partially entrusted. These steps include exploring trial designs with innovative and flexible dosing methodologies, ensuring that participants are aware of and have access to palliative care, and exhibiting compassion and sup-port for participants' hopeful pursuit of better quality of life. In phase III trials in LMICs, researchers can take action before and during trials to maximize host community benefits, in consultation with community leaders, whether or not the trial proves successful. They can also seek support from sponsors of such trials to ensure that sufficient resources exist to create a context where trials are not simply serving the interests of wealthy communities. Doing so can help to show a commitment to trial participants in whose interests they are partially entrusted and help to ensure recognition of the hope for others that often motivates trial participation.

6

Selling Hope

Exploitation and Unproven
Stem Cell Interventions

People with medical needs that cannot be fully addressed through proven medical treatments often look to what is perceived to be the cutting edge of scientific advancement for new treatments. People have long sought enrollment in legitimate clinical trials for new drugs and medical treatments in the hope that they will gain early access to new means of addressing their medical needs and thus stabilizing their health or even preventing death. However, the availability of promising new treatments in clinical trials is limited, and individuals may not be eligible to participate in these trials for a range of reasons.

For those unable to enroll in clinical trials for experimental medical interventions, there are often clinics willing to sell putative experimental or cutting-edge treatments to them for a price. While this is not a new phenomenon, a large global market of stem cell clinics has developed to try to take advantage of the early promise of these treatments. For example, a recent news story described Danny Bullen, a ten-year-old boy with autism living in the Canary Islands.[1] His medical condition was described as severe: he was unable to use the toilet on his own or to communicate verbally. Danny's parents were described as "desperate" and spent years trying, as they saw it, to find a cure for his autism. Through online support groups, Danny's parents found a stem cell intervention that gave them "real reason to hope." The clinic they identified, the Miami-based Art and Science Surgicenter, charged roughly $28,000 for two rounds of stem cell interventions, but Danny's parents felt it was well worth this price, given assertions that the stem cell intervention would cause "all autism symptoms to completely disappear" and that "all symptoms related to ASD [autism spectrum disorder] have completely disappeared in many of the young patients." In short, the severity and weightiness of Danny's condition convinced his parents to take a leap of hope for better health based on the promise of this new intervention.

While Danny's parents' pursuit of an unproven intervention is understandable, given their desperation to help him, evidence supporting stem cell interventions for autism is limited at best. The news article discussing Danny's case references a Duke University study that showed some promise for stem cell intervention for autism. However, this phase I trial was small and did not include a control group, thus limiting its reliability.[2] A more recent study failed to establish the efficacy of this intervention,[3] and critics have called this line of research "more like a 'Hail Mary pass' than a rational therapy."[4] The clinic selling this product to Danny's family also does little to provide assurance that its products are safe and effective. The Art and Science Surgicenter's online presence is limited to a nonfunctioning webpage and Facebook and Instagram pages that haven't been updated for over two and a half years and that focus largely on musculoskeletal and cosmetic treatments. Nonetheless, Danny's parents were thrilled with the results of their first session, saying that Danny spoke his first sentence "just hours" after receiving the intervention, despite being told it would take "several months" before noting any significant changes in his functioning.[5] Danny's parents clearly held a vibrant hope that stem cell interventions would cure his autism, despite a lack of supporting evidence. Were they being exploited in this case, or were they reasonably seeking ways to preserve hope for a better life for their child?

The Promise of Stem Cell Interventions

Stem cells have been proposed as having the promise of curing a range of diseases and reversing degeneration in the human body. This promise is linked to the ability of stem cells to self-renew or make copies of themselves and to differentiate into specialized cell types in the human body. This promise has led to intensive public and private investment in scientific research on stem cells. In many cases, expectations about the applications of stem cells to human health have outpaced the rate that new, effective, and safe stem cell treatments have been developed. Nonetheless, some stem cell treatments have been approved for human use, with many others being researched and tested.

Ethical issues have been associated with the development of stem cells since the early days of research on their application in humans.[6] Much of this initial concern was associated with the use of embryonic stem cells, which are typically harvested from the human blastocyst and involve its destruction. Embryonic stem cells are pluripotent, meaning that they have the capacity to form any type of human cell. Some ethicists and members of the public found the destruction of the blastocyst objectionable, raising concerns about the perceived loss of human life and associations with abortion. These objections led to restrictions on the use and development of embryonic stem cells in some jurisdictions and placed limits on stem cell research.

For this reason, the development of adult stem cells became a way to expand research into and applications for stem cells while avoiding ethical concerns about and public objections to using embryonic stem cells. Adult stem cells, unlike embryonic stem cells, are already somewhat specialized into specific cell types. They are multipotent, meaning that they can develop into multiple cell types—but not every cell type, as with pluripotent stem cells. Despite this limitation, an advantage of adult stem cells from the standpoint of those concerned with the destruction of embryos is that adult stem cells can be derived from humans without significant risk of harm.[7]

Among adult stem cells, mesenchymal stem cells have received considerable attention for their promise as a marketable form of stem cell therapy. These stem cells are found in human bone marrow and can differentiate into bone, cartilage, and fat cells. More recently, some scientists have located these cells more widely in the human body, and they are commonly derived from bone marrow and adipose or fat tissue. Researchers have seen potential for mesenchymal stem cells to be used to treat immune diseases, musculoskeletal issues, cardiac disease, and a range of other illnesses. At this time, research into these uses of mesenchymal stem cells is in early stages, and they are not approved for human use.[8]

When stem cells are harvested from one's own body, they are described as autologous stem cells. Autologous mesenchymal stem cells have been of interest to physicians and entrepreneurs wishing to sell stem cell interventions outside of clinical trials and directly to consumers for several reasons. In addition to their medical potential, the relative ease of harvesting them, and their public acceptability relative to embryonic stem cells, autologous stem cells fall into a regulatory gray area in some jurisdictions. As a result, a direct-to-consumer market for stem cell interventions has developed in many areas of the world, with most of these businesses offering autologous stem cells derived from adipose tissue and bone marrow. While regulations on the practice of medicine vary greatly by country, in the US businesses selling autologous stem cell interventions have claimed that they are exempt from Food and Drug Administration (FDA) oversight.[9]

As I will show in this chapter, there are a number or reasons to object to this practice. One is that there are questions about the efficacy of mesenchymal stem cell interventions or even whether these cells should be described as stem cells. Confusion over how these cells should be defined and mixed evidence on how well they work have allowed entrepreneurs to cherry-pick research to sell the public on their efficacy. As Sipp, Robey, and Turner describe it, confusion over these cells and the willingness of some actors to take advantage of this confusion has led mesenchymal stem cells to "acquire a near-magical, all-things-to-all-people quality in the media and in the public mind—hype that has been easy to exploit."[10] That is, the combination of unsupported hype about the efficacy of these cells as a treatment for a range of medical conditions with a regulatory gray area allowing their sale has created an opportunity for exploitation of patients hoping for better health.

Moreover, significant harms have been reported by those given autologous stem cells. In some cases, patients have developed lesions and tumors after these interventions. A recent review of such cases found thirty-five instances of complications following stem cell injection, eight of which resulted in death.[11] Another study identified three patients who had been blinded as a result of receiving adipose-derived stem cell interventions for macular degeneration.[12] In some cases, patients also travel to countries for care that have higher rates of infection in their healthcare systems and greater exposure to endemic infectious diseases than in their home countries.[13] If these interventions are ineffective, then patients also face financial losses that can be significant. Psychological damage has been hypothesized as well, as when failed treatments result in "dashed hopes."[14]

In many cases, critics charge specifically that those selling unproven stem cell interventions are exploiting their customers' hope for a cure or improved quality of life. For example, the International Society for Stem Cell Research (ISSCR) maintains that clinics offering unproven stem cell interventions "are exploiting patients' hopes by purporting to offer new and effective stem cell therapies for seriously ill patients, typically for large sums of money and without credible scientific rationale, transparency, oversight, or patient protections."[15] Similar concerns have been raised in light of well-publicized cases of people seeking out these alleged cures. For example, doctors capitalizing on publicity around former hockey great Gordie Howe's reported recovery from the effects of a stroke after an unproven stem cell intervention are accused of "exploiting hope" for rapid recovery following treatment.[16] It is clear that unproven stem cell interventions raise significant ethical concerns. What is less clear is what is meant by the charge that hope, specifically, is being exploited in sales of unproven stem cell therapies directly to consumers.

The Business of Selling Stem Cells

The market for unproven stem cell interventions is global, both in terms of the patients seeking these interventions and the businesses willing to offer them. Researchers in 2009 found twenty-three providers of direct-to-consumer stem cell interventions, focused largely in Asia, Europe, and Central America and the Caribbean. These providers most commonly advertised themselves as treating multiple sclerosis, Parkinson's disease, stroke, diabetes, and spinal cord injuries.[17] A 2014 search of the webpages of stem cell clinics found sixty-eight clinics in twenty-one countries across five continents.[18] The US was the largest host country for these businesses, representing a quarter of the total. Notably, however, some of these clinics offered cross-border treatment in Mexico. Other significant destinations were China and India with 12 percent each, Thailand at 11 percent, and Mexico at 9 percent. North American and Asia were the most common regions hosting these businesses, whereas the European Union (EU) countries hosted only 11 percent of the total, possibly because of more stringent regulations governing direct-to-consumer sales of stem cell products there. These businesses most commonly advertised themselves as offering interventions for multiple sclerosis, anti-aging, Parkinson's disease, stroke, and spinal cord injuries.

A 2016 study confirmed the global nature of the direct-to-consumer stem cell market but also reported much larger numbers of businesses.[19] This search of business websites found 417 clinics offering stem cell interventions. As with the prior study, the US was found to host the largest number of these businesses, with Mexico the third most common destination. Again, Asia was well represented, with India, China, Thailand, Malaysia, and Indonesia in the top ten most common destinations. Unlike the previous study, this search found more businesses in the EU, with the UK and Germany in the top ten. This study also demonstrated some overlap and some variability in the conditions these businesses advertised themselves as treating. Anti-aging interventions were by far the most common, followed by diabetes, sports and orthopedic injuries, multiple sclerosis, Parkinson's disease, and spinal cord injuries. Some of this variability is due to these businesses frequently being vague or unclear as to what conditions they claim to treat.

A search for US-based businesses in 2016 identified 351 businesses selling stem cell interventions directly to consumers at 570 clinics.[20] These clinics were located across the US, but with larger clusters in California, Florida, Texas, Colorado, Arizona, and New York. Nearly 80 percent of these businesses advertised autologous stem cell interventions, most commonly derived from bone marrow and adipose tissue. These businesses most commonly marketed themselves as offering interventions for orthopedic conditions, pain management, sports injuries, neurological conditions, immune system conditions, lung and respiratory system problems, urological conditions, and cosmetic treatments. The market for these businesses in the US is showing considerable growth: by 2017, a follow-up study noted 432 businesses selling such products at 716 clinics.[21] This is a long-standing trend— between 2009 and 2014 the number of new US-based stem cell businesses doubled each year, leading to a rate of 90 to 100 new businesses each year between 2014 and 2016.[22]

Though much smaller, a market for direct-to-consumer stem cell interventions exists in Canada as well. A 2018 search for stem cell businesses identified thirty businesses marketing stem cell interventions directly to consumers at forty-three locations.[23] Similar to their US cousins, these companies largely sell autologous stem cells derived from bone marrow and adipose tissue. These interventions were aimed at similar conditions to those in the US as well, including most commonly orthopedic and musculoskeletal conditions, pain relief, sports injuries, cosmetic and hair loss treatments, and neurological conditions.

The rise of businesses selling unproven stem cell products has often been associated with low- and middle-income countries (LMICs) that are thought to have relatively weak regulatory environments in which these businesses can flourish.[24] However, regulatory gaps and gray areas have allowed these businesses to operate in North America, Japan, Australia, and the EU as well. In the US, FDA regulations of medical procedures, devices, and products typically require premarketing oversight, which includes establishing the efficacy and safety of these interventions. An exception to this requirement is made for "same surgical procedures," where the patient's own cells are transferred within their body within the same medical intervention. While many US-based stem cell companies have not made their interpretation of FDA oversight requirements clear, a general trend has been for them to claim that they do not require FDA oversight and in some cases are explicitly exempt from oversight, as autologous stem cell procedures fall under the same surgical procedure exemption.[25] Japan and Australia have also given considerable authority to individual medical practitioners to use autologous stem cell interventions with limited oversight, whereas the EU has been more active in applying its rules against clinics selling stem cell interventions.[26] While stem cell clinics have been expanding in Canada, Health Canada recently announced a clarification of its policy such that it views these clinics as violating its policies.[27]

Hyping Stem Cell Interventions

Businesses selling stem cell treatments directly to consumers use a variety of advertising techniques. Most directly, these businesses typically have websites that include flashy graphics, patient testimonials, and statistics on the claimed efficacy of their products. In addition to these websites, stem cell clinics in the US have used YouTube videos and channels to host advertisements and patient testimonials, advertisements on Google searches, Twitter channels to promote their products, webinars, press releases, advertisements on television and in newspapers, and marketing events at hotels and conference sites.[28] Most websites of clinics across the world have been found to name their specific medical personnel and frequently describe them as "specialists," who are "renowned," "experienced," and "acclaimed."[29]

In some cases, businesses selling these interventions engage in outright fraud or fail to receive informed consent for treatment, as when patients report being misled about the nature, efficacy, and cost of unproven interventions by unscrupulous clinics.[30] Fraud can take place by the seller knowingly misrepresenting the efficacy of the intervention or by not offering the intervention as described. In some cases, fraud around unproven interventions can affect large numbers of people, as when a Winnipeg-based physician enrolled seventy patients in what was claimed to be a clinical trial of an unproven stem cell intervention for multiple sclerosis. In this case, the fraudster lacked the medical credentials he claimed and made false claims about the positive results of his clinical trial being run in India.[31]

This fraud can rob patients of the money paid for the intervention, create opportunity costs when false claims about unproven interventions lead patients to abandon current treatment or not access other promising interventions, and can undermine the legitimacy of well-run clinical trials for new medical interventions. In the Winnipeg case, patients paid up to $45,000 each to participate in the alleged clinical trial, were not given follow-up treatment or testing after completing the trial, and in some cases were removed from the trial after raising concerns about it.[32] In cases like these, fraudulent administration of unproven medical interventions can create clear harms and losses for participants on top of the moral wrong of deception, leading to little controversy over the ethical problems connected with them.

Outside of outright fraud, those selling stem cell products directly to consumers frequently make claims about the efficacy of these interventions that are not supported by good evidence. For example, all businesses included in a review of Canadian stem cell clinics made positive claims about the efficacy of their services.[33] These claims tended to focus on the promise of stem cells and potential for symptom relief rather than the definitive cure of diseases. Most of these claims were not quantified, but five of the thirty reviewed had specific and very optimistic claims about efficacy rates. Efficacy claims are often made using emotionally laden, "hype" language to persuade patients to purchase their goods. A study of 243 websites offering stem cell therapies found that 31.7 percent of these businesses used what the researchers categorized as "hype" language.[34] Examples of this language include references to stem cells as a "fountain of youth," a "revolution in biologics," and "breakthrough healing."

The language of hope factors directly and indirectly into many of these efficacy claims. Petersen and Seear argue that stem cell clinics marketing directly to consumers engage in a "political economy of hope," understood as a biomedical system that promises that better and new treatments are constantly under development and forthcoming, justifying continued investment in these enterprises.[35] After reviewing advertisements by these companies, they found a pattern of presenting patients as having been abandoned by mainstream, evidence-based medicine. These companies then fill a space vacated by mainstream medicine by promising better health to these individuals. As they describe it, the patients are "assumed to have little or no hope—having been abandoned by mainstream healthcare professionals—and yet *hopeful* and actively engaged in the management of their own condition."[36] This understanding of hope, as promoted by direct-to-consumer marketing, is consistent with the understanding of hope presented in Chapter 3. It is not necessarily built on a misunderstanding about the true likelihood of the stem cell intervention to improve the health or well-being of these patients, but it can act as a way for patients to take control over their own health and care and can allow them to engage imaginatively and emotionally in the idea of their disease being treated through a technological breakthrough.

Stem cell companies cultivate the hope of patients in a number of ways. Petersen and Seear note that these companies tend to use patient testimonials, interactive content, and links to scientific studies and news stories to present a narrative of hope, choice, and personal empowerment. Patient testimonials can be a particularly effective part of this hopeful narrative, as they allow patients to imagine themselves in the position of a former customer who has completed the transformation from desperate and ill to cured, healthier, or at least stable—living proof of these interventions' efficacy. For companies operating outside of well-established international markets for medical care, establishing their scientific legitimacy and safety can be part of this process of supporting hope for patients. For example, stem cell clinics in China augment standard advertising techniques with clinical concierges and use former patients as "patient ambassadors" who recruit and support new customers.[37] Patients are frequently asked if their stories can be used as part of online advertising, with clinics carefully selecting success stories to present to the public. In some cases, these stories are coached or edited, and patients may receive compensation for their participation. These stories, including patient blogs and video testimonials, can also be used to assure potential customers that perceived language and cultural barriers to treatment abroad can be bridged and that the care offered is of equal or even greater quality to that offered at home or in more familiar destinations.

In addition to questionable claims about the efficacy of these interventions, businesses selling stem cell interventions directly to consumers have been found to use "tokens of scientific legitimacy" to make their products appear grounded in evidence generated by valid scientific processes. Clinic websites throughout the world have frequently listed affiliations with professional societies and have claimed association with academic institutions. Others frequently claim that they have approval from local regulators, in some cases including the FDA.[38] A study of 100 websites selling anti-aging interventions that used stem cells found these tokens as well, including references to clinical research (31 percent), representations of medical professionals (23 percent), and the perspectives of scientists or academics (12 percent).[39] Canadian businesses selling these products commonly claimed (a) to have received accreditation by external bodies or had their products certified, (b) to have received awards, (c) to employ scientific or medical advisory board members with impressive achievements and credentials, (d) to have received ethics review for their services, (e) to have clinicians practicing in their facilities who are associated with prominent educational institutions and professional associations, (f) to have patent applications under review, and (g) to be publishing or using peer-reviewed research—as well as more generally using technical and scientific language.[40] These tokens of scientific legitimacy are also found in advertisements. For example, at one informational seminar targeting potential customers for a stem cell business, the individuals running the seminar dressed in medical scrubs and circulated a sign-in sheet similar to those used in doctors' offices.[41]

Clinical trial registries such as clinicaltrials.gov are a key means of implying scientific legitimacy as well. These registries typically have not imposed limitations on who can register with them and often include disclaimers that registration should not be understood as evidence that the intervention is efficacious or even that the study is well designed. Thus, while this registry includes information on many legitimate clinical trials, it also includes companies focused on selling a product to consumers rather than overseeing well-designed clinical trials. Inclusion in a government-administered registry can and does send the message of legitimacy, which companies marketing directly to consumers often prominently display. Moreover, the trial descriptions in these registries are often themselves used to advertise treatments being sold directly to consumers and to instill hope in potential customers. One study of early-phase trials for autologous stem cell interventions registered on clinicaltrials.gov found that stem cell studies were more likely than other drug studies to use therapeutic language such as "therapy" or "treatment" when describing their trials.[42] This language can specifically promote a therapeutic misconception around these early-stage trials and more generally can be used to instill hope in new stem cell technologies in advance of evidence to support this hope.

In addition to promoting language that can mislead potential customers and raise their hopes for better health, these businesses typically do not make the risks of medical complications and even death clear in their advertising materials. For example, a review of thirty Canadian businesses selling stem cell interventions directly to consumers found that sixteen of these businesses had no discussion of risks.[43] In some cases, these businesses went so far as to positively state that there were no risks associated with their interventions. The remainder of these businesses made minimal statements about risks, typically limiting these statements to acknowledging the potential for discomfort associated with injections and not discussing the risks specifically of their stem cell products. This failure to address the risks associated with these interventions is particularly concerning, given that the direct-to-consumer nature of these products may make potential customers less likely to consult with their physicians or travel medicine specialists at home. As a result, they may not receive warnings about the risks of these interventions from other, less biased sources.[44] These findings have been confirmed by others who have found that websites offering stem cell interventions often use strong and definitive statements about benefits while downplaying risks, creating the impression that these interventions are safe and effective.[45]

The problem of misleading and unsupported statements about the safety and efficacy of unproven stem cell interventions is compounded on so-called fake news websites. These sources include websites that entirely fabricate or regularly distort information and "junk science" websites that make scientifically dubious claims. A review of articles discussing stem cell interventions on these websites found that they frequently included wildly unsupported claims, including that stem cell interventions could regrow teeth in humans, a vitamin supplement could restore stem cells in adults, and a stem cell injection could be used to bring dead people back to life.[46] These stories were often presented in a conspiratorial manner, claiming that mainstream scientists and drug companies were colluding to keep these interventions from the public. These stories often make reference to real clinical studies or legitimate news sources while greatly exaggerating or misrepresenting their actual claims. As a result, consumers of these misleading news sources may develop both a greatly unrealistic understanding of the state of stem cell interventions and a distrust of more legitimate news sources.

News reporting on unproven stem cell interventions from more legitimate news sources has been found to overstate their safety and efficacy as well. A review of newspaper coverage of stem cell research in Canada, the US, and the UK between 2010 and 2013 found a tendency to present highly optimistic timelines for the translation of stem cell research into treatments.[47] Specifically, 69 percent of these reports stated that the research discussed would be available for human use in the "near future," "just around the corner," or within five to ten years, leading to concerns that these reports were creating unrealistic hope. Chinese newspapers have also been found to produce overly optimistic portrayals of unproven stem cell interventions, including discussing the benefits of these products in 93.8 percent of articles compared with discussing the risks in only 9.3 percent of articles. Moreover, 87 percent of these articles discussed the efficacy of interventions, and 81.4 percent featured providers, both of which would tend to encourage purchase of these interventions.[48] While these studies examined news coverage of unproven stem cell interventions in general, specific types of unproven interventions have been examined as well. Platelet-rich plasma interventions (which are often labeled as stem cell interventions) for sports-related injuries have received considerable news coverage when used by athletes and other celebrities. A study of newspaper coverage of these products in Australia, Canada, Ireland, New Zealand, the UK, and the US found that 23.8 percent of reports called these interventions effective, 22.8 percent noted efficacy was unclear, and only 6.5 percent described them as ineffective (leaving 46.9 percent not discussing efficacy).[49] Just over half of these articles mentioned purported benefits of platelet-rich plasma interventions, whereas just over a quarter discussed risks or limitations of this intervention. This review found that these news stories tended not to use typical "hype" language around unproven stem cell interventions but relied on implicit hype by focusing on elite athlete and celebrity use of these purportedly effective interventions.

Exploiting Stem Cell Hopes

Charges that clinicians selling stem cell interventions exploit the hope of their patients are often not specific about the nature of the alleged wrong or whether the hope being exploited is false or well informed. For example, the ISSCR recommends that clinicians only provide unproven stem cell interventions to their patients under very strict circumstances and not as part of for-profit clinics, because doing otherwise may "exploit the hopes of patients."[50] Why this is the case is unclear, however. In many cases, the fairness of the transaction seems to be at the heart of the concern, as patients receiving these interventions face significant risks and little potential benefit, while clinicians stand to make substantial financial gains from the transaction. For example, Petersen, Seear, and Munsie charge that new stem cell technologies engender hope for better health in patients, especially those with significant and intractable health problems. As a result, "in this context of high, yet unfulfilled expectations, many scientists, clinicians and policymakers fear that desperate patients may submit themselves to clinically unproven SCTs [stem cell treatments] and suffer harm and financial exploitation."[51] Variants of this concern with financially exploiting or profiting from "vulnerable" patients appear regularly in discussion of direct-to-consumer sales of unproven stem cell interventions.

In many cases, stem cell hype leads to misinformed hope about the efficacy of stem cell interventions, which can then be exploited. When misinformed hope is intentionally created by clinicians advertising and selling these interventions, charges of exploiting hope are relatively clear and convincing. This concern seems to be at the heart, for example, of the worry that "doctors and entrepreneurs exploit patient trust and take advantage of the dearth of cell therapy regulations in many countries."[52] More directly, Insoo Hyun charges that "there are some unscrupulous clinicians around the world exploiting the hopes of patients by purporting to provide effective stem cell therapies for large sums of money. These so-called stem cell clinics advance claims about their proffered stem cell therapies without credible rationale, transparency, oversight, or patient protections."[53] The most direct reading of "purporting" here is that the clinicians knowingly mislead their patients about the efficacy of these interventions and then exploit them by receiving "large sums of money" as a benefit. In some cases, this concern focuses on the benefits to those operating these businesses at the expense of misinformed and desperate patients. For example, Murdoch and

Scott charge that stem cell science has been shaped by a "confluence of hype, hope, broad medical potential, and connection to deeply shared desires and cultural values." As a result, "entrepreneurial individuals and companies of low moral regard can now leverage the general cultural authority of science and the furor surrounding stem cell research in particular to their fiscal advantage."[54] A similar concern was voiced by the International Campaign for Cures of Spinal Cord Injury Paralysis about clinics selling unproven stem cell interventions. In this case, advertisements for these clinics are seen as intentionally misleading, and individuals with serious spinal cord injuries (SCI) are particularly vulnerable to being misled: "People with SCI, as with any serious medical conditions, are highly susceptible to advertisements promising recovery, even when the costs are high and potential risks are unknown. It is morally unacceptable to prey on and profit from their hope for a cure."[55]

In other cases, misinformed hope can be generated through well-intentioned actions by those selling these interventions, such as when they are "true believers" in their potential efficacy despite a lack of supporting evidence. For example, a UK doctor was found to have abused his position as a physician by sending his patients to a stem cell clinic in the Netherlands despite a lack of evidence that this intervention would be effective.[56] These patients were all diagnosed with multiple sclerosis and were desperate for a treatment that would address this degenerative neurological condition. The physician in this case seemed to acknowledge that there was no evidence of efficacy for these stem cell interventions, instead using the desperation of the patients as a reason to give stem cell interventions "a try." The panel reviewing this doctor's actions found multiple reasons for concern, including a lack of follow-up care and failure to obtain informed consent to treatment. Some of these concerns focused specifically on exploitation as well, seemingly linked to the physician's gain from these interventions. Specifically, the panel wrote that these patients were "desperate to find some relief for their disease and were prepared to raise large sums of money in the hope that the treatment offered would alleviate their symptoms" and thus the physician "was taking unfair advantage of vulnerable patients and was therefore exploitative of them."[57] Notably, this panel did not find that the physician intentionally misled his patients, as he genuinely felt that the intervention could work for them. However, the panel indicated that the patients were not fully informed of the likelihood of the intervention succeeding or its lack of scientific support. Varieties of "true believing," willful ignorance about the true state of research on stem cell treatments, or systematic misreading of this evidence may be common among providers of these interventions. In other cases, clinicians may have a mix of beliefs about the efficacy of the interventions they are selling and mixed motivations toward their patients.

In addition to these instances of false hope, patients seeking unproven interventions may be aware of the costs and likely consequences of seeking these interventions and yet choose to purchase them anyway. These patients have often been found to downplay the possibility that unproven interventions will produce a "miracle" cure or complete recovery from their medical condition; rather, they seek to improve their health in small, incremental ways or to halt or slow the degeneration of their health.[58] For many of these patients, the appeal of pursuing unproven interventions is that it allows them to take an active role in managing their health, even if the expected positive results are modest or nonexistent. This is particularly true for patients with the most severe and often terminal illnesses, whose lack of other options and sense of desperation are acute.[59] In these cases, the experience of agency and hope for positive outcomes rather than the reality of these outcomes is the most likely benefit—one that they feel is worth the cost of these interventions.[60]

In their interviews with patients who sought unproven stem cell interventions, Petersen, Seear, and Munsie give several examples of patients who seemingly did not base their hopes on a misunderstanding about the likely results of the intervention. In one case, a patient notes that she "never thought it was going to be a miracle ... and people who go with that thought in mind are going to be disappointed every time."[61] Others' expressions of their hope for better health were akin to the understanding of hope presented in Chapter 3 and developed by Adrienne Martin. For example, one patient discussed how hope for better health from unproven stem cell interventions took the form of imaginative engagement about the future: "I feel as though there is some sort of hope, that if I've had these few changes, then you never know what else can happen, and if more research is done using embryonic stem cells then maybe there's something more that's going to be happening in the future."[62] While this individual's hope was tied to developments in embryonic stem cells rather than autologous interventions, it demonstrates how hope can encourage positive thinking about and engagement with the future without being tied to false beliefs about the current state of stem cell research.

These cases present the actions of consenting adults who find value in pursuing this hope for a positive result from unproven stem cell interventions despite understanding that there is little evidence that the interventions they are purchasing will improve their health and that there is some risk of harm. Nonetheless, these patients often pay very large sums of money for these interventions. Those selling them take advantage of this hope despite knowing that they are unable to offer any assurances of benefit and, in fact, have little or no scientific basis supporting the use of the intervention. Even if the clinicians do not act fraudulently and the patients are fully informed, these cases evoke the concern that bad actors are exploiting the hope of sick and desperate people.

It is not obvious, however, if cases involving informed hope are in fact problematically exploitative or whether we are simply conflating these cases with more clearly problematic instances of fraud and lack of informed consent. As I demonstrated in the previous chapter, linking the wrongness of exploitation to the fairness of the distribution of the risks and rewards created through the exchange can miss much of what is concerning about these interactions. Selling unproven stem cell interventions seems deeply unfair. Patients take on all the risks associated with these interventions and have little prospect for medical improvement, while physicians selling these interventions stand to receive significant financial gains. However, well-informed patients may benefit considerably from the hope created by these interventions, especially if their medical prognosis is very poor and they believe they lack viable medical options. Similarly, while the chances of improved health from unproven stem cell interventions will typically be very small, individuals receiving unproven stem cell interventions as part of well-run clinical trials or even outside of these trials have a nonzero chance of medical improvement that may be very valuable to them, especially if they have a degenerative disease or a terminal diagnosis. Finally, focusing solely on the distribution of risks and benefits created through these exchanges misses important elements of what can make these interactions exploitative, including what obligations physicians have to their patients, how these patients are treated, whether purchase of unproven stem cell interventions also serves a larger scientific purpose, and whether charging patients fees for receiving them is justified.

Roles of Physicians

While clinics selling unproven stem cell interventions directly to consumers employ a variety of professionals from varied medical and non-medical fields, I will focus on the roles and responsibilities of—and potential for exploitation by—physicians working in these clinics. The reason for this approach is that physicians tend to play a leading role in the creation and viability of these clinics. For example, a study of websites promoting Canadian stem cell clinics found that twelve of the fifteen sites reviewed featured physicians providing these services.[63] Physician involvement in these clinics has also been observed in the US.[64] In a separate study of US stem cell businesses, 94.6 percent of 166 businesses were found to advertise physician involvement in administering these interventions, including a total of 401 named physicians; 80.5 percent of these physicians had been trained in the US and represented a wide range of specialties.[65]

A cursory look at the websites of large networks of direct-to-consumer stem cell clinics makes the leading role of physicians clear. For example, the website for the Cell Surgical Network, an international network of direct-to-consumer clinics, includes a prominent link to its "Physician Network," describes the founding of the network by two medical doctors, and features images of lab coat–wearing and surgical instrument–wielding medical professionals in its descriptions of its partner sites.[66] Regenexx, another international network of clinics, prominently boasts of the training its physician partners receive.[67] As is typical of smaller clinics, the Ontario Stem Cell Treatment Centre seeks to assure potential customers of the quality and legitimacy of its products by describing the medical credentials ("attended medical school at the University of Toronto"), experience ("has held a myriad of leadership positions"), and links to trusted public institutions ("current member of . . . the Canadian Medical Association") of its physician team.[68]

Professional guidelines for physicians offer a sense of their expected roles in treating their patients and the elements of their care in which they are entrusted. The American Medical Association's code of ethics maintains that "the relationship between a patient and a physician is based on trust, which gives rise to physicians' ethical responsibility to place patients' welfare above the physician's own self-interest or obligations to others, to use sound medical judgment on patients' behalf, and to advocate for their patients' welfare."[69] When introducing innovations into medical practice, they are advised to use "sound scientific evidence and appropriate clinical expertise," be "aware of influences that may drive the creation and adoption of innovative practices for reasons other than patient or public benefit," and to know "what the known or anticipated risks, benefits, and burdens of the recommended therapy and alternatives are."[70]

In the UK, the General Medical Council's Ethical Guidance for Doctors again focuses on a relationship of trust between patients and doctors, stating that "Patients must be able to trust doctors with their lives and health."[71] This trust requires a range of steps relevant to physicians in the business of selling unproven stem cell interventions, including that physicians "make the care of your patients your first concern," "not allow any interests you have to affect the way you prescribe for, treat, refer or commission services for patients," "provide effective treatments based on the best available evidence," "make sure that your conduct justifies your patients' trust in you and the public's trust in the profession," and "be honest and trustworthy in all your communication with patients and colleagues. This means you must make clear the limits of your knowledge and make reasonable checks to make sure any information you give is accurate."

Similarly, the Code of Ethics and Professionalism developed by the Canadian Medical Association notes that the relationship between physicians and patients is "a relationship of trust that recognizes the inherent vulnerability of the patient even as the patient is an active participant in their own care. The physician owes a duty of loyalty to protect and further the patient's best interests and goals of care by using the physician's expertise, knowledge, and prudent clinical judgment."[72] It describes members of the medical profession as being committed and giving primacy to the well-being of patients, taking all reasonable steps to prevent harm to patients and disclose risks of harm, manage financial conflicts of interest, and "never exploit the patient for personal advantage."

The Medical Board of Australia's code of conduct for physicians describes the role of physicians as including giving primacy to the care of their patients, not taking advantage of patients, being truthful, and promoting and protecting the health of patients.[73] It describes several ways that physicians involved in direct-to-consumer marketing of unproven stem cell interventions could adhere to the code, including providing factual advertising, not using testimonials, and not "exploiting patients' vulnerability or fears about their future health, or raising unrealistic expectations";[74] managing and disclosing financial interests that can be perceived to conflict with patients' interests;[75] and "not exploiting patients' vulnerability or lack of medical knowledge when providing or recommending treatment or service."[76]

Outside of national codes, the European Council of Medical Orders presents a similar understanding of the basic responsibilities of physicians in its *Principles of European Medical Ethics*.[77] They include a requirement to favor the needs of one's patients: "In the practice of his or her profession, the doctor commits to giving priority to the patient's healthcare interests. The doctor must only use his or her professional knowledge to improve or maintain the health of those who entrust themselves to his or her care, at their request; the doctor may not, in any case, act to their detriment."[78] These principles distinguish the practice of medicine from that of business and notes that while doctors may make their qualifications known, this "information must be clearly distinguishable from any advertising or any information likely to mislead patients."[79] Other relevant protections for patients include not claiming medical competencies that one lacks.[80] The World Medical Association's *International Code of Medical Ethics* similarly requires that physicians "act in the patient's best interest when providing medical care."[81] It also includes prohibitions around conflicts of interest between the physician and patient ("a physician shall not allow his/her judgment to be influenced by personal profit") and requirements of transparency and honesty ("deal honestly with patients").

Munsie and Hyun also describe professional standards for care that help to establish international norms for the responsibilities of physicians to their patients.[82] They cite the *Physician Charter*, drafted by US- and EU-based groups and published widely.[83] This charter specifies that it is the responsibility of physicians to place their patients' interests above their own interests, including interests in financial benefit. Moreover, physicians are called on to work as a community to ensure practitioner competence and promote patient safety, support the generation of scientific knowledge, and manage financial conflicts of interest. They suggest that the sale of unproven stem cell interventions would violate these responsibilities when they offer and profit from interventions that are not proven to be safe and effective. As they put it, normal market standards of *caveat emptor* are not appropriate to the physician–patient relationship, as it is "a fiduciary bond whereby the doctor has a moral duty to look after the best interests of the patient. This fiduciary relationship, which characterizes all physician–patient relationships, is derived from the power differential that exists between the expert and the non-expert and the non-expert's vulnerability caused by illness and his or her necessary trust in the doctor."[84] That is, the relationship between physician and patient is a relationship of vulnerability and trust that is not present in other market exchanges. The fact that unproven stem cell interventions are sold in the market does not eliminate the partial entrustment generated through this relationship.

Finally, the ISSCR specifically condemns the sale of unproven stem cell interventions directly to consumers as a violation of the "professional ethics" of scientists and clinicians.[85] Their specific concerns are that the efficacy and safety of most of the interventions for the conditions for which these interventions are marketed have not been established. Thus, as with other professional guidelines, the ISSCR is concerned with protecting the interests of patients with whose health clinicians are entrusted. But beyond this, the ISSCR guideline notes that direct-to-consumer sales of unproven stem cell products can undermine scientific progress and the legitimacy of the field. Specifically, these sales "may jeopardize the reputation of the field and cause confusion about the actual state of scientific and clinical development." The perceived mechanism of the threat to the stem cell research community is left vague in this document, but the suggestion is that reputational loss could undermine legitimacy, public support, and public funding of this field. Owing to these patient and reputational risks, the ISSCR recommends that government authorities and professional organizations establish regulations governing the commercialization of unproven stem cell interventions.

What these documents show is a widespread consensus that the relationship between physicians and patients is one of vulnerability, the granting of intimacy and bodily access, and partial entrustment. Patients place their health and safety under the care of their physicians, and this relationship creates obligations on the part of physicians. While the codes of conduct described in the preceding differ in their details and the language used, there is a consensus that physicians must give the health and safety of their patients priority over other concerns. These obligations include requirements of truth and transparency, where physicians must give their patients an accurate accounting of the state of evidence around available medical treatments. Physicians have financial interests, but these must be transparent, and conflicts between the interests of physicians and patients must be managed to protect patients from exploitation. Advertising of services may be permissible, but it must be done so accurately and not used to manipulate prospective patients for the financial interests of physicians. Taken together, these duties to patients mean that physicians arguably fail in their duties and, more specifically, exploit their patients' hope for better health when they take advantage of this hope and partial entrustment for their own financial benefit without providing patients with accurate information and care that serves their best interests.

Regulating Stem Cell Sales

On my account, the exploitation of patients' hope for better health by physicians takes place when these physicians choose to prioritize their own gains from the sale of unproven stem cell interventions rather than being constrained by their responsibilities to their patients. These responsibilities include prioritizing the health and well-being of their patients, providing accurate information about the efficacy and safety of interventions, and managing conflicts between the physician's financial interests and the interests of their patients. The concern here is not that the distribution of benefits and risks is unfair in these relationships; rather, the physician acts to take advantage of the vulnerabilities created by a patient's hope for better health and trust in the physician rather than seeing this partial entrustment as creating responsibilities to the patient.

One consequence of this view is that exploitation is likely a subset of what people object to when unproven interventions are sold directly to consumers. Concerns about fraud and failures of consent are likely at the heart of most of these objections, focusing on cases where physicians intentionally mislead their customers about the efficacy of the intervention or where these patients fail to fully understand the likely outcomes of using these interventions. Existing policies aimed at preventing fraud and informing the choices of customers should be used and potentially expanded to address these important ethical concerns.[86,87]

The exploitation of hope when selling unproven stem cell interventions will often be linked to misinformation as well. As described earlier, advertising of these interventions frequently overstates their efficacy, understates their risks, and uses patient testimonials and hype language to promote hope and drive customers to purchase these interventions. These actions are linked primarily to creating and taking advantage of false hopes. Such exploitation can take place both when physicians knowingly misstate the efficacy and safety of their products, thus engaging in deliberate fraud, and when they are "true believers" in the products' efficacy despite a lack of supporting evidence. While the full moral weight of these cases will differ based on the intentions of the physician, in both they can be said to violate their responsibilities to their patients for their own benefit, thus exploiting the (false) hope of these individuals.

Effective and focused policy responses to the exploitation of hope in this context are difficult. Many countries forbid the sale of unproven stem cell interventions on the grounds that they have not been proven safe and effective through clinical trials submitted to and approved by the relevant regulatory agency.[88] Recently, for example, Health Canada ruled that autologous stem cell products are considered drugs and cannot be sold without approval from Health Canada, something that has been given in only a very few cases.[89] Others have pointed to using regulations around truth in advertising to take action against clinics that make misleading or outright false claims about stem cell interventions online.[90] Prohibiting or restricting the sale of unproven stem cell interventions directly to consumers does come as a cost to patient choice. This loss can be offset by enhancing access to (and thus funding for) well-run clinical trials that may preserve the hope of participants for better health and produce generalizable knowledge while protecting participants from fraud and exploitative pricing. However, increased access to clinical trials is unlikely to offset the number and range of opportunities to purchase unproven interventions. Well-run clinical trials must complete many hurdles before enrolling human participants, meaning that many unproven interventions now being sold will not be able to be offered through clinical trials. And, as argued in the previous chapter, even clinical trials can exploit the hopes of participants.

Professional bodies can also sanction members they see as exploiting the hope of or otherwise acting inappropriately toward vulnerable patients.[91] In many jurisdictions, these bodies are self-regulated on the understanding that the profession, as a community, will oversee the behaviors of its members in the public's interest. These bodies can impose a range of sanctions on their members, in the medical context ranging from fines and restrictions on certain activities to removal from the professional body and prohibition against the practice of medicine. An advantage of this approach is that it would rely on highly informed individuals who have knowledge of the evidentiary basis of stem cell interventions, awareness of the roles and responsibilities of physicians, and strong self-interest in maintaining the public image and autonomy of their profession. On the other hand, sanctioning colleagues can prove difficult, and power differentials within professions can lead to uneven application of sanctions.

The most effective means of reducing the exploitation of hope for better health from unproven interventions is likely to be counseling from disinterested medical caregivers. This approach, already advocated for to reduce incidences of fraud and uninformed decision-making, can be adapted to help ensure that patients' decisions about unproven interventions take into account both the likely outcomes of these interventions and the emotional, social, and financial costs of purchasing them.[92] Help and advice from relatively disinterested and well-informed parties can balance against the self-interested sellers of unproven interventions who are willing to exploit their customers' hope for improved health.

In some cases, patients' hope for better health from unproven stem cell interventions will not be based on false hopes. As described earlier, some patients understand that the evidence supporting the efficacy of these interventions is lacking, but choose to pursue these interventions nonetheless. This choice can be well-informed and rational given the benefits and sustaining character of hope. Moreover, the evidence to support the safety and efficacy of a product does not need to be understood as a binary of proven or unproven; rather, evidence of efficacy can be stronger or weaker, existing on a continuum. As I showed in the previous chapter, clinical trials are designed to answer different research questions and provide different forms and quality of evidence to support the use of medical interventions. As such, some evidence of efficacy in an unproven intervention, even if highly unlikely, should be treated as different from a case of no evidence of safety and efficacy. For example, recent studies of autologous hematopoietic stem cell treatment for multiple sclerosis have provided early evidence that these interventions could be safe and effective.[93],[94] As such, they have raised hopes for patients with multiple sclerosis that this intervention could halt or possibly reverse the deterioration of their health. Sale of these products has greater potential to prevent concerns about exploitation if the limited evidence of safety and efficacy is clear to patients, the health and safety of these patients are prioritized, and conflicts of the physicians' interests are managed, including by avoiding the use of manipulative advertising.

In practice, again, this balance is difficult to strike. For example, Clínica Ruiz, a Mexico-based and physician-run clinic selling this intervention to patients with multiple sclerosis, features patient testimonials and claims of a 0 percent rate of serious infections.[95] Even researchers running the initial clinical trials on this intervention have been the object of criticism from ethicists due to the large fees charged to participate in these trials and the use of language that oversold the intervention's known efficacy.[96] Thus, patients hoping beyond all expectation for better health and taking a leap of hope to access these interventions can do so without being exploited, but the existing and limited evidence of efficacy does not ensure that their hope will not be exploited.

Sarah Chan notes that "when help does not seem to be available, people will look for hope, creating a potential market; as that market gap becomes filled with opportunistic providers, the balance shifts from 'management of hope' to clinics trading in hope."[97] While this may lead to exploitation, she argues that trading in hope is not intrinsically a morally problematic behavior once we recognize that patients may prefer to engage in hope rather than "do nothing." While patients in these cases may be well informed, physicians retain obligations to prioritize their health and safety and to manage the conflict between their financial gain and the good of the patient. Specifying the distinction between supporting hopeful patients while personally benefiting from this hope versus simply exploiting this hope is difficult without knowing the specific context of the situation. In principle, physicians may be able to benefit from their patients' hopes without exploiting them. In practice, the actions taken by physicians selling directly to patients, including their choices of language and imagery when advertising these services, tend to express that the trust and hope of these patients are seen primarily as an opportunity, which is not consistent with physicians' responsibilities to their patients.

Conclusion

If we return to the case of Danny Bullen, his parents' hope that stem cells would reverse or stabilize symptoms of his autism was founded on some clinical evidence. However, they also appear to rule out any contradicting evidence and can reasonably be described as holding false hopes about the likely efficacy of this intervention. Moreover, their statement that this product had led to profound improvements in their son's verbal ability mere hours after treatment runs contrary to any known properties of stem cells, even when they are found to be effective. While their desperation to improve Danny's quality of life is understandable and worthy of sympathy, there is good reason to think that it is being exploited by the physician selling them this product. The physician selling this product is a general surgeon who completed a fellowship in cardiovascular surgery. His website includes typical markers of legitimacy, notes that he is "extra qualified" for surgery, provides patient testimonials, and offers a range of surgeries—but it does not discuss stem cell interventions.[98] Given his apparent lack of expertise in stem cell interventions, lack of transparency about the interventions being offered, and large fees being charged for this service, it is difficult to see this exchange as consistent with physicians' obligations to prioritize the health of their patients and to be transparent about the evidence of safety and efficacy of treatments.

While restrictions on the sale of unproven stem cell interventions directly to consumers are arguably justified as protecting customers from exploitation, individual countries can create and enforce these prohibitions only within their own borders. As a result, the global nature of the trade in unproven stem cell interventions means that physicians and customers can travel to jurisdictions that allow these transactions. Some of the most troubling examples of clinics selling unproven stem cell interventions directly to consumers include cases of clinics offering information sessions or consulting offices in areas with stricter regulatory restrictions and then providing services in countries with looser regulations. In other cases, clinics can relocate or rename themselves in response to bad press or changes in regulations. For example, the Stem Cell Institute, now located in Panama City, Panama, was previously known as the Institute of Cellular Medicine and was based in Costa Rica before being shut down by that country's health ministry.[99] Thus, exploitation in the sale of hope for benefits from unproven medical interventions can and will continue.

Much of the responsibility to avoid exploiting the hopes of patients will fall on physicians—both those providing unproven interventions and those working with patients interested in seeking these interventions. In the latter group, physicians and other healthcare workers can manage hopes by being transparent about the state of stem cell science and quashing false hopes while preserving and managing realistic hope.[100] Those wishing to sell unproven interventions to the hopeful, however, will find it very difficult to do so without exploiting hope, particularly given the deep conflict between financial interests as a seller of these interventions and the responsibility of physicians to their patients.

7

Legislating Hope

Exploitation in "Right-to-Try" Legislation

In 2014, Matt Bellina was diagnosed with amyotrophic lateral sclerosis (ALS), a neurodegenerative disease. ALS disrupts the ability of the brain to communicate with the body's muscles, gradually leading to the loss of the ability to walk, eat, talk, and breathe. There is currently no proven treatment for ALS, and so Bellina was informed that he would eventually die from this disease.

Bellina was a thirty-year-old navy fighter pilot with three children when he was diagnosed with ALS. He expressed a desire to try drugs in the clinical testing phase to try to save his life or at least improve his life expectancy and quality of life. He sought to enroll himself in clinical trials for new treatments for ALS but was told he did not qualify, as he had had the disease for too long to be a good candidate for these trials. He expressed frustration that, as he understood it, the approval process for new treatments could take as long as fifteen years, whereas the life expectancy for people diagnosed with ALS is two to five years. As a result, Bellina stated, "I have no hope of seeing a cure in my lifetime." Thus, he became an advocate for reforms to the regulatory system for new drugs so that terminally ill individuals could have greater access to experimental treatments outside of clinical trials. As he put it, these reforms are "my only hope, my only chance."[1]

Bellina's story is not uncommon among individuals with serious or terminal diseases who have exhausted options to participate in clinical trials. Frustrated by limitations in the clinical trial process, including the use of placebo or other control arms and restrictions on direct benefits to trial participants, some patient advocates have argued for so-called right-to-try laws that allow pharmaceutical companies to distribute experimental drugs that have not yet gained approval from regulatory agencies.[2]

These laws have raised concerns that those providing these interventions may exploit seriously ill people by providing allegedly cutting-edge, "miracle" cures for their medical conditions without evidentiary support. For example, some critics of right-to-try legislation have argued that not only might these laws slow the progress of clinical research by removing the incentive to participate in clinical trials, but permission to distribute unproven interventions and protection from legal liability would allow individuals to "exploit the dying with impunity."[3] Others argue that this legislation will do little to increase access to unproven interventions and thus would "exploit false hope."[4] In this chapter I explore these concerns, examining both the potential of individuals to take advantage of weakened regulatory protections to exploit the hopes of patients and the potential of politicians and interest groups using the rhetoric of right-to-try to exploit hopeful patients for a policy agenda.

Legislating for a Right to Try

US patients seeking access to experimental medical interventions have faced restrictions on their ability to do so as a result of the US Food and Drug Administration's (FDA's) regulatory power over medical treatments. Initially, these patients sought to overturn these restrictions through the courts. After some initial success in pushing for terminally ill patients' right to pursue experimental interventions without restriction, the US Supreme Court in 2008 declined to overturn a lower court ruling in favor of the FDA's right to regulate this access.[5]

Partially as a result of this court decision, in 2014 US states began passing right-to-try laws aimed at giving people with medical needs that could not be addressed through existing, conventional treatments access to experimental interventions that had not received regulatory approval.[6] This legislative push was motivated in part by a public perception that regulators, and especially the FDA, were too slow to approve new medical treatments. For example, the typical timeline for a new treatment to complete clinical testing and receive FDA approval is seven years for drugs in an expedited program and eight years for drugs not in one of these programs.[7] While the FDA can and does grant access to unproven interventions, it was also viewed as imposing too many restrictions on accessing experimental interventions, especially for individuals with terminal illnesses.

This perception of the FDA's reluctance to give individuals access to experimental medical interventions has a basis in truth. As dramatized by the film *Dallas Buyers Club*, advocates for individuals diagnosed with HIV/AIDS found that FDA regulations and actions often prevented them from accessing experimental interventions for their disease. In large part as a response to this pressure, the FDA implemented a series of policies beginning in the 1980s that were designed to increase the availability of unapproved, experimental interventions.[8] These policies have set up a process that is often referred to as "expanded access" to or "compassionate use" of experimental interventions. While these policies have changed over time, the current practice is generally to allow compassionate use of unapproved interventions when (a) patients have a terminal or serious medical condition, (b) they have no access to comparable treatment, (c) they are able to give informed consent to receive the intervention, (d) they have approval from an institutional review board, and (d) access will not interfere with development of and the approval process for the intervention. In addition to these requirements, the manufacturer must be willing to provide access to the intervention, which they may be unwilling to do if they are concerned that offering this access will complicate their ability to eventually receive regulatory approval for the intervention. This process was streamlined in response to concerns that applications for compassionate use were too cumbersome and took too long to complete, resulting in an application process that the FDA states takes forty-five minutes and can include the assistance of a patient "concierge."[9] Nonetheless, significant barriers to the compassionate use of experimental interventions continue to exist, including lack of awareness of this pathway to accessing interventions and the necessity of working with a physician to identify potential interventions.[10]

While state right-to-try laws were aimed at improving access to experimental medical interventions, they were unlikely to achieve this aim, because, first, they did not clearly build on the regulatory changes that the FDA had already implemented to improve compassionate access. In particular, these laws did not compel insurance companies to pay for these interventions, so they remained financially out of reach for many individuals. Further, these laws do not compel manufacturers to make their drugs available to interested patients. Thus, it is not clear that these laws would be able to increase the availability of experimental drugs on a compassionate basis. Most importantly, these state laws did not change federal law regarding the regulation of experimental medical interventions. Under the US Constitution's supremacy clause, federal laws overrule conflicting state laws, meaning that these state right-to-try laws could not compel regulatory changes by the FDA without changes to federal laws.[11] While several patients in Texas were able to gain access to unproven interventions through that state's right-to-try law, no other successful applications of state legislation have been reported.[12,13] For these reasons, a common criticism of state right-to-try laws is that they do not accomplish anything "other than the creation of false hope."[14]

By 2017, thirty-eight US states had passed right-to-try laws.[15] Partly because state right-to-try laws could not trump federal law, energy then shifted to passing a federal version of these laws. As with the push to pass state right-to-try laws, this effort was driven primarily by advocacy from the libertarian Goldwater Institute. On May 30, 2018, the federal version of the right-to-try act was signed into law by President Donald Trump. The federal version of this law is similar in many respects to the state versions, with the crucial difference that it supersedes existing federal requirements for FDA approval before accessing unproven interventions. In addition to limiting FDA oversight of compassionate access to these drugs, the federal right-to-try act does not require approval by institutional review boards. Under the federal version of this law, patients must be diagnosed with a life-threatening condition and not be eligible to participate in a clinical trial involving the intervention they seek. This requirement was designed to address concerns that the right-to-try law would undermine clinical trials and progress in establishing the safety and efficacy of new treatments.[16] After an intervention has completed a phase I clinical trial, companies are allowed to give access to these interventions to consenting patients. In exchange, these companies are given liability protection from harms these patients may experience as a result. However, insurance companies are not required to pay for these interventions, and manufacturers can only recover the direct costs associated with giving access to the intervention. Manufacturers who do grant access to their unproven interventions through the federal right-to-try law must send the FDA an annual report outlining how many patients received how many doses of the intervention and whether any adverse events were experienced as a result.

Right-to-Try and the Rhetoric of Hope and Freedom

The Goldwater Institute drafted the model legislation that was largely adopted in both state and federal right-to-try laws, and it heavily used the language of hope and freedom. While the Goldwater Institute has an ideological emphasis on personal freedom and government deregulation, it also relied on the language of hope to promote passage of this legislation. For example, its report *Dead on Arrival* makes the case for why federal right-to-try legislation is needed and appears on the institute's right-to-try website under the heading "Why We Needed Right to Try."[17] This report does not use the words "liberty" or "freedom," instead relying on the language of hope to make its case. It presents the image of Americans who have received a terminal diagnosis, for whom unproven interventions "may be a faint hope, or even a false one. But it is their only hope."[18] The report includes several stories of terminally ill individuals who, it says, are stymied by the FDA in seeking access to experimental drugs outside of clinical trials. For these individuals, such access is their only hope to prevent death or at least slow down their disease's progress. For example, the report describes Mike DeBartoli, a former firefighter residing in California and diagnosed with ALS. DeBartoli makes the case for right-to-try, saying "I have no hope now. I will take false hope. . . . To live the rest of my life knowing that I'm not even given a shot. What is that? I don't know who the FDA thinks they are protecting. Who are they to tell me what I should be hopeful for or not hopeful for? You're telling me you won't approve me to take a possible medication that doesn't hurt me, that will possibly save my life, because you want to have your fingers in it? I just don't understand it."[19] Here and elsewhere in the report, "false hope" is used to describe experimental interventions that do not turn out to cure these individuals, not the concern that right-to-try legislation will not end up giving access to these interventions. While DeBartoli was turned down from participating in several clinical trials for ALS interventions, the report does not disclose that he did participate in at least one such trial.[20] DeBartoli died from ALS on November 1, 2017, before the federal right-to-try law was passed.

For many of those advocating for these laws, the value of hope is coupled with the freedom to choose how to pursue better health. Wisconsin Senator Ron Johnson, who introduced the federal right-to-try legislation in the US Senate, spoke of this relationship, stating that "what we can and must do is give patients and families the freedom to decide for themselves how to fight their illness. With no other options, they at least have the right to hope."[21] In addition to the Goldwater Institute, a series of other libertarian-leaning groups, including Freedom Partners, Americans for Prosperity, and the LIBRE Initiative expressed support for the federal right-to-try law. As with the Goldwater Institute, these groups used the language of hope to make their case. In a letter urging the leadership of a House committee to approve the bill, they wrote that the committee could "give hope to these families and patients who are facing the most dire circumstances" and deliver "real hope to millions of Americans who are desperately looking for potentially life-saving treatment."[22]

Whereas opponents of right-to-try laws have argued that hopes raised by these laws will be baseless, this criticism may not be concerning to the libertarian and pro-deregulation groups that advocated for these laws. Instead, the freedom and personal liberty language used to support these laws may betray the primary interests of many of their proponents. For example, when introducing the model legislation on which state and federal right-to-try laws were based, the Goldwater Institute justified the need for this legislation claiming, "Patients should be free to exercise a basic freedom—attempting to preserve one's own life. The burdens imposed on a terminal patient who fights to save his or her own life are a violation of personal liberty."[23] The enemy of personal liberty, in this story, is the FDA, which "burdens the rights of terminal patients by claiming the authority to override both the will of the patient and the recommendation of a doctor by bureaucratic veto."[24] In addition to the liberty-dampening effects of the FDA's regulatory powers, the Goldwater Institute specifically objected to the FDA's policy of designing compassionate use to ensure that clinical trials are not disrupted or undermined when individuals seek access to unproven interventions. They charge that this policy indicates that the "FDA puts protection of the clinical-trial process above the lives of terminally ill patients" and that "Right to Try allows a patient to access investigational medications that have passed basic safety tests without interference by the government."[25]

On this view, the FDA is the enemy of personal liberty. It creates unjustified barriers to exercising personal liberty, and it promotes social goods such as determining the efficacy of new medical interventions through clinical trials over the right of individuals to live their lives as they see fit. This focus on individual freedom and, by extension, disempowering the FDA, was explicit in the statements of some of the law's supporters as well. For example, the aforementioned Senator Ron Johnson, in addition to evoking a "right to hope," criticized statements from the FDA commissioner that the right-to-try law would require additional regulation and interpretation. As Johnson put it, "This law intends to diminish the FDA's power over people's lives, not increase it."[26]

This ideological debate takes place between the libertarian views of the Goldwater Institute and its defenders and the FDA and others who favor expert oversight and government intervention to promote the health of the public.[27] This is a long-standing debate in public policy and political theory, and reasonable people can disagree about the right answers to these questions and how to balance these potentially competing interests. However, if this legislation does not genuinely improve individuals' access to unproven medical interventions and give them legitimate reasons to hope for better health, then it serves only the political aim of elevating personal liberty over social goals like advancing medical research. That is, if state and federal right-to-try laws will do little to improve access to experimental interventions, then the hopes engendered by this legislation are false hopes, and the rhetoric of freedom as promoting hope for better health is deceptive. If so, this legislation serves the goal of personal liberty and freedom as ideological ends in themselves.

The Right to Ask: False Hopes and
Real Harms

How, then, will this legislation impact access to experimental interventions? While the rhetoric of hope was heavily used in promoting both state and federal right-to-try laws, there are limitations within these laws that have led critics to charge that any hopes linked to them are false hopes. Defenders of right-to-try legislation can argue that, since patients must receive a terminal diagnosis before accessing experimental interventions, there is no harm in granting these individuals the freedom to at least try to improve their health even if in nearly all cases this hope will not be realized.

However, there are several significant costs associated with accessing experimental interventions, even for terminally ill patients. First, as noted in Chapter 5, patients seeking enrollment in clinical trials may forgo palliative care when doing so. As such, pursuing experimental interventions can come at the cost of accessing palliative care that would improve their quality of life. For example, children diagnosed with cancer already face barriers to timely access to palliative care, and these delays could be worsened by being presented with additional options for possibly curative care that are unlikely in practice to provide any benefits.[28] Second, because the federal right-to-try legislation does not require insurance coverage of these experimental interventions, those pursuing these interventions will need to pay for them out of pocket. These costs are potentially devastating. For example, one researcher who was willing to provide an experimental ALS intervention under the Colorado right-to-try law estimated that it would cost patients $100,000 to undergo this intervention.[29] In addition to payments for the interventions themselves, costs of accessing the intervention can include travel and relocation expenses.[30] The need to pay for these interventions out of pocket also raises questions of fairness: rather than granting access to patients who are the sickest or most likely to benefit from accessing experimental interventions outside of a clinical trial, this system would distribute access based on the ability to afford the intervention, either out of one's own savings or by borrowing from friends and family.[31] Third, accessing experimental interventions is not without health risks, even for terminally ill patients. In some cases, experimental interventions can further shorten patients' lives or subject them to pain and a loss of quality of life that could have been prevented by not partaking in the experimental intervention.[32]

Finally, raising hopes when these hopes will not be realized can be psychologically damaging. Accessing experimental interventions will generally have at least the potential to improve the patient's health if that intervention is in a state of equipoise, where its benefits compared with current therapies are uncertain. However, if right-to-try laws have no potential in practice to increase access to experimental therapies, they risk raising hopes in an already vulnerable and desperate population of terminally ill patients who will then invest their limited time and resources into pursuing experimental interventions that will never be made available to them. This raises the question of whether the hopes raised by right-to-try legislation are well founded or false.

A primary aim of the federal right-to-try legislation is to overcome alleged slowness and unnecessary bureaucracy found in the FDA's compassionate use process. However, in 2016 the FDA processed over 1,000 applications (each of which often includes multiple individuals) for compassionate use of unproven interventions and approved over 99% of them, typically within hours to days.[33] While defenders of the federal right-to-try legislation argue that this timeline could be shortened even more, the FDA is privy to proprietary safety and efficacy data for similar drugs that would not be accessible by individual physicians.[34] Thus, it is not clear that the federal right-to-try legislation would speed access to unproven interventions, and there is reason to think that excluding the FDA from the approval process would come at the cost of access to safety and efficacy data that could be used to protect patients.

Not only is it doubtful that the existing compassionate access program is unnecessarily burdensome to those wishing to access unproven interventions, but there are also significant questions as to whether many drug manufacturers will be willing to use the pathway provided by right-to-try legislation to supply their unproven interventions to patients. While the legislation does give pharmaceutical manufacturers liability protection from any harms caused by their interventions, Joffe and Fernandez Lynch note that threats of litigation have not been a serious impediment to providing access to these interventions in the past.[35] However, adverse events could be used by the FDA to evaluate the safety and efficacy of these drugs, and thus these companies will be motivated to retain control over these products and administer them through controlled clinical trials. The federal right-to-try legislation also prohibits charging more than is necessary to recover costs for providing access to these interventions, meaning that there is no direct financial incentive to make them available. Moreover, these companies may have limited supplies of unproven interventions and prefer to administer them through clinical trials designed to pass the FDA's review process.

In general, the concern is that drug manufacturers will be much more focused on gaining regulatory approval for their unproven interventions than providing access to these interventions outside of this approval process. If providing these interventions through the right-to-try process detracts from that mission by producing evidence of harm, rerouting resources from the approval process, or potentially generating news coverage that could discourage investment in their product, then they would have a strong incentive not to provide access to these interventions.

Critics of the federal right-to-try law expressed concern that it would sabotage the public health mission of the FDA by undermining the principle that access to unproven interventions should wait until these interventions have been proven safe and effective.[36] Importantly, this charge that federal right-to-try legislation will erode the authority of the FDA to regulate new medical treatments already has some signs of being realized. For example, Jaci Hermstad was recently diagnosed with a rare and aggressive form of ALS for which there is no proven effective treatment and that will lead to her death if untreated.[37] Hermstad and her family learned of an experimental intervention for ALS soon after her diagnosis and were eager to try it. However, this intervention had not been previously administered to humans and had not been tested through a phase I clinical trial; as such, Hermstad was not eligible to receive access to this intervention under the federal right-to-try act. While the FDA did not insist on completion of a phase I clinical trial before making the treatment available under compassionate use, they did ask that toxicology testing be completed. Instead, Hermstad and her family began a campaign to be given access to this intervention that culminated in expressions of support from US legislators, including Senator Chuck Grassley and Speaker of the House Nancy Pelosi. The family's own representative introduced a one-sentence piece of legislation directing the FDA to make this intervention available to Hermstad. While this legislation was not formally considered, it resulted in the FDA indicating that they would be more open to granting compassionate access to the drug, even with abbreviated toxicology testing. As Hermstad's physician described it, the political pressure had the effect of putting Congress's foot "on the neck of the FDA."[38]

While this case took place outside of the bounds of the federal right-to-try legislation, the worry is that it opens the process of eroding the FDA's oversight function and makes it more difficult—legally and politically—for the FDA to decline or place restrictions on requests to access experimental interventions. As Florko describes it, "What right to try has done, and what one-patient bills like this will do, is put us back into a position where we have to justify FDA's existence to society. For this patient it seems like an individual decision, but it has long term impact on whether we allow FDA to do its function."[39] This was essentially the view of Hermstad's mother as well, though one that she saw in a much more positive light: "There should be absolutely nothing, no bureaucracy, nothing, to stop the FDA from allowing somebody who is going to die anyway to not try a drug. Period."[40] Thus, the concern that right-to-try creates a slippery slope toward erosion of the FDA's ability to regulate access to experimental interventions is being realized in practice. Taken together, these criticisms of the likely outcomes of and intentions for the right-to-try legislation led one advocacy group to describe it as "false hope legislation" that should be renamed the "False Hope Act of 2017."[41]

Exploiting False Hopes for a Right to Try

There are several reasons to think that patients' hopes associated with right-to-try laws will be based on a misunderstanding and are false hopes. First, the rhetoric around right-to-try laws may encourage misunderstanding about the efficacy and safety of specific experimental interventions and the nature of scientific research more generally. The efficacy of drugs accessed via right-to-try will not have been established, as they will only have been required to have completed phase I safety testing. Thus, the rhetoric around these drugs as potentially life-saving treatments may increase the likelihood of misunderstanding the nature of phase I clinical trials as offering therapy rather than establishing safety.[42]

Second, the rhetoric about right-to-try laws as expanding access to experimental interventions is likely to lead to a false understanding of their actual impacts. Specifically, the very name "right-to-try" is misleading. As discussed previously, these laws empower patients to request access to experimental therapies but do not require researchers or their sponsors to provide them or insurance companies to pay for them. As a result, the entitlement to experimental therapies implied by the notion of a right to try misleads those who are in fact only being given a right to ask for access to these drugs—a right, moreover, that these patients have even in the absence of the federal right-to-try law.[43] Some have worried that this language is intentionally misleading and will inevitably lead to false hopes. As Folkers, Chapman, and Redman put it, "We believe that some patients will misinterpret their 'right to try' to mean that a stakeholder—a drug company, a physician, or the FDA—is under a legal obligation to provide an experimental product as treatment. This misunderstanding may turn patients' and families' hope into disappointment."[44]

When President Trump signed the federal right-to-try legislation, he stated, "We will be saving—I don't even want to say thousands because I think it's going to be much more—thousands and thousands, hundreds of thousands, we're going to be saving tremendous numbers of lives. . . . There were no options, and now you have hope." As I have discussed, the statement that the law was needed because "there were no options" is false. Moreover, this legislation has not led to saving thousands, much less hundreds of thousands, of lives.[45] A year after the federal right-to-try act was passed, charges that this law would not lead to increased access to unproven interventions has largely been proven. Shortly after the law passed, a few companies did announce their intention to pursue the right-to-try pathway to make their interventions available. In a September 2018 press release, the CEO of Therapeutic Solutions International announced that their new stem cell immunotherapy intervention for cancer had completed phase I testing and that they would be "providing patients access to it *now* under the Right to Try Law."[46] This statement read more like an attempt to gain publicity for its product than an actual plan to provide access to the intervention, however, as it came immediately after completing phase I testing and referenced "President Trump's recently passed Right to Try Law." Another company developing a stem cell treatment for cancer-related wasting quoted from President Trump's statement after he signed the federal right-to-try law, and it raised the possibility of providing this unproven intervention under that pathway but, crucially, had not yet completed phase I testing of the intervention.[47]

Despite these public statements of interest by some medical companies, a year after the law passed only seven people were publicly known to have accessed interventions via the right-to-try pathway.[48,49] Moreover, it seems that at least one of these people could have accessed unproven interventions via existing FDA pathways.[50] Another case of an individual using right-to-try—a story enthusiastically tweeted out by President Trump—appears to have been off-label use of an FDA-approved drug, not access via right-to-try.[51] Defenders of the law suggest that people will use right-to-try in the near future, however.[52]

There is good reason to think that legislators' willingness to pass both state and federal right-to-try laws is based on wanting to offer some kind of a response to public pressure to provide faster access to effective medical treatments. Such moves will be purely symbolic, come at no cost to the politician, and have no real effect but may garner public support. As Zettler and Greely describe state right-to-try legislation, "Lawmakers have little to lose politically by supporting these laws. Companies, seeing their ineffectiveness, have no powerful reasons to oppose them. And libertarians can celebrate an attack on big government."[53] Thus, public officeholders and interest groups have engaged in different forms of misrepresentation in the right-to-try debate, ranging from intentional lying to serve ideological ends to disinterested willingness to allow this misrepresentation to take place to avoid the perceived political costs of standing up to these misrepresentations.

Much of the rhetoric used to promote both state and federal right-to-try legislation misled the public about the true aims of this legislation. As I've shown, much of the promise about the outcomes of this legislation for ill patients intentionally or unintentionally misrepresents the true likely outcomes and reasons for barriers to accessing unproven interventions. A cynic might note that politicians and policymakers have always lied and misrepresented the truth, so it should hardly be shocking that they also misrepresented the truth in the debate over right-to-try legislation. The norms of public debate could be said to include an assumption of misrepresentation, where the rhetoric and promises of politicians, policymakers, and interest groups are assumed to be misleading at best.

While there is some truth to the cynical position, there is good reason to think that in the case of the federal right-to-try debate these politicians and policy advocates went beyond the range of expected misrepresentation and instead failed in their obligations to the public; as a result, the hopes of desperately ill patients were exploited for political ends. First, public officeholders take on a public trust that includes an obligation to serve the public's interests—the kind of partial entrustment with the welfare of others that creates an opportunity for exploitation that was discussed in Chapter 4. This entrustment can be seen as a form of fiduciary duty or duty of loyalty to those they represent, such that they are entrusted to pursue the best interests of the public and not their own benefit.[54] Insofar as support for right-to-try legislation was a cheap political win for politicians built on unfulfilled hopes that this legislation would meaningfully improve access to effective experimental interventions, then this duty to the public was violated. When politicians and other government representatives engage in large-scale self-interested lying, they violate the loyalty owed to the public by virtue of their role as agents entrusted with the public's interests.[55]

To some extent, lying and misrepresentation are expected and can even serve the public interest, especially in times of emergency and external threat. For example, lying to prevent a public panic during a disease outbreak or to preserve morale in times of war can serve the public good.[56,57] However, the public interest does not seem to be served in the right-to-try debate. While there are genuine reasons for concern about the role of the FDA in providing access to unproven interventions and legitimate debates over the clash between personal control over one's health and the role of government in protecting the public's health, changes to the regulatory system were not a public health emergency and did not require misrepresentation to overcome impediments to public deliberation. This debate could have taken place on the grounds of personal liberty, but transforming it into a question of saving the lives of hundreds, thousands, or tens of thousands of people creates a false basis for this debate. Rather than upholding the trust placed in them by being elected or appointed to public office and as specified by their public roles and obligations, these individuals contributed to creating false and dashed hopes, rewarded those misrepresenting the true aims and outcomes of this legislation, and contributed to increased cynicism and distrust that undermines the public good of democracy.

Moreover, the strongest advocates for right-to-try legislation—namely, the ill patients and their families who hoped to benefit from this legislation—were not acting based on the understanding that public officeholders misrepresented their promise. Rather, those most invested in this debate and most likely to be harmed by misrepresentation about its aims and outcomes hoped deeply that under a right-to-try pathway they, their loved ones, and others in their communities of desperately ill patients would gain access to new treatments that could save their lives and that would not otherwise be available. This was clearly the understanding of the parents of Jordan McLinn, a child with Duchenne muscular dystrophy who appeared on stage with President Trump during the right-to-try signing ceremony. As they describe it in a YouTube video shortly after the federal law was signed, "that's what right-to-try does—it just gives that extra layer of hope for patients that have exhausted every other pathway and every other option that exists."[58] In this way, the public's trust in the words of public officeholders—and specifically the trust of the ill individuals that this law promised to help—was violated. Rather, these advocates, knowingly and unknowingly, exploited the false hopes of desperately ill patients to achieve other political ends.

Exploiting Informed Hope

Most concern with the exploitation of hope in connection to right-to-try laws is rightfully linked to the exploitation of false hope by lawmakers and policy groups. However, there is also good reason for concern that these laws could be used to exploit hopes that unproven interventions may improve the patients' health or at least provide them with the benefits of emotional engagement with a possible future in which their health is improved. This form of exploiting hope largely reflects and expands on the issues discussed in the previous chapter around stem cell clinics selling unproven interventions directly to consumers. In fact, some of these clinics have adopted the rhetoric of right-to-try even without using the new federal right-to-try pathway. For example, the Texas-based stem cell clinic Ambrose Cell Therapy prominently discusses the right-to-try law on its website marketing its interventions directly to consumers. While making no claims to be using the federal right-to-try pathway, they promote a fundamental right of individuals to access experimental interventions without government interference that, they claim, is endorsed by this "enlightened and extraordinary humanitarian" legislation: " 'Right to Try' is a relatively new way to express our fundamental human 'right to life' and the 'right to health.' "[59]

Kasper Raus discusses this concern in compassionate use programs more generally, worrying that "there seems to be a risk that seriously ill patients could be used for financial gain or as cheap and easy research subjects."[60] Regarding the first avenue for exploitation highlighted by Raus, he worries that if manufacturers can charge for access to their unproven drugs through right-to-try or another compassionate use pathway, then they will essentially be able to gain from these products without being able to offer any real assurance of benefit to hopeful patients who are purchasing these unproven interventions. Raus is not clear about how he uses the concept of exploitation or what he takes to be morally problematic about it. However, it seems likely that the concern motivating this use of exploitation is that it would be unfair to allow those researching new treatments to sell unproven interventions when the benefit for patients is unknown or unlikely. As discussed in detail in the previous chapter, this understanding of exploiting hope is problematic because it may undervalue the benefits of hope and miss features in the relationship between those selling unproven interventions and seriously ill patients. Nonetheless, he is correct that the sale of unproven interventions does raise concerns around exploitation.

Regardless of how Raus does or should understand exploitation in this context, this specific concern is not clearly relevant to the federal right-to-try legislation. Recall that in the federal legislation, manufacturers choosing to make their products available to patients through the right-to-try pathway are limited to recovering "direct costs" of the intervention, which are understood as the costs of manufacturing the drug in the quantities needed for that patient and some of the administrative costs of making the drug available.[61] As a result, not only does the right-to-try pathway (along with other compassionate use pathways) not allow for manufacturers to profit from making these drugs available through these means, but they could lose money by doing so through the indirect costs of administering these drugs. As Fernandez Lynch, Zettler, and Sarpatwari note, this requirement speaks directly to the likelihood of exploitation—of hope or otherwise—taking place through right-to-try: "rigorously monitoring and enforcing the statutory requirement that manufacturers may charge only for the direct costs of their drugs under Right to Try also may help to deter those who would seek to exploit vulnerable patients."[62]

The example of BrainStorm Cell Therapeutics, one of the few companies that had publicly announced plans to make its products available through the right-to-try pathway, demonstrates how this requirement works in practice. Shortly after passage of the federal right-to-try legislation, BrainStorm announced that it would be making its unproven stem cell intervention for ALS available through this pathway. Because this intervention requires harvesting stem cells from the bone marrow of each patient and requires highly personalized care, cost for this intervention was estimated at over $300,000. While it was not clear that this amount would go over the allowed direct costs of providing this product through right-to-try, it was reported that the CEO of BrainStorm presented this plan as "a semicommercial enterprise with modest profits that wouldn't exploit patients' desperation." He defended the cost of the intervention by saying, "Companies cannot be NGOs [non-governmental organizations]. We have to have an incentive."[63]

Despite this claim that BrainStorm would not exploit desperate patients, the eye-popping $300,000 price tag for the intervention and reference to "modest profits" led to confusion about how this would be allowable under right-to-try's restriction on indirect costs. Critics linked this plan to exploitation, again based on the seeming unfairness of charging large sums of money—including some profit—for an intervention with no proof of efficacy: "the very fact that his company will be selling an unproven treatment to patients with a terminal illness based on a marginally promising phase 2 trial indicates that the company will be exploiting desperate patients. . . . So what we're talking about here is the possibility that terminally ill patients with ALS could be paying the cost of a house for a treatment that hasn't even been shown to be effective in anything resembling a convincing manner yet."[64] This sentiment was shared in a variety of articles condemning BrainStorm's proposal. Likely in response to this backlash, BrainStorm soon announced that it would not be pursuing the plan to make its product available through right-to-try, citing its inability to find a way to subsidize the cost of its product for those unable to afford it.[65] Instead, it has allowed US patients to travel to Israel to purchase this intervention for the originally advertised $300,000 fee.[66]

In the case of BrainStorm, limits to its ability to make money from right-to-try and public objections to its seeking to do so proved a barrier to using this legislation. Nonetheless, some worry that the right-to-try pathway could be used by unscrupulous physicians, researchers, or other medical providers to bypass FDA regulation and sell their products directly to consumers. Bateman-House and colleagues, for example, note that when state right-to-try laws rely on physicians to declare that an individual is terminally ill and could benefit from an experimental therapy, this can create a conflict of interest for physicians, especially if they are involved in the development of the experimental therapy. As they note, right-to-try laws rely on physicians "being intelligent, virtuous, and devoted to their patients' well-being to the extent that they will not be guided by considerations of personal gain, publicity, or curiosity." But when oversight by other bodies such as the FDA is weakened, these laws open the door "for the unscrupulous or inept to prey on desperately ill patients and their families."[67] In cases where these physicians and others press their own interests over those of their patients, they may engage in the exploitation of hope similar to that discussed in the previous chapter around direct-to-consumer sales of unproven stem cell interventions. As a result, right-to-try legislation will "strip patients of crucial protections from exploitation, quackery, and malfeasance."[68]

There are several hypothetical ways in which such exploitation could take place through the right-to-try pathway. The federal right-to-try law only allows access to interventions that have gone through phase I clinical trials and where the patient is not eligible to enter a clinical trial. These requirements are meant to ensure that basic safety and dosing testing has been completed for the intervention and that pursuing it through the right-to-try pathway will not disrupt the conduct of clinical trials meant to test the efficacy and safety of the intervention. However, they also create an opportunity for an exploitative actor, after completing phase I testing for an intervention, to design the eligibility criteria for phase II testing so restrictively as to create a large population of individuals who could access the intervention via right-to-try.[69] In this scenario, the researcher may not even intend to complete phase II testing, aiming instead to use the right-to-try pathway to distribute an unproven intervention without FDA oversight.

In other cases, researchers might use right-to-try to recruit and pay for continued clinical study of their interventions. While ethicists have noted that the reporting requirements of the federal right-to-try legislation are limited, Raus suggests that researchers could treat patients accessing interventions through this pathway as research participants and package their participation as providing clinical trial data. Raus's worry is that patient safety and reporting requirements are weaker in compassionate use programs than in typical clinical trials, leading to the same benefits to researchers with greater risks for what are effectively research participants. Moreover, clinical trial participants typically do not pay to take part in these studies and may be compensated for participation. However, patients accessing unproven interventions through right-to-try can be charged for the direct costs of doing so and effectively pay for at least part of the costs of the study. For Raus, this possibility raises concerns around transactional fairness–based exploitation, as right-to-try and other compassionate use programs could increase the safety risks and financial costs of trial participation while providing as many or more benefits to researchers and their employers: "If one indeed justifies compassionate use programs [by] reference to the principle of beneficence, they should be designed to provide maximum benefit and minimal risks. If pharmaceutical companies are allowed to charge patients money or use them as research participants for the company's benefit, there is significant risk of exploitation."[70]

Again, as I argued in Chapter 5, this concern around researchers exploiting the hopes of clinical trial participants is better understood in terms of exploitation as a specified responsibility of researchers rather than an issue of fairness. While Raus is correct that right-to-try and other pathways to accessing unproven medical interventions may further shift the balance of benefits and risks in the favor of researchers and away from participants, it is not clear that this shift makes these transactions unfair, all things considered. As I've noted, fully informed hope has a value in and of itself, and the small chance of improving one's health or curing a terminal disease is of incredible value to desperate and seriously ill individuals. Rather, the issue here is that right-to-try may allow researchers to use the hopes of patients to avoid protections in patients' interest and to fund research, which, in some cases, would constitute a failure of these researchers to act in the best interests of the research participants and to manage their own conflicts of interest. As noted in the previous chapter, these issues are especially concerning when these researchers are also the research participants' physicians.

Preserving Hope without Exploitation

Right-to-try legislation is directed toward individuals with weighty hopes for better health and longer lives who are willing to take leaps of hope seeking unproven medical interventions. In doing so, they give researchers and their sponsors considerable access to and control over their bodies and place trust in the words of politicians and policymakers enacting these laws. Right-to-try laws exploit hope in two ways. First, they exploit false hope by misleading desperately ill patients to believe that this legislation will significantly increase their access to unproven interventions and save many lives. This is a false hope both because the legislation has not been effective in increasing access to experimental interventions and because there is little reason to think that accessing unproven interventions will save many lives. These claims are not substantiated but are used to promote an agenda of personal freedom and governmental deregulation. Whatever the value of that agenda, it is distinct from that of giving hope for better health that is used, in part, to promote it. Second, the right-to-try pathway may be used to promote or sell unproven interventions directly to consumers. As discussed previously, claims around the efficacy of these interventions are often misleading, creating false hopes. Even when they are not misleading, these unproven and potentially risky interventions exploit the hopes of patients when they are sold despite physicians' and researchers' entrustment with patients' and participants' interests.

The most straightforward way to address these concerns with exploitation would be to repeal the right-to-try laws that make them possible. However, doing so is likely not currently politically viable in the US, especially given the effectiveness of the rhetoric of hope used to promote its passage in the first place. Repealing these laws might have the added effect of shifting blame for limited access to unproven interventions on regulators rather than the ineffectiveness of right-to-try legislation. Moreover, desperately ill patients can reasonably hope for greater access to unproven interventions, through either clinical trials or other means, than was available before the federal right-to-try law was passed in the US. One positive impact of the debate over and passage of this law is arguably that it has increased pressure on the FDA to continue streamlining its compassionate use pathway while seeking to protect the public's interests.

One of the primary reasons that the federal right-to-try law and other compassionate use programs have limited efficacy is that pharmaceutical developers are not required to make their unproven interventions available outside of clinical trials. Even when these interventions are made available, these companies may charge for direct costs of providing these potentially very expensive products, and insurance companies are not required to pay for them. New legislation could address both of these limitations, vastly increasing access to unproven interventions. However, there is good reason to think that doing so would be hugely problematic, as it would decrease willingness to engage in clinical trials needed to prove safety and efficacy of new treatments, expose patients to risky and often ineffective interventions, undermine insurers' fiduciary responsibility to spend members' contributions effectively, and provide unscrupulous suppliers with a massive new revenue stream that would incentivize the exploitation of hopeful patients.

Instead, several steps could support seriously ill patients in their hopes for better health while protecting them from exploitation. First, many of these patients want to enter legitimate clinical trials but are unable to. They may be restricted from participating for a range of reasons, including past participation in clinical trials that might obscure the results of new trials, other health complications, or even insufficiently advanced disease. In other cases, however, trial participation is limited because trials are underfunded and cannot enroll sufficient numbers of participants, the trial is geographically distant and participants cannot afford to travel to the trial or take time away from work, or the research that would lead to new clinical trials and, potentially, treatments is not funded. Increased funding for research and clinical trial participation and use of "virtual" trials not requiring relocation would address some of these concerns, increasing options for hopeful patients.[71] While keeping in mind that clinical trial participation might still lead to patients' hopes being exploited, these would-be participants can be protected from this exploitation if they are well informed and are given more opportunities for later-stage trial participation.

In addition, these trials can in some cases be designed to respond to the concerns of potential participants. Specifically, some ill patients have expressed reluctance to participate in clinical trials because of their use of a placebo arm.[72] Their interest in participating in these trials is based on the hope that they will receive effective treatment for their illness; if they might receive a placebo, then the chances that their hopes will not be realized is higher. Increased funding for clinical trials could be tied to promoting trial designs that increase the number and variety of people participating in these trials and, where reasonable, ensure that all participants receive the unproven intervention.[73]

The FDA can also continue addressing concerns with its compassionate access program by continuing to streamline the application and approval process to reduce the amount of time and paperwork required to use this pathway.[74] More can be done also to promote and increase familiarity with this pathway, which, ironically, may be encouraged through publicity surrounding right-to-try legislation. One perceived advantage of the right-to-try pathway is that it prohibits the FDA from using outcomes from access to these drugs through right-to-try to determine their safety and efficacy. Thus, the FDA could further clarify a policy of not using clinical outcomes from compassionate use to potentially disadvantage these companies in the approval process. Going even further, the FDA could use the greater reporting requirements of compassionate access to contribute to the approval process.[75]

Finally, while the FDA has been the target of much of the anger from patient groups seeking greater access to unproven interventions, the FDA's power to increase such access is limited. For example, a group of individuals with ALS recently launched protests against the FDA for not approving new treatments fast enough. These patients are disappointed that they have not received access to unproven interventions through right-to-try and so want to pressure the FDA for more reforms in the style of ACT UP protesters fighting the FDA for faster access to HIV/AIDS treatments in the 1980s. But as one former ACT UP member noted, members of this group were eventually able to convince the FDA to respond to their concerns and create pathways for compassionate access. But now, they argue, the FDA is not slowing access to safe and effective treatments. Thus, continued pressure on the FDA when it is not the institution blocking access to unapproved interventions may simply undermine patient protections and slow the development of new treatments: "I'd do exactly what we did in HIV, I just wouldn't make the same mistakes we made with thirty years of hindsight. As we dug deeper, our targets changed. . . . Hopefully people living with ALS can learn those lessons quickly."[76]

As noted earlier, right-to-try has been rightly criticized as being more a right-to-ask researchers and drug manufacturers for access to unproven interventions outside of clinical trials. While right-to-try legislation seeks to encourage researchers and drug manufacturers to give access to their unproven interventions by granting them liability protection and reducing reporting requirements, granting individuals access to unproven interventions is still well outside their central mission of developing effective and safe treatments. They may be reasonably wary of diverting resources from this mission and legitimately concerned with the ethical issues raised by distributing unproven interventions, including worries about exploiting the hopes of these individuals. Thus, some researchers and drug manufacturers have partnered with bioethicists, physicians, and patient groups to create compassionate use advisory committees to help navigate these issues and facilitate access to unproven interventions when this can be done so safely and ethically.[77]

Conclusion

This chapter began with the story of Matt Bellina, the navy veteran and father with ALS who sought access to unproven interventions for his disease outside of clinical trials. Bellina actively lobbied on behalf of right-to-try groups, including the Goldwater Institute, and his name appears on the version of the bill that was signed into law, along with the names of other advocates. In addition to lending his voice and name to this cause, Bellina appeared on stage with President Trump during the signing ceremony for the right-to-try law.

Two of the other people named on this legislation—including Frank Mongiello, who also has ALS—have not been able to access unproven interventions through this pathway, joining many others whose hopes for access have not been realized. As Mongiello's wife, Marilyn, put it, "We had a lot of hope that if the right to try was passed it would give an incentive for the drug companies to make available the drugs. But now it doesn't seem as though the drug companies are giving away their drugs either." However, Matt Bellina is one of the few individuals who have received access to an intervention through right-to-try. Specifically, Bellina has been given access to BrainStorm Cell Therapeutics's unproven ALS intervention—the only person given this opportunity after BrainStorm reversed its decision to make its product more widely available through the right-to-try pathway. Bellina has expressed regret that others have not received this intervention and reports improved health that he attributes to it.[78]

It does not appear that Bellina's hope was exploited. While the hopes of the vast majority of people supporting the right-to-try pathway have thus far been false hopes, reporting suggests that Bellina received access to an unproven intervention that he would not have received otherwise. This access was likely due in large part to his prominence as a right-to-try advocate, and others may not be able to replicate his experience. Moreover, while Bellina advocated for the right-to-try legislation in terms of his hope for better health, the language of personal freedom was prominent in his own advocacy, suggesting that he supported the ideological aim of legislators pushing for this bill and was willing to serve this aim.[79] This is a happy result for Bellina, and we can hope with him that his health improves because of this intervention.

However, outside of a few isolated cases, thus far the federal right-to-try law is a story of exploiting false hope for better health, given that it has not significantly increased access to unproven treatments for terminally ill patients. Instead, it was a means of using the hopes of terminally ill patients for better health to push forward an agenda of deregulating federal oversight of drug approvals. Where individuals have accessed unproven interventions and invoked the right to try, there is the further danger of providers using the rhetoric of hope to profit from selling unproven interventions without proof of safety or efficacy.

8

Networks of Hope

Exploitation in Crowdfunding Campaigns

While pregnant, Gemma Nuttall was diagnosed with ovarian cancer. She chose to put off chemotherapy to treat this disease until after the birth of her child. Before she could receive treatment, the cancer spread to her brain. She was told that no curative treatment was available and that she would only live a few months more. Her family responded to this news by searching for alternative medical interventions online. One website for a German clinic included patient testimonials that Nuttall's mother, Helen Sproates, found compelling. However, services at this clinic would cost £93,000 for one trip, with additional visits necessary. This was much more money than Nuttall and her family could afford, even after taking out loans and selling a house.

For this reason, Sproates began a crowdfunding campaign to raise money for this intervention. After raising an initial £16,000, her appeal caught the attention of actress Kate Winslet, who contributed to the campaign and promoted it in the media.[1] As Nuttall's mother described it to potential donors on her campaign page, this is a "proven treatment and has worked for many patients in the past" and so "we hope [it] can save her life." Whereas Nuttall would not have been able to access this service without the help of crowdfunding, she was able to make seven trips for unproven cancer interventions after raising over £340,000.[2] After completing these trips, she was told that she was "cancer-free," which her family described as a "miracle."[3]

This story received widespread, international news coverage, which included claims of the unproven interventions as being life-saving and glowing descriptions of the clinic offering this service. As I discussed in Chapter 6, businesses selling unproven medical interventions directly to consumers are widespread internationally. In this chapter I will discuss how crowdfunding campaigns like Gemma Nuttall's can greatly increase the financial accessibility of these interventions, expand the pool of potential customers, serve as a means of marketing these interventions, and spread misinformation about their safety and efficacy. When these businesses exploit the hopes of their customers, crowdfunding and other social networks expand the scope of this exploitation to campaign donors and a wider audience of people exposed to these marketing messages. As such, crowdfunders and crowdfunding platforms may partake and be complicit in the exploitation of hope by these businesses.

Medical Crowdfunding

Crowdfunding is the practice of seeking financial resources from groups of people. While group fundraising is hardly a new practice, online platforms have made the process of seeking and giving contributions much easier. Moreover, these online platforms, combined with virtual social networks, have allowed individual crowdfunders to reach a much larger potential audience than they would have if they relied only on proximate personal connections to raise funds.

The earliest users of online crowdfunding were entrepreneurs seeking investment for entire businesses or specific products. These forms of entrepreneurial crowdfunding do not typically depend fully on the charity of donors to provide funding. Rather, they typically provide supporters with some form of reward for donations, such as an equity stake in a new business or early access to a product under development. Thus, entrepreneurial crowdfunding mimics traditional forms of fundraising for businesses and product developers but uses the accessibility and visibility of online crowd-funding platforms to expand the range of potential supporters to include nontraditional, smaller supporters and to increase the geographic reach of potential supporters. Many crowdfunding platforms specialize in this form of crowdfunding, including Kickstarter and IndieGoGo. This form of online crowdfunding using platforms that facilitate giving is relatively new: IndieGoGo was founded in 2008 and Kickstarter in 2009.

After online crowdfunding platforms were developed for entrepreneurs, some platforms began including or specializing in fundraising for individuals' personal needs. These charitable crowdfunding platforms raise funds for a wide range of causes, including education, pet care, and housing. Nonprofit groups use these platforms to raise money on others' behalf, and individuals use them for themselves and friends and family members. As opposed to entrepreneurial crowdfunding, which often rewards supporters and thus provides more of a traditional business relationship between supporter and recipient, charitable crowdfunding typically relies on the goodwill of donors rather than the promise of some benefit.

While many platforms host crowdfunding campaigns for individuals seeking charitable contributions, this form of crowd-funding is increasingly dominated by GoFundMe in North America and, to a lesser extent, worldwide. As with other online crowdfunding platforms, GoFundMe is relatively new, having been founded in 2010. In 2015 it was purchased by a private invest-ment fund from its original founders and was valued at $600 mil-lion.[4] It has dominated the charitable crowdfunding sector in part by being one of the earliest such platforms and by acquiring competitors. In 2017 it purchased the charitable crowdfunding platform CrowdRise, and in 2018 it purchased its largest compet-itor, YouCaring. GoFundMe has grown rapidly in the charitable crowdfunding sector, to the point of dominating this practice. By 2016, GoFundMe was growing by 300 percent per year and raising money from 25 million donors through 2 million crowdfunding campaigns.[5] In 2017, it was reported that it had raised $3 billion since 2010 and was raising $140 million per month in donations, with $100 million in revenues in 2016.[6] At that time, these revenues were generated through a 5 percent fee on donations through its platform. More recently, and following the lead of other charitable crowdfunding platforms, GoFundMe has dropped this fee and instead relies on donors giving optional tips to GoFundMe; credit card fees still apply to donations, however, at the rate of 2.9 percent. More recently, the total raised by GoFundMe was reported as $5 billion and growing.[7]

The most common form of charitable crowdfunding is fundraising for health-related purposes, or medical crowdfunding. Medical crowdfunding is the single largest crowdfunding category on GoFundMe.com, and these campaigns spill over to other categories, such as Emergency, as well. In 2018 one-third of all GoFundMe campaigns were for health-related expenses, totaling 250,000 such campaigns and raising $650 million.[8] At present, GoFundMe describes itself as "the leader in online medical fundraising," with over 250,000 campaigns per year raising over $750 million annually.[9]

People use medical crowdfunding for a variety of reasons. As one would expect, these include receiving essential medical services such as cancer care and emergency treatment. Studies have found that, among Canadian crowdfunders, cancer is the most common underlying health condition motivating crowdfunding.[10,11] This is the case in the US as well, where a review of 200 crowdfunding campaigns found that 31 percent were related to cancer, with acute events and chronic needs like diabetes, musculoskeletal disorders, and congenital malformations also common.[12] Canadian crowdfunders generally have access to public health insurance but still sought help paying for lost income due to illness, specific medical treatments not available through the public health system, or quicker access to care.[13,14] Similar reasons for crowdfunding are often cited in the US context as well, including general, health-related financial difficulties, lost wages due to illness, the high cost of care, unpaid debts, and increased indirect expenses such as travel to access care. Even those individuals with private health insurance faced costs due to gaps in coverage, high deductible payments, and high copayments.[15]

Crowdfunders use different kinds of language and rationales to make the case that they deserve donations. Friends or family members writing about recipients, for example, may describe them as positive members of their communities.[16] Deserving attributes can include a history of giving to others in the community, implying a duty of reciprocity for community members to give back to this individual. Family connections are also sometimes emphasized, implying a relational obligation on the part of friends and family to help a loved one.[17] In other cases, the depth of need is highlighted as a way of stressing the good that will be done by donating to this individual. These cases are thus often presented as crises rather than chronic needs, making this kind of rationale a better fit for emergency, acute medical needs rather than chronic illness.[18] Others stress characteristics like being a hard worker, striving to earn the money needed for surgery, or having been previously harmed by family, society, or bad luck to convey that they deserve donations, good luck, and social support.[19]

Medical crowdfunding can often have an enormously positive impact on the lives of people who use it.[20] Most obviously, medical crowdfunding can mean the difference between accessing and not accessing life-changing or even life-saving treatment. For individuals with no health insurance or personal savings, crowd-funded financing can be the only means of paying for essential medical care. For example, stories of individuals paying for gender-affirming surgeries with crowdfunding are common. In these cases, crowdfunding can allow individuals facing gender dysphoria and depression faster access to these treatments, which can vastly improve their quality of life and, in some cases, decrease chances of experiencing violence or self-harm.[21]

Medical bankruptcy—that is, being forced to declare bankruptcy in large part because of health-related debts—is also a significant concern for individuals lacking adequate health insurance. This problem is particularly acute in the US, where health costs are high and insurance coverage is not universal. For example, one study found that in 2007, 62.1 percent of all bankruptcies in the US were related to medical debts, even though most of these individuals had health insurance.[22] Another study found that half of all debt-collection activities on consumer credit reports in the US were related to medical bills.[23] This problem has persisted in the US even after the Affordable Care Act was passed and implemented. A survey of US bankruptcy filings from 2013 to 2016 found that in 58.5 percent of cases medical expenses contributed to bankruptcy, amounting to 530,000 bankruptcies annually.[24] Importantly, medical crowdfunding has been found to have a positive impact on avoiding medical bankruptcy. Specifically, it has been estimated that in the US, every 10 percent increase in funds raised through medical crowdfunding amounts to a .04 percent reduction in chapter 13 bankruptcy filings.[25]

Despite these benefits, medical crowdfunding is also associated with several ethical issues that have led to widespread criticism of its expanded use. These issues are much broader than the specific worry about crowdfunding for unproven medical interventions that is the focus of this chapter, but a brief survey of them will help to explain the more general context of and concerns with this practice and show how responses to crowdfunding for unproven interventions may impact other ethical concerns. An overarching concern with medical crowdfunding is that it is a deeply problematic response to the issue of inadequate funding for essential medical care and barriers to accessing this care. If access to essential medical care is an entitlement or human right, then medical crowdfunding is useful in improving access to this entitlement. However, it does not do so universally and should be seen as more of a response than solution to the problem of health system failures.

Notably, GoFundMe CEO Rob Solomon acknowledged this issue, stating that "there are people who are not getting relief from us or from the institutions that are supposed to be there. We shouldn't be the solution to a complex set of systemic problems. They should be solved by the government working properly, and by health care companies working with their constituents. We firmly believe that access to comprehensive health care is a right and things have to be fixed at the local, state and federal levels of government to make this a reality."[26] Of particular concern in this context is the potential for medical crowdfunding to be portrayed as a solution to systemic problems in the distribution of healthcare when it only—and imperfectly—addresses some of the symptoms of this problem.[27] This concern has been borne out in practice, as crowdfunding campaigns do not tend to justify donations based on systemic failings, and positive messaging in these campaigns has been associated with higher rates of giving.[28,29] More generally, critics worry that a shift to crowdfunding normalizes the private provision of essential medical services and can shift public perceptions around the commodification of healthcare.[30]

A key problem with portraying crowdfunding as a solution to healthcare access is that it distributes resources inequitably. While people can reasonably differ about how health resources should be distributed, the most plausible views argue that individuals should receive care according to the degree of their need, the amount of good that can be done through the care, or some mix of the two. The problem with crowdfunding is that it likely does not do this, instead distributing resources according to other factors such as the size and wealth of one's social networks, the amount of sympathy the public has with one's story, the ability to craft a compelling narrative of need, and social connections that can increase the visibility of a campaign, including through the media. If these factors are associated with higher levels of income, education, and socioeconomic status, then there is reason to think that medical crowdfunding will be most useful to and benefit relatively privileged people, albeit those with unmet healthcare needs. My and colleagues' research of Canadian medical crowdfunders suggests that this is the case, finding that crowdfunding for cancer-related care is more common in areas with higher income, educational attainments, and home ownership.[31] Studies of crowdfunding campaigns for gender-affirming treatments also found that (a) receiving more Facebook shares is correlated with raising more money, (b) trans men raise significantly more money than trans women, and (c) young, white, and transgender men perform better than other groups.[32,33] Others have shown that the number of a campaign's social media shares and "likes" is correlated with successfully meeting its financial goals.[34]

Another key concern with the practice of medical crowdfunding is that it comes at a significant cost to medical and personal privacy. To raise money via medical crowdfunding, campaigners are encouraged to share personal details about their family, medical needs, and financial situation. This information can include details of medical records, images and videos of the recipient in their hospital room and under medical care, and images and information about third parties such as minor children. This disclosure of private information can be particularly challenging and personally costly when the campaign recipient is a member of a stigmatized group or is seeking treatment related to a stigmatized need, such as gender-affirmation treatment.[35] While such information is not strictly required by crowdfunding platforms, it is typically encouraged to establish the legitimacy of the campaign and worthiness of the recipient. In some cases, campaigners have indicated comfort with this transfer of information, as it encourages emotional bonds with donors, many of whom already have close relationships with the recipient. But these recipients must also calculate how much information to divulge to encourage others to give.[36] While this decision is in a sense voluntary, campaigners typically face significant medical needs and financial pressures that may leave them with no other option than to display their medical and family information online. Moreover, these campaigns may include the information of third parties, minor children, and incapacitated adults who do not or cannot give consent to having their information shared online.[37]

Crowdfunding for Unproven Medical Interventions

In addition to the previously noted general ethical concerns with medical crowdfunding, this practice has been found specifically to raise money to allow for the purchase of a range of medical interventions that have not been established to be safe and effective. In general, the motivation for using medical crowdfunding to access these unproven interventions is because (a) public and private insurance will not pay for them, (b) they require international travel because they are not available locally, possibly owing to regulatory restrictions, or (c) some mix of the two.

In some cases, these interventions are locally available and even approved by local regulators but not paid for by public or private insurance because of a lack of proven efficacy. A prime example of such crowdfunding is for homeopathic and some naturopathic medical interventions, or what can more generally be categorized as complementary and alternative medicine (CAM). A wide variety of interventions fall under the CAM label, and some show evidence of efficacy in specific contexts or are, at the very least, harmless to those pursuing them. However, researchers have established reasons for concern with crowdfunding for CAM interventions of medical conditions that threaten the health and survival of patients—specifically cancers that are treatable through conventional medicine.

For example, one review of campaigns on the crowdfunding platforms GoFundMe and YouCaring identified 474 campaigns originating in the US and Canada for homeopathic or naturopathic remedies for cancer. These campaigns sought over $12.5 million and raised 27.5 percent of this amount, or over $3.4 million. These campaigns sought these interventions both in the US and abroad. This same study noted another alternative intervention, hyperbaric oxygen therapy for brain injury, appearing in 190 campaigns and raising $785,000 of over $4 million requested.[38] Similarly, my own and colleagues' review of campaigns for homeopathic cancer interventions on GoFundMe found 220 campaigns. These campaigns were mostly from the US (85 percent) but also from Canada, the UK, and the European Union. They requested nearly $5.8 million and raised over $1.4 million, or 24 percent of the amount requested.[39] These campaigns also sought a range of other CAM interventions, including vitamin supplements, naturopathy, pH balancing, and energy healing. Finally, a review of the UK-based crowdfunding platform JustGiving and GoFundMe identified £8 million in contributions to campaigns for CAM cancer interventions since 2012.[40]

In addition to CAM treatments, unproven stem cell interventions are a major source of activity on crowdfunding platforms. As discussed in Chapter 6, businesses selling these interventions often take advantage of regulatory loopholes in the US, Canada, and elsewhere to sell stem cell products derived from the patient's own body. In other cases, campaigners seek interventions abroad, because specific stem cell interventions are restricted locally, they are not available locally, the price is lower abroad, or the quality of services is perceived to be better abroad. These studies are varied but tell a consistent story of stem cell interventions raising significant sums of money. For example, the previously discussed study of CAM cancer treatments and hyperbaric oxygen interventions for brain injury on GoFundMe and YouCaring also identified unproven stem cell interventions for brain and spinal cord injury.

The 281 campaigns identified requested over $8 million and were pledged nearly $1.85 million.[41] In my own work, my colleagues and I searched GoFundMe and YouCaring specifically for US businesses that had been identified as selling unproven stem cell interventions. This study found 408 campaigns requesting nearly $7.5 million and receiving pledges for just over $1.45 million.[42] These campaigns were dominated by two businesses—StemGenex, which has received a warning letter from the Food and Drug Administration (FDA) and is the subject of a class-action law-suit by former patients, and the Lung Institute, which actively suggests that potential patients crowdfund for their services and is being sued by former patients.[43,44] Finally, my study of unproven stem cell interventions for neurological diseases on GoFundMe found 1,030 campaigns initiated during a one-year period. These campaigns requested nearly $33.5 million and were pledged just over $5 million. These interventions were intended for a range of neurological conditions and diseases, but most commonly multiple sclerosis, autism, spinal cord injuries and paralysis, cerebral palsy, and stroke. Again, specific clinics dominated these campaigns, in-cluding Panama's Stem Cell Institute, StemGenex in California, and Mexico's Clínica Ruiz.[45]

In addition to these businesses marketing unproven stem cell interventions directly to consumers, crowdfunding is also being used to access clinical trials for unproven interventions (see Chapter 5) and compassionate access to unproven interventions (see Chapter 7). The previously mentioned study of unproven stem cell interventions for neurological diseases and injuries identified two academic centers—Northwestern and Duke Universities—as the intended destinations for at least thirty-four campaign recipients raising over $340,000 for unproven interventions for multiple sclerosis, autism, and cerebral palsy.[46] This kind of fund-raising has been reported elsewhere as well. For example, the Ilinetsky family had twins with Canavan disease, a currently in-curable condition that leads to degeneration of brain tissue and death in childhood. The Ilinetskys learned of a proposed gene-replacement therapy for Canavan disease that had not yet entered phase I trials and needed $3.5 million in funding to begin. They initiated a crowdfunding campaign for $2 million to fund this trial. Their campaign fell well short of this goal, but another campaign for a Canavan intervention has raised over $1.3 million. Other crowdfunding campaigns funding clinical research are common at GoFundMe and, in fact, one of that company's conference rooms is named in honor of a campaign that raised over $2 million for clinical research into Sanfilippo syndrome.[47] These fundraisers have the potential to boost research funding and increase access to experimental interventions. At the same time, they bypass normal peer review of research proposals and thus may expose participants to the dangers of early trial participation discussed in Chapter 5, with even less potential for success and thus more danger of false and exploited hope.

While there is little to no evidence of efficacy for most of these interventions, they can be defended as harmless, an expression of patient autonomy, or a way to preserve patients' hope—especially for those with a terminal cancer diagnosis. For example, one crowdfunding campaigner included in these studies reported that the campaign "gave her hope at a point when we had none." Seeking this intervention gave her a sense of control over her treatment and "empowerment" that was "so useful" and thus "was not false hope."[48] Despite these potential benefits, studies of crowdfunding campaigns for unproven interventions show that they can have significant harms as well. For example, my research found that at least 28 percent of campaigners seeking homeopathic cancer remedies had died by the time data was collected on these campaigns. This number likely underestimates the poor health of this groups, because many campaigns had not been running for long, some closed upon death and so were not reviewed, and many did not report the recipient's outcome. This same study noted that 38 percent of campaigners used homeopathy as an intervention to complement conventional cancer treatments and thus were likely not harmed by it. However, 31 percent pursued homeopathic remedies because curative care was not available and, in doing so, may have forgone effective palliative treatment. Most concerning, 29 percent chose to forgo conventional, evidence-based treatment in favor of CAM interventions and may have deprived themselves of curative treatment.[49] Thus, any benefits of CAM interventions for serious illnesses, including providing hope and empowerment, must be balanced against the danger that such interventions will replace effective curative and palliative care.

Misinformation and Viral Hype

As seen in the previous section and in Chapter 6, crowdfunding helps recipients access unproven interventions that can waste financial resources, expose recipients to risky interventions, raise false hopes, and make it less likely that recipients pursue effective curative or palliative care. In addition to providing the financial resources that allow recipients to pursue these interventions, crowdfunding can take misinformed hope on the part of the crowdfunding campaigner and spread it virally through false claims repeated in the campaign. Thus, not only is the campaigner's hope exploited in these cases, but they may be unintentionally responsible for spreading this misinformation to many others and opening them up to exploitation.

In studies of crowdfunding campaigns for unproven medical interventions, these campaigns frequently make unsupported claims about the safety and efficacy of these interventions. For example, my study of campaigns for homeopathic cancer interventions found that 29 percent made unsupported claims about the efficacy of these interventions, whereas only 1 percent acknowledged a lack of supporting evidence.[50] Similarly, my study of 408 campaigns for stem cell interventions from US businesses selling these treatments directly to consumers found that 43.6 percent of these campaigns made definitive statements about the efficacy of these interventions despite a lack of supporting evidence and an additional 30.4 percent made optimistic or hopeful statements. Few of these campaigns discussed the interventions' risks and, when they did, they declared that there were no risks or fewer than in proven treatments.[51] These campaigns also use the language of scientific research to try to establish their legitimacy. Among these 408 campaigns, 78 discussed the desired intervention using the language of clinical research: 71.8 percent used references to research as a signifier of scientific credibility (e.g., "government-approved clinical trials"), 51.3 percent cited the "experimental" nature of stem cell interventions as a reason why they were not covered by insurance (e.g., "As long as the FDA calls these procedures 'Experimental' the Insurance companies will do the same"), and 26.9 percent claimed that the recipient would be contributing to the advancement of scientific knowledge by receiving the proposed intervention (e.g., "the results will be shared with the FDA in the fight for approval").[52] A separate study of crowdfunding campaigns for unproven stem cell interventions found narratives of scientific breakthroughs to be common, as well as discussion of these interventions as being "experimental" or "promising," or situating them as part of clinical studies or research.[53]

Crowdfunding works by leveraging social networks to expand the campaigner's network of potential donors to both immediate social connections and the connections of those individuals as well. By sharing campaigns online via social networks like Facebook and Twitter, the campaigner hopes to exponentially increase the visibility of their campaign and network of potential donors. Thus, a single campaign can have a very large influence by being exposed to very large groups of individuals. In the case of the 408 campaigns for services at US-based stem cell businesses, 13,050 people (averaging 32 per campaign) donated to these campaigns, and they were shared at least 111,040 times (averaging 272 per campaign) on Facebook and Twitter.[54] Similarly, my previously discussed study of 1,030 campaigns for unproven interventions for neurological diseases and injuries found that they had 38,713 donors (averaging 37.6 per campaign) and were shared 199,490 times on Facebook (averaging 193.7 per campaign).[55] The 220 campaigns for homeopathic cancer remedies were supported by 13,621 donors (averaging 61.9 per campaign) and were shared on Facebook 112,353 times (averaging 510.7 per campaign).[56]

Not only are these campaigns viewed by large groups of people through being shared on social networks, but the format of these campaigns is especially effective for conveying misinformation about the safety and efficacy of unproven medical interventions. Specifically, these campaigns take the form of personal testimonials that are particularly convincing when compared with other means of marketing. Personal narratives have been found to be more persuasive to readers than presentations that rely on statistical information.[57] Personal narratives may help the audience relate to specific elements of the story and develop a sympathetic relationship with the campaigner.[58] Rather than coming from an impersonal source or from the marketing arm of a business, personal testimonials have the advantage of taking on the voice of someone similar to and identifiable with the reader. This is particularly true with testimonials in crowdfunding campaigns, where the reader may personally know the campaigner or have close social connections.[59]

These campaigns, and the misinformation they contain, are also frequently spread through media coverage. Media coverage is an important means of increasing the visibility of crowdfunding campaigns and, thus, the range of potential donors. Through this coverage, crowdfunding campaigns can go "viral," as in the case of a campaign to support the victims of a bus crash in Canada that received extensive media coverage and raised over $15 million.[60] While such viral campaigns are the exception rather than the rule in medical crowdfunding, even modest and local media coverage can significantly increase donations to a campaign. For this reason, GoFundMe suggests seeking out press coverage to increase the likelihood of reaching one's campaign goal. Specific tips include identifying journalists who have written similar stories about crowdfunding campaigns, giving journalists a "newsworthy hook," and writing a press release to distribute to journalists.[61] A study of newspaper coverage of medical crowdfunding campaigns found that they tend to portray them positively (43.75 percent) or neutrally (47.92 percent) but rarely negatively (4.76 percent). Of the articles reviewed, over 20 percent were for unproven interventions, and these articles included references to where contributions could be made 80 percent of the time and hyperlinks to the campaign in over half of all cases. In some instances, these news stories did not make it clear that the interventions were not scientifically proven to be safe and effective, and news coverage more generally can lend legitimacy to unproven medical interventions.[62]

Hyping Hope

Even when campaigners have a good understanding of the likelihood of an unproven intervention to improve their health, they face pressure to exaggerate the efficacy of these interventions to encourage giving. The reason for this, as discussed earlier, is that medical crowdfunding favors the distribution of financial resources for health according to how popular and visible the campaign is, how sympathetic the recipient and their medical need are to the public, how deserving the recipient is perceived to be, and how likely the money is to transform the recipient's life. Conversely, individuals who have difficulties telling their story in an engaging and sympathetic way or have health needs that are stigmatized or less engaging to the public are less likely to be rewarded in what can be reduced to an online popularity contest. As a result, campaigners have strong incentives to tell their stories in ways that will lead to donations, including by making unrealistic promises about the potential of the unproven interventions they are seeking.

GoFundMe explicitly urges its users to develop their campaigns in ways that engage with readers and increase the likelihood of reaching their fundraising goals. Campaign titles should be "inspiring" and make "people want to learn more about and share your cause." The story itself should be "compelling" and "inspire empathy and compel readers to care enough to make a donation."[63] Campaigners raising money for medical issues are specifically told that "people will be more willing to support your cause if they have a full understanding of the financial, physical and emotional trouble you're experiencing" and to be specific about the "recommended treatment" and how the funds will "help you or your beneficiary." Updates are also flagged as being important for medical crowdfunding campaigns, as donors will "be eager to know how you're doing and how the funds are being used." They note that updates "with a positive spin are wonderful" but that even medical setbacks are an opportunity to "be sure to let your supporters know if you need additional help."[64]

Positivity is an important part of engaging with potential donors, and GoFundMe recommends that individuals raising funds for in vitro fertilization expenses, for example, "share messages of hope."[65] For individuals raising money to participate in clinical trials for new cancer interventions, one example campaign is praised as doing an "amazing job" of telling readers "why we're so hopeful."[66] For a time, GoFundMe even gave advice to individuals seeking funding for unproven stem cell interventions, stating, "If you've exhausted your options and are looking for an alternative to traditional methods, there's hope yet. While this course of treatment is still in the early stages of research, plenty of GoFundMe community members have found considerable success with it."[67] This page includes approving links to two campaigns, including one for a child stating, "The neurologist told mom this is likely as good as she'll ever get—please help her if you're able. We believe in miracles, and umbilical stemcells are Hope for Hay."[68]

Former crowdfunders post similar advice online for those raising money for medical services, and books have been published to guide successful crowdfunding. Campaigners are advised to tell "a great tale" and to give regular updates because donors "want to see what their previous donations have accomplished."[69,70] Given the size of the medical crowdfunding sector and its importance to the health and well-being of so many individuals, it isn't surprising that a community of for-profit crowdfunding advisors has developed to give counsel to would-be medical crowdfunding campaigners. For example, Roy Morejon, the president and cofounder of crowd-funding consulting company Enventys Partners, notes that good storytelling is essential for a successful campaign.[71] Thus, both the structural incentives and online advice given to crowdfunding campaigners push them in the direction of producing positive, hopeful stories that will draw the public into their campaign and motivate giving.

This message is borne out in crowdfunding campaigns for unproven interventions. A quick look at GoFundMe's list of "trending" medical campaigns any day will confirm this. For example, one trending campaign describes a woman diagnosed with stage IV breast cancer for whom no conventional treatment is available. Under the heading "Hope and Possibility," she describes "a promising treatment plan in Germany" that uses "cutting edge" treatments. Despite an update to the campaign that indicates that the cancer has spread to her liver, she writes "that we have never once thought that the road was hopeless."[72] Similarly, another cam-paign for a recipient with stage IV cancer and no conventional treatment options seeks alternative interventions. This campaign is hopeful and optimistic throughout, calling the recipient "a moun-tain that is refusing to bow to the wind" and stating that giving to the campaign will show her that "we have faith in her ability to not only attack this disease using natural and western medicine, but also using the power of positivity." The campaign concludes with an update that the recipient has been battling infection but will now be able to pursue these alternative interventions. As a result, "the future is looking GREAT and POSITIVE."[73]

Hoping for Others

Crowdfunding campaigns can and often do spread misleading information about the efficacy and safety of unproven interventions. The structure of crowdfunding incentivizes this misinformation, as crowdfunding campaigners must compete with other campaigns for attention, motivate giving through a sympathetic story, and demonstrate that donating is worthwhile, including by claiming that the donations will likely have a positive impact. This is true whether the individual writing and organizing the crowdfunding campaign is also the intended recipient of the medical interventions or if the campaigner is writing on behalf of another person.

Friends and family of individuals who need medical treatment often start crowdfunding campaigns on their behalf because the campaigner has more of the skills needed to organize an effective crowdfunding campaign, the ill individual is reluctant to directly ask others for financial help, or the recipient's illness makes it difficult for them to create and maintain the campaign. In some cases, well-intentioned people seek access to unproven medical interventions on behalf of others who are not able to give informed consent to their own medical care. These campaigns are often initiated through family relationships, as in cases where a parent makes medical decisions on behalf of a young child or a son or daughter makes decisions for a parent facing cognitive decline. Campaigning for unproven interventions on behalf of individuals who have limited autonomy and medical decision-making capacity raise many ethical issues, including the spread of misinformation about the safety and efficacy of unproven interventions, as discussed earlier. Another, distinct worry is that advocating on behalf of another with limited autonomy raises special concerns about engendering and exploiting hope in others.

This issue arose in the case Charlie Gard, whose parents sought to transfer him from a London hospital to a US-based facility for an unproven intervention. Charlie was diagnosed with a mitochondrial disease that led to progressive muscle deterioration and brain damage; as a result, he was hospitalized from eight weeks after birth. For five months, his parents sought to transfer him abroad for care, whereas his local medical team felt that doing so would only prolong his suffering.[74] Because the UK National Health Service would not pay for this unproven intervention, Charlie's parents set up a campaign on GoFundMe. Charlie's mother, Connie Yates, wrote of Charlie's condition, saying that they "watched our poor baby get weaker and weaker, he now needs a ventilator to breathe but we have never lost hope throughout all this time." After searching for treatment for Charlie, they "found hope" in a US doctor willing to provide him with an experimental nucleoside bypass therapy that, while "it hasn't been tried on anyone with his gene before," "had success with another mitochondrial depletion syndrome called TK2 which is similar." In the campaign, Yates is clear that the intervention is not guaranteed to work but expresses hope throughout. She notes that this is hope not just for her son but for other children, too: "If Charlie receives this treatment and it does work like the Dr in America thinks, it won't be just Charlie's life that has been saved, it will be many more children in the future, who are born with this horrible disease and it will open up other trials on other mitochondrial depletion syndrome's [sic]." She sees the campaign as charting a path for others: "We need to give other people hope." After Charlie's parents lost their legal case to transfer him to the US, he was placed in hospice care and died; the donated money was used to set up a charitable fund to aid research into mitochondrial diseases.[75]

While gaining less media attention, crowdfunding campaigns for adolescents and adults with cognitive limitations are common as well. In one campaign, the daughter of Malgosia Wolanski explains that her mother was experiencing mild cognitive impairment that was worsened by a head injury, which led to a diagnosis of early-onset Alzheimer's disease, for which "her only hope of possibly preserving and even recovering some cognitive abilities is Stem Cell Therapy."[76] Wolanski's daughter supports a claim that the intervention is effective with links to the clinic website and a documentary that has been described as an evidence-free series of one-sided patient testimonials.[77] The crowdfunding campaign does not include Wolanski's perspective or words or any indication that she has expressed an interest in this intervention or that she is able to consent to it on her own behalf.

These cases are similar in that a family member's hope for a cure for a loved one led to public campaigning on their behalf, strongly expressed hope for better health, and unsupported claims about the promise and potential efficacy of these interventions. When they broadcast their own hopes for better health for another person through crowdfunding campaigns, they frequently mix this hope, knowingly or unknowingly, with substantial misinformation about the likely outcomes of the intervention and the evidence base for donating. When people in close relationships seek unproven medical care on behalf of minors or incompetent adults, they may do so with the genuine best interests, or perceived best interests, of the patient in mind. However, these relationships raise the possibility that they are protecting their own hopes and emotional interests at the cost of prolonging suffering in another. In the case of Charlie Gard, his medical team expressed that seeking unproven interventions would only prolong his suffering with no real potential for better health. Similarly, in the case of Wolanski, seeking unproven stem cell interventions would involve financial cost and some risk, coupled with a trip abroad that could be especially stressful for an individual with memory impairment. In these cases, the decision-maker's hope for better health may conflict with the best interests of the patient.

Sympathetic medical needs, and especially those of children, also create an opportunity for individuals and political interest groups to exploit others' hope for a cure for the patient to advance their own agendas. In these cases, the patient's interests and public's hope become entangled in debates over larger political and policy issues. As Charlie Gard's case received more media coverage, a range of public officials used his illness to support their own views, including right-to-life and anti-euthanasia campaigners and critics of public insurance for healthcare in the US.[78] Thus, the needs of dependents can be used to generate hope that can then be exploited by a range of actors.

Networks of Exploitation

Crowdfunding specifically, and social media more generally, provide a means by which information about unproven interventions can be quickly or "virally" spread to large audiences. In many cases, the information about the safety and efficacy of these interventions is misleading or outright false, possibly because the campaigners hold false beliefs about the interventions they are seeking for themselves or on behalf of others. Moreover, the structure of crowdfunding creates a strong incentive to create or build on misinformation by exaggerating claims of efficacy, making false claims or omitting information about the risks of interventions, and linking to company websites and quoting the claims of businesses providing these interventions. This misinformation is packaged in the form of emotionally charged testimonials that are effective in transmitting misinformation and persuading readers to make donations and potentially seek out such interventions themselves. These campaigns can spread an unsupported message of hope, ensure that this message takes root in a network of donors and readers, and help the campaigners to fund their interventions; as such, they can reasonably be charged with creating false hopes in others and, by encouraging pledges of financial support, they may be complicit in the exploitation of these false hopes by those selling these interventions.

Participation by crowdfunding campaigners in the exploitation of hope can take two forms. First, campaigners can act as conduits for exploitation by enabling exploiters to reach a larger audience of potential exploitees. As I have shown, they do so by providing the means of reaching a larger financial base through donors who will finance the unproven interventions. As a result of requesting funding from their social networks, campaigners provide paying customers to businesses selling unproven interventions. Moreover, these campaigners increase the number of potential customers for businesses selling unproven interventions by transmitting marketing messages for them in the form of powerful personal testimonials that emphasize the supposed efficacy and safety of these interventions or at least underemphasize any doubts about the likely outcome of the intervention.

Serving as a conduit for exploitation in this way is morally distinct from exploiting hope directly. As discussed in Chapter 6, businesses selling unproven interventions exist and exploit hope in the absence of crowdfunding campaigns. Campaigners widen the scope of exploitation by these businesses by enabling access to a larger population of potential exploitees. This is the case even if the campaigner genuinely believes in the misleading marketing messages of businesses selling unproven interventions and even if, as is likely, the recipient is also a victim of exploitation. That is, campaigners and recipients may have their hopes exploited by those selling these interventions and, at the same time, make potential donors vulnerable to exploitation. Whether or not they intend to do so or do so knowingly, these campaigners frequently are part of the process of exploitation and worsen the scope and impacts of those exploiting the hopes of seriously ill individuals.

It may seem strange to say that individuals campaigning for funding for medical interventions can be culpable in the exploitation of potential donors in cases that do not constitute outright fraud (such as when medical needs are fabricated or the identify of a person in need is stolen). When examining culpability for the exploitation of hope in medical crowdfunding, the greatest criticism is owed to clinics like those described in Chapter 6 whose entire business model is based on promoting unproven and potentially dangerous interventions to sick customers. However, crowdfunding serves as an important means of funneling resources to these companies and greatly magnifies their reach and credibility.

Second, campaigners may directly participate in the exploitation of hope through their crowdfunding campaigns—particularly when campaigners exaggerate unsupported statements of the safety and efficacy of the interventions they are seeking, fail to disclose questions or uncertainties about safety and efficacy, or otherwise mislead potential donors. In these situations, the actions of the campaigners follow the hallmarks of exploiting false hope, where the hopes of potential donors are used to benefit the recipient. Here the specific concern is that the campaigner plays on and amplifies donors' hopes for better health for the campaign recipient in a misleading manner, allowing and encouraging giving to the recipient on a false basis. Doing so can violate a partial entrustment of the donors' financial and emotional well-being to the crowdfunder, created by the relationship between donor and crowdfunder. Most generally, fundraising relationships are ones of trust where the fundraiser assumes responsibilities of promise-keeping that the funds will be used for the advertised purpose, truth telling around the need for the funds and ability of the funds to address this need, and transparency throughout the fundraising process and disposal of these funds.[79] This entrustment by donors of their financial resources and their hopes to help others is inconsistent with crowdfunders misleading potential donors about the efficacy and safety of unproven interventions. This general relationship of trust between fundraiser and funder will be even stronger and more open to exploitation in certain circumstances, as when potential donors are friends and family members placing greater hope—and thus emotional and financial vulnerability—in the hands of the crowdfunder.

Potential donors act based on trust that the information being given to them is accurate. Commentators on medical crowdfunding have suggested that potential donors have an obligation to educate themselves about the evidence base of any intervention they may be supporting to fulfill an obligation to be well informed about the efficacy, need for, and likely impact of any intervention.[80] While these donors should inform themselves from independent sources as well as the word of the campaigner, campaigners actively undermine the ability of donors to be well informed when they provide them with misinformation, lead them to biased or untrustworthy sources of information, and willfully obscure key details around safety and efficacy. By intentionally manipulating the hopes of potential donors to benefit the recipient, campaigners effectively exploit these hopes by failing in an obligation to allow potential donors to make informed decisions.

Crucially, crowdfunders in these cases generally act in the genuine hope that these interventions may improve their own health or that of a loved one. This aim is, of course, importantly different from that of enriching oneself. Nonetheless, crowdfunders may violate the trust of donors—often close friends and family—to use their hopes and receive an unproven medical intervention. Their actions will amount to exploiting the hopes of those donating to and otherwise supporting these campaigns. More broadly, campaigners will be complicit in the exploitative and deeply ethically problematic practices of companies selling unproven medical interventions.

Crowd Control

I have argued that crowdfunding campaigners raising funds for un-proven medical interventions can be complicit in the exploitative actions of those providing these interventions and may even them-selves exploit donors' hopes of improving the recipient's health. However, attempts to address the contribution of crowdfunding to networks of exploitation should not start with the crowdfunders themselves. While there is room to try to educate campaigners on the best evidence of the safety and efficacy of a range of unproven med-ical interventions, fundamentally these are individuals hoping to improve the health of themselves or loved ones. This fact does not ex-cuse complicity in exploitation or exploitative acts but does create a context in which these individuals and their advocates are themselves vulnerable to exploitation and have few ways to act on their own hopes for better health. Interventions against these crowdfunders, beyond attempts at better education and improving their options, es-pecially for palliative care, may simply worsen their already difficult situations without greatly protecting potential donors.

Actions can and should be taken against those businesses and individuals directly providing these interventions, particularly when they misrepresent their safety and efficacy, as discussed in Chapter 6. However, while regulations on direct-to-consumer pro-vision of unproven interventions are essential, there are limitations in how effective they would be. Prohibitions on false or misleading advertising by these businesses are important, but crowdfunding campaigners will likely continue to build on and exaggerate mar-keting messages that are carefully crafted not to violate existing regulations against false advertising. Specific jurisdictions can and should limit or prohibit the direct provision of unproven medical interventions to guard against the exploitation of hope and other ethical concerns like direct harm and fraud. However, given the global nature of this practice, businesses can and will relocate to jurisdictions with more permissive laws or less oversight. Affordability of these interventions will limit how many people access them, but crowdfunding increases the number of people who can access these interventions, the number of people financially harmed by doing so, the scope of the exploitation of the hopes of these funders, and the audience for the marketing messages of these businesses.

Thus, crowdfunding platforms should also limit or prohibit the use of their platforms to fund these interventions. The least restrictive means of doing so would be to provide warnings about specific unproven interventions and general guidance on how to assess the efficacy and safety of medical interventions. While crowdfunding platforms could develop these guides on their own, patient advocacy and expert groups have already done so for specific intervention types, and crowdfunding platforms could draw from these guides or partner with these groups to try to better educate campaigners and potential donors. To take one example, the International Society for Stem Cell Research has developed a patient guide that could be linked to or drawn from to balance against the unsupported claims common in crowdfunding campaigns for unproven stem cell interventions.[81]

One limitation of this approach is that campaigners and, especially, donors may be unlikely to carefully read and consider such guidelines, particularly if they are located among frequently asked questions (FAQ) pages or otherwise buried among various resources on crowdfunding platforms. Moreover, campaigners will typically have settled on a treatment plan, including communicating with providers, before establishing a crowdfunding campaign. As a result, any such countervailing information would have to work to dislodge already developed beliefs in and hopes for the success of specific unproven interventions. Thus, a more restrictive approach of prohibiting some types of campaigns for unproven medical interventions could be justified based on the impact of these campaigns, their role in enabling the exploitation of the hopes of recipients and donors, and the lack of effective but less coercive approaches.

GoFundMe has shown some limited willingness to take this route. In March 2019 it announced a ban on fundraisers for services at the Hallwang Clinic in Germany, which offers a range of unproven interventions for cancer, including vitamin infusions and ozone therapy alongside immunotherapy. While immunotherapy shows promise in treating some forms of cancer, Hallwang also uses it for solid tumor cancers where efficacy is not well established. Reports of former patients suggest that they were told by Hallwang (or interpreted messages from the clinic as promising) very high rates of success with its products.[82]

GoFundMe presented the decision to ban campaigns for services at Hallwang as temporary while it consulted with experts and users. It also indicated an interest in balancing the preferences of users against concerns about misleading information on these interventions, stating that "GoFundMe respects the decisions of patients and their loved ones about what they choose to fundraise for. We also recognize the tension between that openness and the need to make sure people are equipped to make well-informed decisions, and we're doing more to help with that."[83] Following that action, GoFundMe also announced it was prohibiting campaigns raising money for groups spreading unfounded concerns about the safety and efficacy of vaccines. Again, misinformation linked to these campaigns served as the rationale for this action: "Campaigns raising money to promote misinformation about vaccines violate GoFundMe's terms of service and will be removed from the platform."[84]

As these actions show, prohibitions on certain campaigns on GoFundMe have been justified by how they spread misinformation about medical interventions and that doing so violates the terms of service of that platform. Specifically, at the time these actions were taken, GoFundMe prohibited campaigns for "pharmaceuticals or other products that make health claims that have not been approved or verified by the applicable local and/or national regulatory body."[85] This language would not prohibit campaigns for all unproven interventions, but those that made unsupported marketing claims or skirted local regulations on medical interventions could be targeted.

The creation and exploitation of false hopes, as I have argued, create a strong ethical case for crowdfunding platforms like GoFundMe to prohibit some or all of these campaigns. As Rob Solomon, the CEO of GoFundMe, put the concern, "We shouldn't be a regulator, and we're not equipped to be one. But a clinic that is creating false hope and charging exorbitant amounts?"[86] However, policy position does raise the question of how far these platforms should go in determining which campaigns for unproven interventions should be allowed. In addition to this question of whether it is appropriate for a crowdfunding platform to serve as a regulator and the potential technical and practical roadblocks of its doing so, these limits could come at a cost to individual autonomy and the well-informed and rational hopes of patients and their supporters for better health in the face of serious illness. To recognize this concern and to respect the genuine hopes of some patients, GoFundMe could develop a blacklist of problematic companies who clearly exploit the hopes of crowdfunders and donors or engage in other problematic behaviors, just as was done with the Hallwang Clinic. Such a list could be developed using data on crowdfunding campaigns for unproven interventions, research on marketing activities by academics, reports by patient advocacy groups, and actions by health and marketing regulators.

Instead, GoFundMe and other, smaller crowdfunding platforms have failed to restrict campaigns for unproven interventions. In fact, GoFundMe followed its limited restrictions by changing its terms of service to allow more campaigns for unproven interventions. Rather than prohibiting campaigns for medical products that haven't been approved or verified by regulators as in the past, now the prohibition is against "pharmaceuticals or similar products or therapies that are either illegal, prohibited, or enjoined by an applicable regulatory body; ... or other products, medical practices, or any related equipment or paraphernalia that have been found by an applicable regulatory body to cause consumer harm."[87] Instead of requiring that campaigns limit themselves to products and claims that have been actively approved or verified by regulators, this change now shifts the burden of proof. Those concerned with these campaigns for unproven medical interventions must now show that these interventions are specifically prohibited by regulators or found to be harmful. This standard is much more difficult to meet than showing that the claims of these companies raise false hopes or are unproven; as a result, they create ample room for crowdfunding to continue to serve as a means for businesses selling unproven interventions to exploit the hopes of their customers and, to a lesser extent, campaigners to exploit the hopes of their donors. While crowdfunding platforms do not directly exploit hope in this way, the failure to act against such campaigns leaves them active and necessary participants in such exploitation.

Conclusion

This chapter began with the story of the viral, celebrity-aided crowdfunding campaign for Gemma Nuttall. This campaign raised hundreds of thousands of pounds and allowed Nuttall to undergo unproven interventions for her ovarian cancer. After receiving multiple rounds of these interventions, Nuttall was declared cancer free, and her celebrity supporter Kate Winslet was credited with having saved her life.[88]

Sadly, Nuttall's cancer returned, and she died a year later. Her mother, Helen Sproates, has since questioned whether she should have initiated a crowdfunding campaign for her daughter. She reports that Nuttall was initially against the idea of crowdfunding, because she preferred to keep her life and medical condition private and discussions about using crowdfunding led to "quite big rows." Pursuing this unproven intervention was a source of stress in both of their lives. Even after being declared cancer free, the clinic suggested returning regularly for expensive "maintenance" interventions. Despite raising huge sums of money through the crowdfunding campaign, Nuttall chose not to return. She was concerned that traveling frequently for care would exact too much of a physical toll and that additional interventions would use up all her financial resources. While Sproates believes that this intervention extended Nuttall's life, she questions whether they should have pursued it at all given the time and emotional costs of doing so. As she put it, "You do not do anything else except get on the plane, go have treatment, come back on the plane. . . . I ask myself should we have done the bucket list and spent the last few months of Gemma's life with her daughter, trying to be happy and make memories?"[89]

The cancer clinic that Nuttall crowdfunded for and received services from was the Hallwang Clinic. This is the same clinic that was prohibited from using GoFundMe's platform, and had Nuttall and her family tried to raise money for this intervention more recently, they would have been unable to do so. Nuttall's crowdfunding campaign served as a significant means of advertising for this business. In addition to frequent claims that this intervention was a "miracle" and had saved Nuttall's life, contemporary reporting on her campaign stated credulously that the intervention "is working" and that additional interventions will "strengthen her position even more."[90] Before her cancer returned, Nuttall's crowdfunding page also included enthusiastic reports of the effects of Hallwang's interventions. The clinic took up Nuttall's story to promote its interventions, including a video of her among its many patient testimonials on its website.[91] Nuttall's mother has requested that the clinic remove this video and those of other former patients who have died, as "she's inspired a lot of people. But Gemma hasn't turned out well."[92]

While GoFundMe has blocked campaigns for services at the Hallwang Clinic, campaigns for many unproven interventions and for businesses that encourage unsupported claims about the safety and efficacy of these interventions remain. Moreover, other crowd-funding platforms still allow donations to the Hallwang Clinic. These campaigns greatly encourage the reach of these marketing messages and, because of the competitive nature of crowdfunding, exaggerate these claims and build on the hopes of potential donors. Crowdfunding increases the viability of the direct-to-consumer marketplace for unproven interventions and greatly expands the number of patients and donors whose financial resources and hopes are exploited by these groups. While other social networks like Twitter do not directly participate in crowdfunding, they help spread crowdfunding messages. More generally, social networks serve as means to encourage misinformation about the safety and efficacy of a range of unproven medical interventions, raising hopes in them and creating a large market of interested patients. Addressing the direct exploitation of hope by sellers of unproven interventions, then, will also require addressing the networks of exploitation through which they now operate.

Conclusion

Exploiting Hope

In this book I have developed an account of exploiting hope and have applied it to cases of people seeking better health through unproven medical interventions. Drawing on examples from the press, I noted that everyday use of the charge that someone has exploited the hope of another person typically involves *weighty* hopes, meaning hopes central or very important to one's well-being or sense of self. These weighty hopes can involve individuals who lack the means to a minimally decent life, including cases where they are hoping for basic safety, a decent income, or good health. In other instances, individuals have their basic needs met but hope for a better than good life, seeking to realize their hopes for wealth or public recognition of their talents.

Whether these weighty hopes are for a decent minimum or something more, they involve making oneself vulnerable, risk-taking, and placing some aspects of one's well-being in the hands of another—what I call *leaps of hope*. In some cases, these leaps entrust one's life to another person, as when refugees pay smugglers to deliver them safely abroad or patients engage physicians to look after their health. Other cases are seemingly more trivial, as when would-be pop and literary stars hire agents to develop their careers. But even here, these leaps of hope leave individuals vulnerable to both significant financial losses and lost hope, with the potential for emotional and psychological damage.

Accounts of exploitation have tended to locate its wrongness in the distribution of benefits created by exchanges between exploiter and exploitee. These fairness-based accounts argue that exploitation is enabled by special opportunities for unusual and unfair benefits in specific transactions or systemic opportunities for unfair benefits against a backdrop of injustice. While these accounts are effective in explaining some cases of exploitation, I argued that they are not the best fit for the context of exploiting hope or even exploitation more generally. Rather, I proposed and defended a respect-based account, where relationships between individuals specify a general duty of beneficence. When individuals choose to benefit from transactions with others in violation of a specified duty to them, they exploit them.

Largely adopting Adrienne Martin's account of hope, I argued that the leaps of hope in typical examples of exploiting hope are not necessarily ill-informed or irrational.[1] Even in cases where the hoped-for outcome is extremely unlikely, *hoping against all expectation* of the hoped-for outcome being realized can be well informed and rational. What is needed in these cases is for the hopeful person to be attracted to the hoped-for outcome, think it possible, take a stance toward that possible outcome that gives them reason to think, feel, or plan around it in certain ways, and treat the positive features of the hoped-for outcome as giving sufficient reason for these thoughts, feelings, and plans. Hope in this sense can include acting or fantasizing as if the hoped-for outcome will occur, even in cases where one understands that this is very unlikely.

Taken together, I argued that exploiting hope entails interactions where the exploiter takes advantage of hope in the preceding sense to benefit, in violation of a specified duty of beneficence to the exploitee. More specifically, leaps of weighty hope can create a relationship of partial entrustment, where the potential exploiter becomes entrusted with specific elements of the potential exploitee's well-being. Fairness-based theories of exploitation fail to give an adequate account of these relationships, as they cannot explain the importance of the distinctive features of exploiting hope and struggle to explain the ethical dimensions of exploiting hope for better health.

In practice, this respect-based account should lead individuals to ask the following questions: (1) *Should this interaction happen at all or the partial entrustment be accepted*? Interactions with vulnerable people entail moral entanglements that include partial entrustment with dimensions of others' well-being. While a moral life is not one devoid of all such entanglements, and they are not always matters of choice, caution and forethought are needed when seeking interactions with others, especially when respectful, non-exploitative interactions are not possible. (2) If the entrustment is accepted, *how can the hopeful relationship be managed most respectfully*? Once partial entrustment with another's well-being is given, questions of how to manage that entrustment, including when and how to restrict one's demands on and benefit from that person, are raised and need answering. (3) As these relationships develop, new information is gained, and conditions change, one must regularly ask, *should the hopeful relationship be continued*? While hope beyond all expectation might be reasonable and sustaining at one point in time and allow for a non-exploitative interaction, changes to one's hope, physical well-being, emotional state, and financial well-being might all impact whether and how the relationship should be continued. Thus, a relationship founded on hope might be non-exploitative initially but evolve into a relationship that exploits hope later.

Exploiting Hope for Better Health

In the applied chapters of this book I showed how my account of exploiting hope helps to illuminate how exploitation can take place in transactions involving unproven medical interventions. These applications help to demonstrate the explanatory power and fit of my theoretical approach while providing insights into when and how the exploitation of hope takes place.

In all these cases, the hoped-for outcome—typically better health, better quality of life, or potentially a cure—is clearly weighty. The first case examines terminally ill people with cancer seeking to enroll in phase I clinical trials for cancer treatments and individuals in low- and middle-income countries (LMICs) seeking to enroll in phase III clinical trials. In both situations, the hoped-for outcome is certainly weighty—longer lives or better health for people with cancer, and better health and access to medicines for LMIC research participants and their communities. In the second case, people may seek unproven stem cell interventions for a range of reasons, but in most cases they are tied to weighty hopes for better health and quality of life. Similarly, the third case explores individuals with terminal illnesses who hope to be allowed access to experimental interventions through compassionate use pathways, including the much-hyped right-to-try pathway in the US. Finally, while crowdfunding is used for many purposes, the fourth case shows that often it involves individuals with weighty medical needs seeking a range of unproven interventions that they hope will improve their health.

These weighty hopes lead to leaps of hope that make these individuals vulnerable to exploitation. In the first case, research participants become vulnerable to clinical researchers who are trusted to convey full and accurate information about the trials, to design the trials, and to manage trial outcomes. Those seeking unproven stem cell interventions do so at substantial financial cost and put their health and bodily integrity at risk by receiving these interventions. People seeking compassionate access to unproven interventions through the right-to-try pathway face heightened expectations and the danger of dashed hopes. Finally, crowdfunders wishing to purchase unproven interventions face similar financial and health vulnerabilities as those purchasing unproven stem cell treatments and spread the vulnerabilities created by heightened hope and misinformation to their networks of supporters.

Acting on these weighty hopes creates relationships of partial entrustment of the hopeful person's well-being. As I have argued, the parameters of this partial entrustment with the health of trial participants and their communities will be shaped by factors such as the depth of the relationship, complicating factors such as the dual roles of physician-researchers, and the ability of researchers to manage the research design, and the availability of any resulting treatments to benefit participants and their communities. In the second case, patients entrust physicians with their health and rely on them to provide unbiased advice on how best to pursue medical treatment. Physicians selling unproven stem cell interventions create a conflict between this role and the pursuit of financial gain, violating this trust by presenting misleading information to their patients and providing interventions for which there is little evidence of efficacy. Hope for better health through right-to-try has been encouraged by the rhetoric of politicians, policymakers, and interest groups who promised that this legislation would make a range of potential cures available and save thousands of lives. These promises created false hopes that were exploited by politicians seeking to appear to address health needs and by interest groups with deregulatory agendas that this legislation serves. Political promises—despite the fact that many people are rightfully skeptical of them—can create a relationship of vulnerability, obligation, and expectation that, when unfulfilled, leads to exploitation. Finally, crowdfunders are entrusted with aspects of funders' financial and emotional well-being when these donors give crowdfunders their financial resources and entrust them with their hopes for the recipient's health. These relationships create obligations of truth telling, promise keeping, and transparency that can be violated when crowdfunders base their campaigns on misinformation about the safety and efficacy of unproven interventions.

Exploiting Hope beyond Health

This book focused on applying my account of exploiting hope to cases of seeking better health through unproven medical interventions. As my survey of popular discussion of exploiting hope showed, this concern is also applied to a broad range of cases not directly related to health. Concerns with the exploitation of hope are often linked to smuggling persons across borders, employment schemes, politicians promising economic opportunities, gamblers pursuing winnings, would-be novelists and pop stars pursuing their dreams, and many other contexts. These examples show that hope for a better life, not just hope for better health, creates a vulnerability that can be exploited when those entrusted with these vulnerabilities violate this trust.

As my detailed discussion of cases of exploiting hope for better health showed, each case is importantly different and creates different vulnerabilities and relationships of partial entrustment with specific dimensions of the exploitee's well-being. These contexts matter greatly for identifying relationships of exploitation and developing responses to patterns of exploitation. Cases of exploiting hope for better health are distinctive, then, in terms of the special characteristics of vulnerability and entrustment found in hope for better health and relationships with those entrusted to protect and help improve health. But they are also part of a larger pattern of ethical duties where hopes create vulnerabilities and relationships of trust that can be violated by exploiters who place their own interests above their responsibilities to specific others. The entrusted responsibilities of people smugglers, employers, politicians, talent agents, and others create opportunities for the exploitation of hope and deserve their own separate considerations. The account of exploiting hope developed here is not limited to exploiting hope for better health and, as such, can and should be applied to illuminate the ethical dimensions of these other cases.

Exploitations or Exploitation?

In Chapter 2 of this book I surveyed various theories of exploitation with the aim of identifying an account of exploitation best suited to the context of exploiting hope for better health. Using the example of sweatshop labor, I presented a respect-based account of exploitation that understands exploitation to be a failure to fulfill a specified duty of beneficence. Such an understanding of exploitation can account for much of what is taken to be problematic with employers choosing to offer low wages to their employees, especially when they could offer higher wages or better working conditions.

As I noted, this respect-based account is not the only plausible account of exploitation available. Transactional fairness accounts of exploitation have dominated discussion of theories of exploitation in the context of sweatshop labor and elsewhere. These theories can account for a common perception that it is unfair for employers to gain far more—or disproportionately—from transactions with workers who cannot meet their basic needs. At the same time, structural fairness accounts of exploitation rightly emphasize the relevance of structural factors in creating conditions under which unfair transactions become possible and normalized. Therefore, one could reasonably take the position that "exploitation" describes multiple distinct types of unethical transactions and that all of these accounts of exploitation are needed to give a full account of the wrongness of exploitation.

I believe that this approach is worth considering. However, my exploration of exploiting hope and application of a specific respect-based account of exploitation makes a strong case for either emphasizing respect-based accounts of exploitation above the fairness-based accounts or arguing that exploitation should be interpreted *solely* as a failure of respect. There are three primary reasons for doing so. First, the fairness-based accounts are limited in their application. While Alan Wertheimer is clear that his understanding of fairness is not tied only to a hypothetical fair-market price, transactional fairness–based accounts struggle to give a clear account of exploitation outside of the marketplace and when involving non-divisible and non-commodifiable goods.[2] This limitation is clearest when discussing exploitation in intimate relationships, where even looking to a fair division of benefits seems to mistake the character of the relationship. Moreover, my discussion of exploiting hope showed that such exploitation often involves parties outside of the central transaction, as when crowdfunding creates networks of exploitation. While a respect-based account of exploitation can make sense of how vulnerability and partial entrustment with this vulnerability extends across such networks, a transactional account would struggle to do so, as these networks extend beyond the scope of specific transactions involving an exchange of benefits. In other respects, transactional fairness accounts of exploitation can apply to too wide a range of cases, as their understanding of fairness is not limited to the weighty goods that motivate most concerns with exploitation. Structural fairness–based accounts do well in highlighting how injustice creates a vulnerability that can be exploited. However, they are not applicable outside of that context and lack the ability to illuminate other types of vulnerability.

Second, the account of exploitation presented here encompasses and extends the advantages and range of the fairness-based accounts. As demonstrated in the cases presented here, this account can explain the wrongness of transactions in the marketplace, as with direct-to-consumer sales of unproven stem cell treatments. It also succeeds in explaining the wrongness of exploitation in nonmarket settings, as with exploitation by physicians, researchers, and politicians. While the exploitation of hope against a backdrop of structural injustice was not a major theme of these cases, it was present in the context of exploiting the hopes of clinical trial participants in LMICs and, to a lesser extent, in the context of compassionate access to experimental medical interventions. This respect-based account can explain how relationships specify general duties to combat structural injustice similarly to a political account of responsibility, encompassing the advantages of this understanding of structural exploitation.

Third, this account allows for a specificity to context lacking in the other accounts. As the cases discussed in this book show, the specific dimensions of hope are important to understanding the kind of vulnerability created in specific cases. The nature of the relationship between individuals matters to understanding what dimensions of one's well-being are entrusted to another and, therefore, what potential for exploitation is present. We can discuss generalities around the duties of, for example, researchers overseeing phase I cancer trials. But a full understanding of relationships of partial entrustment must include the specific relationship between the researcher and research participant, the structure of the trial, and the goals of all parties, among other factors. Simply examining the division of benefits is not a replacement for this emphasis on the particularity of each case.

Thus, I will conclude by advocating for the benefits of respect-based accounts of exploitation and, specifically, the version tethered to the partial entrustment of vulnerabilities developed here. I hope to have shown that this understanding of exploitation is a powerful tool for understanding how hope can be exploited in the context of unproven medical interventions and beyond. Moreover, this account is generalizable to much of what is popularly charged as exploitative and can help diagnose both what is wrong with these instances of exploitation and how to reduce their regularity.

Notes

Introduction

1. Emily Dickinson, "'Hope' Is the Thing with Feathers," *The Complete Poems of Emily Dickinson* (Boston: Back Bay Books, 1976).
2. William Shakespeare, *Richard II: The Oxford Shakespeare* (Oxford: Oxford University Press, 2011), II.2.
3. John Steinbeck, *The Grapes of Wrath* (New York: Penguin, 2006).
4. Karl Marx, *Karl Marx: Selected Writings*, ed. David McLellan (Oxford: Oxford University Press, 2000).
5. Gerald A. Cohen, "The Labor Theory of Value and the Concept of Exploitation," *Philosophy and Public Affairs* 8, no. 4 (1979): 338–60.
6. Allen E. Buchanan, "Marx, Morality, and History: An Assessment of Recent Analytical Work on Marx," *Ethics* 98, no. 1 (1987): 104–36.
7. Jon Elster, "Exploring Exploitation," *Journal of Peace Research* 15, no. 1 (1978): 3–17.
8. Allen E. Buchanan, *Marx and Justice: The Radical Critique of Liberalism* (London: Methuen, 1982), 40.
9. Buchanan, *Marx and Justice*, 43.
10. Alan Wertheimer, *Exploitation* (Princeton, NJ: Princeton University Press, 1999).
11. Ruth J. Sample, *Exploitation: What It Is and Why It's Wrong* (Lanham, MD: Rowman and Littlefield, 2003).
12. Adrienne M. Martin, "Hope and Exploitation," *Hastings Center Report* 38, no. 5 (2008): 49–55.
13. Adrienne M. Martin, *How We Hope: A Moral Psychology* (Princeton, NJ: Princeton University Press, 2016).

Chapter 1

1. Office of the Commissioner, Food and Drug Administration, "FDA Seeks Permanent Injunctions against Two Stem Cell Clinics," news release,

May 9, 2018, http://www.fda.gov/news-events/press-announcements/fda-seeks-permanent-injunctions-against-two-stem-cell-clinics.

2. Lizzy Davies, "Italy Boat Wreck: Scores of Migrants Die as Boat Sinks off Lampedusa," *Guardian*, October 3, 2013, https://www.theguardian.com/world/2013/oct/03/lampedusa-migrants-killed-boat-sinks-italy.

3. Sheena McFarland, "Victims Face Deportation," *Salt Lake Tribune*, May 10, 2009, https://archive.sltrib.com/story.php?ref=/ci_12339001.

4. Mike Roberts, "A Wedding Party Hijack," Series: Abandoned Brides, *Province*, October 17, 2005.

5. United States Department of Justice, "California Man Arrested, Charged for Adult Adoption Scheme to Defraud Undocumented Immigrants," news release, February 11, 2016, https://www.justice.gov/opa/pr/california-man-arrested-charged-adult-adoption-scheme-defraud-undocumented-immigrants.

6. Brian Bauer, "Mine Jobs Scam," letter to the editor, *Cairns Sun*, July 20, 2011.

7. "Jobhunters Exploited in Mining," *Cairns Sun*, June 26, 2008.

8. Randy B. Williams, "Sorry, Get in Line," letter to the editor, *Edmonton Journal*, September 14, 2010.

9. Jayantha Dhanapala and Savitri Goonesekere, "'Torch of Awareness' for Voters," *Daily Mirror*, September 5, 2013, http://www.dailymirror.lk/opinion/torch-of-awareness-for-voters/172-34912.

10. Douglas Anele, "Deconstructing Buharimania," *Vanguard Nigeria*, March 8, 2015, https://www.vanguardngr.com/2015/03/deconstructing-buharimania/.

11. Cassandra Szklarski, "Plan to End Immigrant Backlog Gets $700 Million," *Vancouver Sun*, November 25, 2005.

12. "4 File a Class-Action Suit against Sweepstakes Firm," *St. Louis Post-Dispatch*, January 31, 1998.

13. "Mystery Call Offers Prize," *Wiltshire Gazette and Herald*, June 19, 2002, https://www.gazetteandherald.co.uk/news/7347542.mystery-call-offers-prize/.

14. Wendy Murphy, "When We Exploit Hope, Feed Greed," *Patriot Ledger*, December 3, 2011.

15. Patrick Hosking, "Publishing Outfit That Is Aiming to Make Vanity Fair," *Evening Standard*, February 18, 1999.

16. Caroline Weber, "Holiday Books: Fashion," *New York Times*, December 3, 2006.

17. David Livingston, "Beyond Hats and Bags: How Clothes Look and What They May (or May Not) Mean," *Globe and Mail*, February 13, 1982.

18. "Waging War against a Deadly Disorder," *New Zealand Herald*, February 4, 2006.

19. John Kerry, "Remarks at the 2015 Trafficking in Persons Report Ceremony," US Embassy in the Dominican Republic, July 27, 2015, https://do.usembassy.gov/remarks-2015-trafficking-persons-report-ceremony/.

20. "Utterly Wrong to Exploit the Hope of Those Wanting a Baby," *Bath Chronicle*, July 20, 2016.

21. "The Government as Bookie," editorial, *Globe and Mail*, May 23, 1995.

22. Murphy, "When We Exploit Hope, Feed Greed."

23. "Sex Ring Smashed," *Sunday Tasmanian*, July 3, 2005.

24. Norbert J. Krieg, "Perils of Illegal Entry into the United States," letter to the editor, *Independent*, September 20, 1990.

25. Gordon Gibson, "Gaming or Gambling: By Any Name It Exploits the Hopes and Dreams of Losers," *Calgary Herald*, February 14, 1998.

26. Andrew Penman and Nick Sommerlad, "Visas Scam Rides Again," *Mirror*, February 19, 2009.

27. "Refugees Wait as Camp's Future Is Decided," *Birmingham Post*, July 13, 2002.

28. "Emulate Scottish Approach on Stem Cells," *Palm Beach Post*, July 1, 2007.

29. John Rolfe and Rosemarie Lentini, "Bond Was Her Word: Subletting Opportunity That Proved Too Good to Be True," *Daily Telegraph*, April 26, 2012.

30. "Model Dreams," *South China Morning Post*, August 11, 1998.

31. Jefferson Morley, "Hoop Dreamer," *Washington Post*, March 26, 1995.

32. Lidia Revello, "Shows 'Exploit' People Says Star," *Aberdeen Evening Express*, May 6, 2014.

33. Katie Begley, "Axed Acts Blast Twist," *Scottish Star*, October 11, 2011.

34. Jane Bakowski, "Hazel's Star Rises in Her Bollywood Roles," *Kent and Sussex Courier*, July 10, 2009.

35. Fiona O'Cleirigh, "It's Time to Pay Interns What They Are Worth," *Guardian*, October 11, 2010.

36. Yves Lavigne, "Groups Demand Tobacco Licencing," *Globe and Mail*, September 23, 1987.

37. Paul Brady, "Debate on Stem-Cell Research," letter to the editor, *Irish Times*, December 3, 2003.

38. Rex Martinich, "Broad Wants Exemptions for Asylum Seeker Ban," *Wimmera Mail-Times*, November 9, 2016.

39. Tracey Kaplan, "DA Launches Effort Warning Obama-Plan Applicants of Scams," *Mercury News*, February 9, 2015, https://www.mercurynews.com/2015/02/09/da-launches-effort-warning-obama-plan-applicants-of-scams/.

40. Kari Johnstone, "The Power of Local Communities in the Fight against Human Trafficking," DipNote, June 28, 2018, https://blogs.state.gov/stories/2018/06/28/en/power-local-communities-fight-against-human-trafficking.

41. Tony Pugh, "Supplements Stuff of Fraud, Senators Told," *Philadelphia Inquirer*, September 11, 2001.

42. Henry Porter, "Crowd Control," *Guardian*, October 12, 1995.

43. William Thorsell, "Games Governments Play," *Globe and Mail*, January 15, 1994.

44. "The Government as Bookie."

45. Terry Sweetman, "After 13 Years, the Australian Writers-Authors Group Has Packed Up Its Quills and Closed Its Doors," *Sunday Mail*, March 1, 1998.

Chapter 2

1. Don van Natta, "Sweatshop Job Abuse Worsening, Workers Say," *New York Times*, September 13, 1995, https://www.nytimes.com/1995/09/13/nyregion/sweatshop-job-abuse-worsening-workers-say.html.

2. Tina Rosenberg, "Globalization," *New York Times*, August 18, 2002, https://www.nytimes.com/2002/08/18/magazine/globalization.html.

3. Allen R. Myerson, "In Principle, a Case for More 'Sweatshops,'" *New York Times*, June 22, 1997, https://www.nytimes.com/1997/06/22/weekinreview/in-principle-a-case-for-more-sweatshops.html.

4. Nicholas D. Kristof and Sheryl WuDunn, "Two Cheers for Sweatshops," *New York Times*, September 24, 2000, https://www.nytimes.com/2000/09/24/magazine/two-cheers-for-sweatshops.html.

5. Nicholas D. Kristof, "Where Sweatshops Are a Dream," *New York Times*, January 14, 2009, https://www.nytimes.com/2009/01/15/opinion/15kristof.html.

6. Denis G. Arnold, "Exploitation and the Sweatshop Quandary," *Business Ethics Quarterly* 13, no. 2 (2003): 243–56, 255.

7. Benjamin Pimentel, "Temporary Workers Sue HP over Overtime Pay," *SFGate*, January 22, 2003, https://www.sfgate.com/business/article/Temporary-workers-sue-HP-over-overtime-pay-2639704.php.

8. Alan Wertheimer, *Exploitation* (Princeton, NJ: Princeton University Press, 1999), 10.

9. Chris Meyers, "Wrongful Beneficence: Exploitation and Third World Sweatshops," *Journal of Social Philosophy* 35, no. 3 (2004): 319–33.

10. Mikhail Valdman, "A Theory of Wrongful Exploitation," *Philosopher's Imprint* 9, no. 6 (2009): 1–14.

11. Robert Mayer, "What's Wrong with Exploitation?," *Journal of Applied Philosophy* 24, no. 2 (2007): 137–50.

12. Wertheimer, *Exploitation*, 232.

13. Wertheimer, *Exploitation*, 230.

14. Hillel Steiner, "A Liberal Theory of Exploitation," *Ethics* 94, no. 2 (1984): 225–41.

15. Valdman, "A Theory of Wrongful Exploitation."

16. Mikhail Valdman, "Exploitation and Injustice," *Social Theory and Practice* 34, no. 4, (2008): 551–572.

17. Matt Zwolinski, "Sweatshops, Choice, and Exploitation," *Business Ethics Quarterly* 17, no. 4 (2007): 689–727, 706.

18. Edd S. Noell, "Bargaining, Consent and the Just Wage in the Sources of Scholastic Economic Thought," *Journal of the History of Economic Thought* 20, no. 4 (1998): 467–78.

19. Zwolinski, "Sweatshops, Choice, and Exploitation," 693.

20. Zwolinski, "Sweatshops, Choice, and Exploitation," 694.

21. Zwolinski, "Sweatshops, Choice, and Exploitation," 695.

22. Zwolinski, "Sweatshops, Choice, and Exploitation," 710.

23. Ruth J. Sample, *Exploitation: What It Is and Why It's Wrong* (Lanham, MD: Rowman and Littlefield, 2003), 57.

24. Sample, *Exploitation*, 165.

25. Matt Zwolinski, "Structural Exploitation," *Social Philosophy and Policy* 29, no. 1 (2012): 154–79.

26. Mayer, "What's Wrong with Exploitation?," 145.

27. Wertheimer, *Exploitation*, 234.

28. Wertheimer, *Exploitation*, 289.

29. Meyers, "Wrongful Beneficence."

30. C. D. Meyers, "Moral Duty, Individual Responsibility, and Sweatshop Exploitation," *Journal of Social Philosophy* 38, no. 4 (2007): 620–26.

31. Meyers, "Moral Duty, Individual Responsibility, and Sweatshop Exploitation," 625.

32. Iris Marion Young, *Responsibility for Justice* (Oxford: Oxford University Press, 2010).

33. Young, *Responsibility for Justice*, 42.
34. Young, *Responsibility for Justice*, 105.
35. Young, *Responsibility for Justice*, 144.
36. Young, *Responsibility for Justice*, 145.
37. Pierre-Yves Néron and Wayne Norman, "Citizenship, Inc.: Do We Really Want Businesses to Be Good Corporate Citizens?," *Business Ethics Quarterly* 18, no. 1 (2008): 1–26.
38. Andrew Crane and Dirk Matten, "Incorporating the Corporation in Citizenship: A Response to Néron and Norman," *Business Ethics Quarterly* 18, no. 1 (2008): 27–33.
39. Andreas Georg Scherer, Guido Palazzo, and Dorothée Baumann, "Global Rules and Private Actors: Toward a New Role of the Transnational Corporation in Global Governance," *Business Ethics Quarterly* 16, no. 4 (2006): 505–32.
40. Andreas Georg Scherer and Guido Palazzo, "Toward a Political Conception of Corporate Responsibility: Business and Society Seen from a Habermasian Perspective," *Academy of Management Review* 32, no. 4 (2007): 1096–120.
41. Gerard Hanlon, "Rethinking Corporate Social Responsibility and the Role of the Firm—On the Denial of Politics," *The Oxford Handbook of Corporate Social Responsibility* (New York, NY: Oxford University Press, 2008).
42. J. (Hans) van Oosterhout, "Corporate Citizenship: An Idea Whose Time Has Not Yet Come," *The Academy of Management Review* 30, no. 4 (2005): 677–81.
43. Helen Popper, "Bolivians See Dreams Fade In Argentina," *Washington Post*, May 21, 2006, https://www.washingtonpost.com/archive/politics/2006/05/21/bolivians-see-dreams-fade-in-argentina-span-classbankheadexploitation-widespread-in-clothing-sweatshopsspan/de589d80-98f9-4b63-a809-8a38afc7e56a/.
44. Immanuel Kant, *Groundwork of the Metaphysics of Morals*, ed. Christine M. Korsgaard, 2nd ed. (Cambridge: Cambridge University Press, 2012).
45. Tara J. Radin and Martin Calkins, "The Struggle against Sweatshops: Moving toward Responsible Global Business," *Journal of Business Ethics* 66, no. 2 (2006): 261–72, 263.
46. Norman E. Bowie, *Business Ethics: A Kantian Perspective* (Cambridge: Cambridge University Press, 2017).
47. Denis G. Arnold and Norman E. Bowie, "Sweatshops and Respect for Persons," *Business Ethics Quarterly* 13, no. 2 (2003): 221–42.

48. Onora O'Neill, *Constructions of Reason: Explorations of Kant's Practical Philosophy* (Cambridge: Cambridge University Press, 1990).
49. Thomas E. Hill, *Dignity and Practical Reason in Kant's Moral Theory* (Ithaca, NY: Cornell University Press, 1992).
50. Arnold and Bowie, "Sweatshops and Respect for Persons."
51. Bowie, *Business Ethics*, 70.
52. Immanuel Kant, *The Metaphysics of Morals*, ed. Mary J. Gregor, 2nd ed. (Cambridge: Cambridge University Press, 1996).
53. Thomas E. Hill, *Human Welfare and Moral Worth: Kantian Perspectives* (Oxford: Oxford University Press, 2002).
54. Barbara Herman, *Moral Literacy* (Cambridge, MA: Harvard University Press, 2007).
55. Sample, *Exploitation*, 57.
56. Sample, *Exploitation*, 165.
57. Sample, *Exploitation*, 71.
58. Jeremy C. Snyder, "Needs Exploitation," *Ethical Theory and Moral Practice* 11, no. 4 (2008): 389–405.
59. Jeremy Snyder, "Exploitation and Demeaning Choices," *Politics, Philosophy and Economics* 12, no. 4 (2013): 345–60.
60. Sample, *Exploitation*, 165.
61. James Dwyer, "What's Wrong with the Global Migration of Health Care Professionals? Individual Rights and International Justice," *Hastings Center Report* 37, no. 5 (2007): 36–43.
62. Donna S. Kline, "Push and Pull Factors in International Nurse Migration," *Journal of Nursing Scholarship* 35, no. 2 (2003): 107–11.
63. Jeremy Snyder, "What's the Matter with Price Gouging?," *Business Ethics Quarterly* 19, no. 2 (2009): 275–93.
64. Barry C. Lynn, "Breaking the Chain," *Harper's Magazine*, July 2006, https://harpers.org/archive/2006/07/breaking-the-chain/.
65. Thomas W. Pogge, *World Poverty and Human Rights*, 2nd ed. (Cambridge: Polity, 2008).
66. Thomas Pogge, "Access to Medicines," *Public Health Ethics* 1, no. 2 (2008): 73–82.
67. Snyder, "Needs Exploitation."
68. Sample, *Exploitation*.
69. Wertheimer, *Exploitation*.
70. Robert Mayer, "Sweatshops, Exploitation, and Moral Responsibility," *Journal of Social Philosophy* 38, no. 4 (2007): 605–19, 616.

71. Ian Maitland, "The Great Non-Debate over International Sweatshops," in *Ethical Theory and Business*, ed. Tom L. Beauchamp and Norman E. Bowie, 7th ed. (New York: Pearson Education, 2004): 579–590.

72. Gordon G. Sollars and Fred Englander, "Sweatshops: Kant and Consequences," *Business Ethics Quarterly* 17, no. 1 (2007): 115–33.

73. Denis G. Arnold and Norman E. Bowie, "Respect for Workers in Global Supply Chains: Advancing the Debate over Sweatshops," *Business Ethics Quarterly* 17, no. 1 (2007): 135–45.

74. Denis G. Arnold and Laura P. Hartman, "Moral Imagination and the Future of Sweatshops," *Business and Society Review* 108, no. 4 (2003): 425–61.

75. Denis G. Arnold and Laura P. Hartman, "Beyond Sweatshops: Positive Deviancy and Global Labour Practices," *Business Ethics* 14, no. 3 (2005): 206.

76. Denis G. Arnold and Laura P. Hartman, "Worker Rights and Low Wage Industrialization: How to Avoid Sweatshops," *Human Rights Quarterly*, 2006, 676–700.

Chapter 3

1. Adrienne M. Martin, *How We Hope: A Moral Psychology* (Princeton, NJ: Princeton University Press, 2016).

2. Martin, *How We Hope*, 4.

3. Thomas Hobbes, *Leviathan: Or The Matter, Forme, and Power of a Common-Wealth Ecclesiasticall and Civill* (New Haven, CT: Yale University Press, 2010).

4. David Hume, *A Treatise of Human Nature: Being an Attempt to Introduce the Experimental Method of Reasoning into Moral Subjects* (Auckland: The Floating Press, 2009), 2.3.9.

5. Martin, *How We Hope*, 5.

6. Andrew Norris, "Becoming Who We Are: Democracy and the Political Problem of Hope," *Critical Horizons* 9, no. 1 (2008): 77–89.

7. Martin, *How We Hope*, 14–15.

8. Martin, *How We Hope*, 5.

9. Luc Bovens, "The Value of Hope," *Philosophy and Phenomenological Research* 59, no. 3 (1999): 667–81, 674.

10. Martin, *How We Hope*, 18.

11. Philip Pettit, "Hope and Its Place in Mind," *The Annals of the American Academy of Political and Social Science* 592, no. 1 (2004): 152–65.

12. Philip Pettit, "Hope and Its Place in Mind."

13. Martin, *How We Hope*, 22.

14. Martin, *How We Hope*, 23.
15. Martin, *How We Hope*, 62.
16. Michael Milona and Katie Stockdale, "A Perceptual Theory of Hope," *Ergo: An Open Access Journal of Philosophy* 5, no. 8 (2018): 203–22.
17. Milona and Stockdale, "A Perceptual Theory of Hope."
18. Adrienne M. Martin, "Hopes and Dreams," *Philosophy and Phenomenological Research* 83, no. 1 (2011): 148–73.
19. Martin, "Hopes and Dreams," 167.
20. Martin, "Hopes and Dreams, 167–68.
21. Pettit, "Hope and Its Place in Mind."
22. Martin, "Hopes and Dreams," 168.
23. Sam Horng and Christine Grady, "Misunderstanding in Clinical Research: Distinguishing Therapeutic Misconception, Therapeutic Misestimation, and Therapeutic Optimism," *IRB: Ethics and Human Research* 25, no. 1 (2003): 11–16.
24. Paul S. Appelbaum, Loren H. Roth, and Charles Lidz, "The Therapeutic Misconception: Informed Consent in Psychiatric Research," *International Journal of Law and Psychiatry* 5, no. 3–4 (1982): 319–29.
25. Horng and Grady, "Misunderstanding in Clinical Research."
26. James A. Shepperd et al., "A Primer on Unrealistic Optimism," *Current Directions in Psychological Science* 24, no. 3 (2015): 232–37.
27. Neil D. Weinstein, "Unrealistic Optimism about Future Life Events," *Journal of Personality and Social Psychology* 39, no. 5 (1980): 806.
28. Lynn A. Jansen, "Two Concepts of Therapeutic Optimism," *Journal of Medical Ethics* 37, no. 9 (2011): 563–66.
29. Martin, *How We Hope*.
30. Charles R. Snyder et al., "The Will and the Ways: Development and Validation of an Individual-Differences Measure of Hope," *Journal of Personality and Social Psychology* 60, no. 4 (1991): 570.
31. Jenny Y. Lee and Matthew W. Gallagher, "Hope and Well-Being," *The Oxford Handbook of Hope*, ed. Matthew W. Gallagher and Shane J. Lopez (Oxford: Oxford University Press, 2017), 287–98.
32. Heather N. Rasmussen et al., "Hope and Physical Health," *The Oxford Handbook of Hope*, ed. Matthew W. Gallagher and Shane J. Lopez (Oxford: Oxford University Press, 2017), 159–68.
33. Carla J. Berg et al., "The Role of Hope in Engaging in Healthy Behaviors among College Students," *American Journal of Health Behavior* 35, no. 4 (2011): 402–15.
34. Rasmussen et al., "Hope and Physical Health."

35. C. R. Snyder et al., "Hope against the Cold: Individual Differences in Trait Hope and Acute Pain Tolerance on the Cold Pressor Task," *Journal of Personality* 73, no. 2 (2005): 287–312.
36. Andrew J. Howell, Ryan M. Jacobson, and Denise J. Larsen, "Enhanced Psychological Health among Chronic Pain Clients Engaged in Hope-Focused Group Counseling," *The Counseling Psychologist* 43, no. 4 (2015): 586–613.
37. Carla J. Berg et al., "The Relationship of Children's Hope to Pediatric Asthma Treatment Adherence," *Journal of Positive Psychology* 2, no. 3 (2007): 176–84.
38. Julie M. Maikranz et al., "The Relationship of Hope and Illness-Related Uncertainty to Emotional Adjustment and Adherence among Pediatric Renal and Liver Transplant Recipients," *Journal of Pediatric Psychology* 32, no. 5 (2006): 571–81.
39. Annette L. Stanton, Sharon Danoff-burg, and Melissa E. Huggins, "The First Year after Breast Cancer Diagnosis: Hope and Coping Strategies as Predictors of Adjustment," *Psycho-Oncology: Journal of the Psychological, Social and Behavioral Dimensions of Cancer* 11, no. 2 (2002): 93–102.
40. Rodrigo A. Bressan et al., "Hope Is a Therapeutic Tool," *BMJ* 359 (2017): j5469.
41. Horng and Grady, "Misunderstanding in Clinical Research."
42. Jansen, "Two Concepts of Therapeutic Optimism."
43. Hesiod, *Works of Hesiod and the Homeric Hymns*, trans. Daryl Hine (Chicago: University of Chicago Press, 2008).
44. Friedrich Nietzsche, *Human, All Too Human: A Book for Free Spirits* (Cambridge: Cambridge University Press, 1996).
45. Norris, "Becoming Who We Are."
46. Maria Francesca Drews, "The Evolution of Hope in Patients with Terminal Illness," *Nursing* 47, no. 1 (2017): 13–14.
47. Douglas L. Hill and Chris Feudtner, "Hope in the Midst of Terminal Illness," in *The Oxford Handbook of Hope*, ed. Matthew W. Gallagher and Shane J. Lopez (Oxford: Oxford University Press, 2017), 191–206.
48. Saint Thomas Aquinas, *Summa Theologiae*, trans. Timothy McDermott (Allen, TX: Thomas More Press, 1991).
49. Christy Simpson, "When Hope Makes Us Vulnerable: A Discussion of Patient–Healthcare Provider Interactions in the Context of Hope," *Bioethics* 18, no. 5 (2004): 428–47.
50. Alan Wertheimer, *Exploitation* (Princeton, NJ: Princeton University Press, 1999).

51. Alan Petersen, Casimir MacGregor, and Megan Munsie, "Stem Cell Tourism Exploits People by Marketing Hope," *The Conversation*, July 15, 2014, http://theconversation.com/stem-cell-tourism-exploits-people-by-marketing-hope-29146.

52. Carlos Novas, "The Political Economy of Hope: Patients' Organizations, Science and Biovalue," *BioSocieties* 1, no. 3 (2006): 289–305.

53. Jeremy Snyder et al., "'I Knew What Was Going to Happen If I Did Nothing and so I Was Going to Do Something': Faith, Hope, and Trust in the Decisions of Canadians with Multiple Sclerosis to Seek Unproven Interventions Abroad," *BMC Health Services Research* 14, no. 1 (2014): 445.

Chapter 4

1. Stephen Benet, *John Brown's Body* (Toronto, ON: Aegitas, 2015).

2. Alan Wertheimer, *Exploitation* (Princeton, NJ: Princeton University Press, 1999).

3. Wertheimer, *Exploitation*, 232.

4. Wertheimer, *Exploitation*, 236.

5. Alan Wertheimer, *Rethinking the Ethics of Clinical Research: Widening the Lens* (Oxford: Oxford University Press, 2010).

6. Adrienne M. Martin, "Hope and Exploitation," *Hastings Center Report* 38, no. 5 (2008): 49–55.

7. Martin, "Hope and Exploitation," 53.

8. I. Glenn Cohen, *Patients with Passports: Medical Tourism, Law, and Ethics* (Oxford: Oxford University Press, 2014).

9. Thomas Pogge, "Testing Our Drugs on the Poor Abroad," in *Exploitation and Developing Countries: The Ethics of Clinical Research*, ed. Jennifer S. Hawkins and Ezekiel Emanuel (Princeton, NJ: Princeton University Press, 2008), 112.

10. Pogge, "Testing Our Drugs on the Poor Abroad," 113.

11. Wertheimer, *Exploitation*.

12. Iris Marion Young, *Responsibility for Justice* (Oxford: Oxford University Press, 2010).

13. Martin, "Hope and Exploitation," 54–55.

14. Shelley Wilcox, "The Open Borders Debate on Immigration," *Philosophy Compass* 4, no. 5 (2009): 813–21.

15. Gillian Brock, *Global Justice: A Cosmopolitan Account* (Oxford: Oxford University Press, 2009).

16. Simon Caney, "International Distributive Justice," *Political Studies* 49, no. 5 (2001): 974–97.

17. Daryl Pullman, Amy Zarzeczny, and André Picard, "Media, Politics and Science Policy: MS and Evidence from the CCSVI Trenches," *BMC Medical Ethics* 14, no. 1 (2013): 6.

18. Oguzhan Omer Demir, Murat Sever, and Yavuz Kahya, "The Social Organisation of Migrant Smugglers in Turkey: Roles and Functions," *European Journal on Criminal Policy and Research* 23, no. 3 (2017): 371–91.

19. Paolo Campana, "Out of Africa: The Organization of Migrant Smuggling across the Mediterranean," *European Journal of Criminology* 15, no. 4 (2018): 481–502.

20. Joshua Preiss, "Global Labor Justice and the Limits of Economic Analysis," *Business Ethics Quarterly* 24, no. 1 (2014): 55–83.

21. Michael Kates, "The Ethics of Sweatshops and the Limits of Choice," *Business Ethics Quarterly* 25, no. 2 (2015): 191–212.

22. Ruth J. Sample, *Exploitation: What It Is and Why It's Wrong* (Lanham, MD: Rowman and Littlefield, 2003).

23. Jeremy C. Snyder, "Needs Exploitation," *Ethical Theory and Moral Practice* 11, no. 4 (2008): 389–405.

24. "Penticton Teen Hopes to Have Experimental Cancer Treatment in Texas," *Global News*, March 5, 2015, https://globalnews.ca/news/1867313/penticton-teen-hopes-to-have-experimental-cancer-treatment-in-texas/.

25. Arla Bull, "Supporters Rally to Raise Cancer Treatment Funds for Teacher," *Kitsap Sun*, September 25, 2105, http://www.kitsapsun.com/news/local/mason/supporters-rally-to-raise-cancer-treatment-funds-for-teacher-ep-1288128229-354418171.html.

26. Joanna Frketich, "Family Raising $100,000 for Experimental Treatment for Teen's Lyme Disease," *Hamilton Spectator*, April 16, 2015, https://www.therecord.com/news-story/5562614-family-raising-100-000-for-experimental-treatment-for-teen-s-lyme-disease/.

27. Jeremy Snyder et al., "'I Knew What Was Going to Happen If I Did Nothing and so I Was Going to Do Something': Faith, Hope, and Trust in the Decisions of Canadians with Multiple Sclerosis to Seek Unproven Interventions Abroad," *BMC Health Services Research* 14, no. 1 (2014): 445.

28. Alan Petersen, Kate Seear, and Megan Munsie, "Therapeutic Journeys: The Hopeful Travails of Stem Cell Tourists," *Sociology of Health and Illness* 36, no. 5 (2014): 670–85.

29. Sindia Madan and Kenneth I. Pakenham, "The Stress-Buffering Effects of Hope on Adjustment to Multiple Sclerosis," *International Journal of Behavioral Medicine* 21, no. 6 (2014): 877–90.

30. Henry S. Richardson and Leah Belsky, "The Ancillary-Care Responsibilities of Medical Researchers: An Ethical Framework for Thinking about the Clinical Care That Researchers Owe Their Subjects," *Hastings Center Report* 34, no. 1 (2004): 25–33.

31. Richardson and Belsky, "The Ancillary-Care Responsibilities of Medical Researchers."

32. Henry S. Richardson, *Moral Entanglements: The Ancillary-Care Obligations of Medical Researchers* (Oxford: Oxford University Press, 2012), 70.

33. Richardson, *Moral Entanglements*, 90.

34. Another, comparable example of exploiting hope is the relationship between a gambler and a casino or lottery corporation where the gambler hopes, despite unfavorable odds, to win money needed to erase a debt or otherwise improve their life. Those providing these services are often seen to have a duty to restrict gambling that becomes self-destructive or is otherwise problematic even when it occurs between fully informed and consenting adults. This example is less clear when compared with the previous cases, however, as problematic gambling often demonstrates an element of psychological compulsion, undermining claims that the exchange is consensual.

35. Sam Horng and Christine Grady, "Misunderstanding in Clinical Research: Distinguishing Therapeutic Misconception, Therapeutic Misestimation, and Therapeutic Optimism," *IRB: Ethics and Human Research* 25, no. 1 (2003): 11–16.

Chapter 5

1. Robert Temple and Susan S. Ellenberg, "Placebo-Controlled Trials and Active-Control Trials in the Evaluation of New Treatments. Part 1: Ethical and Scientific Issues," *Annals of Internal Medicine* 133, no. 6 (2000): 455–63.

2. E. A. Eisenhauer et al., "Phase I Clinical Trial Design in Cancer Drug Development," *Journal of Clinical Oncology: Official Journal of the American Society of Clinical Oncology* 18, no. 3 (2000): 684–92.

3. Ciara O'Brien et al., "Novel Early Phase Clinical Trial Design in Oncology," *Pharmaceutical Medicine* 31, no. 5 (2017): 297–307.

4. David B. Resnik, "Therapeutic Misconception, Unrealistic Optimism, and Hope in Phase I Oncology Trials," *Journal of Clinical Research Best Practices* 14, no. 8 (2018): 1–6.

5. Elizabeth Horstmann et al., "Risks and Benefits of Phase 1 Oncology Trials, 1991 through 2002," *New England Journal of Medicine* 352, no. 9 (2005): 895–904.

6. A. Italiano et al., "Treatment Outcome and Survival in Participants of Phase I Oncology Trials Carried Out from 2003 to 2006 at Institut Gustave Roussy," *Annals of Oncology* 19, no. 4 (2007): 787–92.

7. Jeffrey S. Weber et al., "American Society of Clinical Oncology Policy Statement Update: The Critical Role of Phase I Trials in Cancer Research and Treatment," *Journal of Clinical Oncology* 33, no. 3 (2015): 278.

8. Diane A. van der Biessen et al., "Understanding How Coping Strategies and Quality of Life Maintain Hope in Patients Deliberating Phase I Trial Participation," *Psycho-Oncology* 27, no. 1 (2018): 163–70.

9. Gail E. Henderson et al., "Therapeutic Misconception in Early Phase Gene Transfer Trials," *Social Science and Medicine* 62, no. 1 (2006): 239–53.

10. Christopher Daugherty et al., "Perceptions of Cancer Patients and Their Physicians Involved in Phase I Trials." *Journal of Clinical Oncology* 13, no. 5 (1995): 1062–72.

11. Saoirse O. Dolly et al., "A Study of Motivations and Expectations of Patients Seen in Phase 1 Oncology Clinics," *Cancer* 122, no. 22 (2016): 3501–8.

12. Rebecca D. Pentz et al., "Therapeutic Misconception, Misestimation, and Optimism in Participants Enrolled in Phase 1 Trials," *Cancer* 118, no. 18 (2012): 4571–78.

13. Joshua Crites and Eric Kodish, "Unrealistic Optimism and the Ethics of Phase I Cancer Research," *Journal of Medical Ethics* 39, no. 6 (2013): 403–6.

14. Lynn A. Jansen et al., "Perceptions of Control and Unrealistic Optimism in Early-Phase Cancer Trials," *Journal of Medical Ethics* 44, no. 2 (2018): 121–27.

15. Daniel P. Sulmasy et al., "The Culture of Faith and Hope: Patients' Justifications for Their High Estimations of Expected Therapeutic Benefit When Enrolling in Early Phase Oncology Trials," *Cancer* 116, no. 15 (2010): 3702–11.

16. Pentz et al., "Therapeutic Misconception, Misestimation, and Optimism in Participants Enrolled in Phase 1 Trials."

17. Manish Agrawal et al., "Patients' Decision-Making Process Regarding Participation in Phase I Oncology Research," *Journal of Clinical Oncology* 24, no. 27 (2006): 4479–84.

18. Sulmasy et al., "The Culture of Faith and Hope."
19. Weber et al., "American Society of Clinical Oncology Policy Statement Update."
20. Manish Agrawal and Ezekiel J. Emanuel, "Ethics of Phase 1 Oncology Studies: Reexamining the Arguments and Data," *JAMA* 290, no. 8 (2003): 1075–82.
21. Agrawal et al., "Patients' Decision-Making Process Regarding Participation in Phase I Oncology Research."
22. Rebecca Dresser, "First-in-Human Trial Participants: Not a Vulnerable Population, but Vulnerable Nonetheless," *Journal of Law, Medicine and Ethics* 37, no. 1 (2009): 38–50.
23. Manish Agrawal and Marion Danis, "End-of-Life Care for Terminally Ill Participants in Clinical Research," *Journal of Palliative Medicine* 5, no. 5 (2002): 729–37.
24. S. Catt et al., "Reasons Given by Patients for Participating, or Not, in Phase 1 Cancer Trials," *European Journal of Cancer* 47, no. 10 (2011): 1490–97.
25. Steven Joffe et al., "Quality of Informed Consent in Cancer Clinical Trials: A Cross-Sectional Survey," *Lancet* 358, no. 9295 (2001): 1772–77.
26. Franklin G. Miller and Steven Joffe, "Phase 1 Oncology Trials and Informed Consent," *Journal of Medical Ethics* 39, no. 12 (2013): 761–64.
27. Agrawal and Emanuel, "Ethics of Phase 1 Oncology Studies."
28. van der Biessen et al., "Understanding How Coping Strategies and Quality of Life Maintain Hope in Patients Deliberating Phase I Trial Participation."
29. Carine Nierop-van Baalen et al., "Hope Dies Last . . . A Qualitative Study into the Meaning of Hope for People with Cancer in the Palliative Phase," *European Journal of Cancer Care* 25, no. 4 (2016): 570–79.
30. Pia Dellson et al., "Patients' Reasoning Regarding the Decision to Participate in Clinical Cancer Trials: An Interview Study," *Trials* 19, no. 1 (2018): 528.
31. Matthew Miller, "Phase I Cancer Trials: A Collusion of Misunderstanding," *Hastings Center Report* 30, no. 4 (2000): 34–43, 36.
32. Miller, "Phase I Cancer Trials," 37.
33. Valerie Jenkins et al., "What Oncologists Believe They Said and What Patients Believe They Heard: An Analysis of Phase I Trial Discussions," *Journal of Clinical Oncology* 29, no. 1 (2011): 61–68.
34. Agrawal et al., "Patients' Decision-Making Process Regarding Participation in Phase I Oncology Research."
35. Sulmasy et al., "The Culture of Faith and Hope."

36. Barron H. Lerner, *The Breast Cancer Wars: Hope, Fear, and the Pursuit of a Cure in Twentieth-Century America* (Oxford: Oxford University Press, 2003).
37. Sulmasy et al., "The Culture of Faith and Hope."
38. Miller, "Phase I Cancer Trials."
39. Jaklin A. Eliott and Ian N. Olver, "Hope and Hoping in the Talk of Dying Cancer Patients," *Social Science and Medicine* 64, no. 1 (2007): 138–49.
40. Adil E. Shamoo and David B. Resnik, "Strategies to Minimize Risks and Exploitation in Phase One Trials on Healthy Subjects," *American Journal of Bioethics* 6, no. 3 (2006): W1–W13, W9.
41. Shamoo and Resnik, "Strategies to Minimize Risks and Exploitation in Phase One Trials on Healthy Subjects."
42. Dresser, "First-in-Human Trial Participants," 43.
43. Steven Joffe and Franklin G. Miller, "Bench to Bedside: Mapping the Moral Terrain of Clinical Research," *Hastings Center Report* 38, no. 2 (April 2008): 30–42.
44. Gail McBride, "Phase One Trials Can Exploit Terminally Ill Patients," *British Medical Journal* 308, no. 6930 (1994): 679–80, 679.
45. George J. Annas, "The Changing Landscape of Human Experimentation: Nuremberg, Helsinki, and Beyond," *Health Matrix* 2 (1992): 119–40.
46. Justine Seidenfeld et al., "Participants in Phase 1 Oncology Research Trials: Are They Vulnerable?," *Archives of Internal Medicine* 168, no. 1 (2008): 16–20.
47. Miller, "Phase I Cancer Trials."
48. Gillian Nycum and Lynette Reid, "The Harm-Benefit Tradeoff in 'Bad Deal' Trials," *Kennedy Institute of Ethics Journal* 17, no. 4 (2007): 321–50, https://doi.org/10.1353/ken.2008.0004.
49. Nycum and Reid, "The Harm-Benefit Tradeoff in 'Bad Deal' Trials," 341.
50. Jatin Y. Shah et al., "What Leads Indians to Participate in Clinical Trials? A Meta-Analysis of Qualitative Studies," *PloS One* 5, no. 5 (2010): e10730, https://doi.org/10.1371/journal.pone.0010730.
51. Adeline M. Nyamathi et al., "Perceptions of a Community Sample about Participation in Future HIV Vaccine Trials in South India," *AIDS and Behavior* 11, no. 4 (2007): 619–27, https://doi.org/10.1007/s10461-006-9173-8.
52. Harris Interactive, "Participation in Clinical Trials Lower in Europe and India than in the United States," *Healthcare News*, 5 (2005): 38.

53. David Wendler et al., "Why Patients Continue to Participate in Clinical Research," *Archives of Internal Medicine* 168, no. 12 (2008): 1294–99, https://doi.org/10.1001/archinte.168.12.1294.

54. Joyce L. Browne et al., "The Willingness to Participate in Biomedical Research Involving Human Beings in Low- and Middle-Income Countries: A Systematic Review," *Tropical Medicine and International Health* 24, no. 3 (2019): 264–79, https://doi.org/10.1111/tmi.13195.

55. Jennifer S. Hawkins and Ezekiel J. Emanuel, *Exploitation and Developing Countries: The Ethics of Clinical Research* (Princeton, NJ: Princeton University Press, 2008).

56. Peter Lurie and Sidney Wolfe, "The Developing World as the 'Answer' to the Dreams of Pharmaceutical Companies: The Surfaxin Story," in *Ethical Issues in International Biomedical Research: A Casebook*, ed. Ezekiel J. Emanuel, Christine Grady, and Elizabeth Wahl (Oxford: Oxford University Press, 2007): 159–170.

57. Marcia Angell, "Investigators' Responsibilities for Human Subjects in Developing Countries," *New England Journal of Medicine* 342, no. 13 (2000): 967–69, https://doi.org/10.1056/NEJM200003303421309.

58. Hawkins and Emanuel, *Exploitation and Developing Countries*.

59. Leonard H. Glantz et al., "Research in Developing Countries: Taking 'Benefit' Seriously," *Hastings Center Report* 28, no. 6 (1998): 38.

60. Segun Gbadegesin and David Wendler, "Protecting Communities in Health Research from Exploitation," *Bioethics* 20, no. 5 (2006): 248–53, https://doi.org/10.1111/j.1467-8519.2006.00501.x.

61. Angela Ballantyne, "HIV International Clinical Research: Exploitation and Risk," *Bioethics* 19, no. 5–6 (2005): 476–91, https://doi.org/10.1111/j.1467-8519.2005.00459.x.

62. David Orentlicher, "Universality and Its Limits: When Research Ethics Can Reflect Local Circumstances," *Journal of Law, Medicine and Ethics* 30, no. 3 (2002): 403–10, https://doi.org/10.1111/j.1748-720X.2002.tb00409.x.

63. Maged El Setouhy et al., "Moral Standards for Research in Developing Countries from 'Reasonable Availability' to 'Fair Benefits,'" *Hastings Center Report* 34, no. 3 (2004): 17–27, https://doi.org/10.2307/3528416.

64. Ruth J. Sample, *Exploitation: What It Is and Why It's Wrong* (Lanham, MD: Rowman and Littlefield, 2003).

65. Alan Wertheimer, *Rethinking the Ethics of Clinical Research: Widening the Lens* (Oxford: Oxford University Press, 2010), 239.

66. Thomas Pogge, "Testing Our Drugs on the Poor Abroad," in *Exploitation and Developing Countries: The Ethics of Clinical Research*, ed. Jennifer S. Hawkins and Ezekiel Emanuel (Princeton, NJ: Princeton University Press, 2008): 105–141.

67. David B. Resnik, "Exploitation in Biomedical Research," *Theoretical Medicine and Bioethics* 24, no. 3 (2003): 233–59, https://doi.org/10.1023/A:1024811830049.

68. Hillel Steiner, "A Liberal Theory of Exploitation," *Ethics* 94, no. 2 (1984): 225–41, https://doi.org/10.1086/292529.

69. Pogge, "Testing Our Drugs on the Poor Abroad," 113.

70. Iris Marion Young, *Responsibility for Justice* (Oxford: Oxford University Press, 2010).

71. Thomas Pogge, "World Poverty and Human Rights," *Ethics and International Affairs* 19, no. 1 (2005): 1–7, https://doi.org/10.1111/j.1747-7093.2005.tb00484.x.

72. Thomas Pogge, "Access to Medicines," *Public Health Ethics* 1, no. 2 (2008): 73–82.

73. Benjamin Freedman, "Equipoise and the Ethics of Clinical Research," *New England Journal of Medicine* 317, no. 3 (1987): 141–45, https://doi.org/10.1056/NEJM198707163170304.

74. David B. Resnik, "The Clinical Investigator-Subject Relationship: A Contextual Approach," *Philosophy, Ethics, and Humanities in Medicine* 4, no. 1 (2009): 16, https://doi.org/10.1186/1747-5341-4-16.

75. Franklin G. Miller and Howard Brody, "Clinical Equipoise and the Incoherence of Research Ethics," *Journal of Medicine and Philosophy: A Forum for Bioethics and Philosophy of Medicine* 32, no. 2 (2007): 151–65, https://doi.org/10.1080/03605310701255750.

76. Henry S. Richardson, *Moral Entanglements: The Ancillary-Care Obligations of Medical Researchers* (Oxford: Oxford University Press, 2012).

77. Henry S. Richardson and Leah Belsky, "The Ancillary-Care Responsibilities of Medical Researchers: An Ethical Framework for Thinking about the Clinical Care That Researchers Owe Their Subjects," *Hastings Center Report* 34, no. 1 (2004): 25–33, https://doi.org/10.2307/3528248.

78. Resnik, "The Clinical Investigator-Subject Relationship."

79. Resnik, "The Clinical Investigator-Subject Relationship."

80. Miller, "Phase I Cancer Trials."

81. Miller, "Phase I Cancer Trials," 41.

82. Alex Dubov, "Moral Justification of Phase 1 Oncology Trials," *Journal of Pain and Palliative Care Pharmacotherapy* 28, no. 2 (2014): 138–51, https://doi.org/10.3109/15360288.2014.908994.
83. Kenneth Kipnis, "Vulnerability in Research Subjects: A Bioethical Taxonomy," in *Ethical and Policy Issues in Research Involving Human Participants*, vol. 2 (Bethesda, MD: National Bioethics Advisory Commission, 2001): G1–G13.
84. Resnik, "Therapeutic Misconception, Unrealistic Optimism, and Hope in Phase I Oncology Trials."
85. Resnik, "The Clinical Investigator-Subject Relationship."
86. Nancy S. Jecker, "Exploiting Subjects in Placebo-Controlled Trials," *American Journal of Bioethics* 2, no. 2 (2002): 19–20.

Chapter 6

1. Alexandra Thompson, "Parents of Autistic Boy Hope to Raise £26,500 for Stem Cell Treatment," *Daily Mail*, January 23, 2019, https://www.dailymail.co.uk/health/article-6623311/Parents-non-verbal-autistic-boy-hope-raise-26-500-pay-stem-cell-treatment-Miami.html.
2. Geraldine Dawson et al., "Autologous Cord Blood Infusions Are Safe and Feasible in Young Children with Autism Spectrum Disorder: Results of a Single-Center Phase I Open-Label Trial," *Stem Cells Translational Medicine* 6, no. 5 (2017): 1332–39.
3. Michael Chez et al., "Safety and Observations from a Placebo-Controlled, Crossover Study to Assess Use of Autologous Umbilical Cord Blood Stem Cells to Improve Symptoms in Children with Autism," *Stem Cells Translational Medicine* 7, no. 4 (2018): 333–41.
4. Nidhi Subbaraman, "Experts Balk at Large Trial of Stem Cells for Autism," *Spectrum* (blog), July 14, 2014, https://www.spectrumnews.org/news/experts-balk-at-large-trial-of-stem-cells-for-autism/.
5. Alexandra Thompson, "Parents of an Autistic Boy, 11, Claim He Spoke His First Full Sentence," *Daily Mail*, April 11, 2019, https://www.dailymail.co.uk/health/article-6912381/Parents-non-verbal-autistic-schoolboy-11-claim-spoke-sentence.html.
6. Insoo Hyun, "The Bioethics of Stem Cell Research and Therapy," *Journal of Clinical Investigation* 120, no. 1 (2010): 71–75.
7. Gerhard Bauer, Magdi Elsallab, and Mohamed Abou-El-Enein, "Concise Review: A Comprehensive Analysis of Reported Adverse Events in

Patients Receiving Unproven Stem Cell-Based Interventions," *Stem Cells Translational Medicine* 7, no. 9 (2018): 676–85.

8. Megan Munsie and Insoo Hyun, "A Question of Ethics: Selling Autologous Stem Cell Therapies Flaunts Professional Standards," *Stem Cell Research* 13, no. 3 (2014): 647–53.

9. Leigh Turner, "The US Direct-to-Consumer Marketplace for Autologous Stem Cell Interventions," *Perspectives in Biology and Medicine* 61, no. 1 (2018): 7–24.

10. Douglas Sipp, Pamela G. Robey, and Leigh Turner, "Clear up This Stem-Cell Mess," *Nature* 561, no. 7724 (2018): 455–57.

11. Bauer, Elsallab, and Abou-El-Enein, "Concise Review."

12. Ajay E. Kuriyan et al., "Vision Loss after Intravitreal Injection of Autologous 'Stem Cells' for AMD," *New England Journal of Medicine* 376, no. 11 (2017): 1047–53.

13. Ruairi Connolly, Timothy O'Brien, and Gerard Flaherty, "Stem Cell Tourism: A Web-Based Analysis of Clinical Services Available to International Travellers," *Travel Medicine and Infectious Disease* 12, no. 6 (2014): 695–701.

14. Paul S. Knoepfler and Leigh G. Turner, "The FDA and the US Direct-to-Consumer Marketplace for Stem Cell Interventions: A Temporal Analysis," *Regenerative Medicine* 13, no. 1 (2018): 19–27.

15. International Society for Stem Cell Research, *Guidelines for the Clinical Translation of Stem Cells* (Skokie, IL: International Society for Stem Cell Research, 2008), 4.

16. Judy Illes and Fabio Rossi, "Opinion: No Miracle Therapy for Stroke," *Vancouver Sun*, February 12, 2015, http://www.vancouversun.com/health/Opinion+miracle+therapy+stroke/10787468/story.html.

17. Alan C. Regenberg et al., "Medicine on the Fringe: Stem Cell-Based Interventions in Advance of Evidence," *Stem Cells* 27, no. 9 (2009): 2312–19.

18. Connolly, O'Brien, and Flaherty, "Stem Cell Tourism: A Web-Based Analysis of Clinical Services Available to International Travellers."

19. Israel Berger et al., "Global Distribution of Businesses Marketing Stem Cell-Based Interventions," *Cell Stem Cell* 19, no. 2 (2016): 158–62.

20. Leigh Turner and Paul Knoepfler, "Selling Stem Cells in the USA: Assessing the Direct-to-Consumer Industry," *Cell Stem Cell* 19, no. 2 (2016): 154–57.

21. Turner, "The US Direct-to-Consumer Marketplace for Autologous Stem Cell Interventions."

22. Knoepfler and Turner, "The FDA and the US Direct-to-Consumer Marketplace for Stem Cell Interventions."

23. Leigh Turner, "Direct-to-Consumer Marketing of Stem Cell Interventions by Canadian Businesses," *Regenerative Medicine* 13, no. 6 (2018): 643–58.

24. Turner, "The US Direct-to-Consumer Marketplace for Autologous Stem Cell Interventions."

25. Knoepfler and Turner, "The FDA and the US Direct-to-Consumer Marketplace for Stem Cell Interventions."

26. Douglas Sipp, "The Malignant Niche: Safe Spaces for Toxic Stem Cell Marketing," *NPJ Regenerative Medicine* 2, no. 1 (2017): 33.

27. Health Canada, "Health Canada Policy Position Paper—Autologous Cell Therapy Products," May 15, 2019, https://www.canada.ca/en/health-canada/services/drugs-health-products/biologics-radiopharmaceuticals-genetic-therapies/applications-submissions/guidance-documents/cell-therapy-policy.html.

28. Paul S. Knoepfler, "The Stem Cell Hard Sell: Report from a Clinic's Patient Recruitment Seminar," *Stem Cells Translational Medicine* 6, no. 1 (2017): 14–16.

29. Connolly, O'Brien, and Flaherty, "Stem Cell Tourism: A Web-Based Analysis of Clinical Services Available to International Travellers."

30. Liz Szabo, "Doctor Accused of Selling False Hope to Families," *USA Today*, November 15, 2013, https://www.usatoday.com/story/news/nation/2013/11/15/stanislaw-burzynski-cancer-controversy/2994561/.

31. Melissa Martin and Mary Agnes Welch, "City Man Who Ran Stem-Cell Trial for MS Patients Fabricated Credentials, Overstated Results," *Winnipeg Free Press*, January 13, 2015, https://www.winnipegfreepress.com/breakingnews/Sufferers-feel-swindled-288496041.html.

32. Martin and Welch, "City Man Who Ran Stem-Cell Trial for MS Patients Fabricated Credentials, Overstated Results."

33. Turner, "Direct-to-Consumer Marketing of Stem Cell Interventions by Canadian Businesses."

34. Blake Murdoch, Amy Zarzeczny, and Timothy Caulfield, "Exploiting Science? A Systematic Analysis of Complementary and Alternative Medicine Clinic Websites' Marketing of Stem Cell Therapies," *BMJ Open* 8, no. 2 (2018): e019414.

35. Alan Petersen and Kate Seear, "Technologies of Hope: Techniques of the Online Advertising of Stem Cell Treatments," *New Genetics and Society* 30, no. 4 (2011): 329–46.

36. Petersen and Seear, "Technologies of Hope," 334.

37. Alan Petersen et al., "Selling Hope in China," in *Stem Cell Tourism and the Political Economy of Hope*, ed. Alan Petersen et al. (London: Palgrave Macmillan, 2017), 121–54.

38. Berger et al., "Global Distribution of Businesses Marketing Stem Cell-Based Interventions."

39. Christen M. Rachul, Ivona Percec, and Timothy Caulfield, "The Fountain of Stem Cell-Based Youth? Online Portrayals of Anti-Aging Stem Cell Technologies," *Aesthetic Surgery Journal* 35, no. 6 (2015): 730–36.

40. Turner, "Direct-to-Consumer Marketing of Stem Cell Interventions by Canadian Businesses."

41. Knoepfler, "The Stem Cell Hard Sell."

42. Christopher Thomas Scott, Mindy C. DeRouen, and LaVera M. Crawley, "The Language of Hope: Therapeutic Intent in Stem-Cell Clinical Trials," *AJOB Primary Research* 1, no. 3 (2010): 4–11.

43. Turner, "Direct-to-Consumer Marketing of Stem Cell Interventions by Canadian Businesses."

44. Connolly, O'Brien, and Flaherty, "Stem Cell Tourism: A Web-Based Analysis of Clinical Services Available to International Travellers."

45. Darren Lau et al., "Stem Cell Clinics Online: The Direct-to-Consumer Portrayal of Stem Cell Medicine," *Cell Stem Cell* 3, no. 6 (2008): 591–94.

46. Alessandro R. Marcon, Blake Murdoch, and Timothy Caulfield, "Fake News Portrayals of Stem Cells and Stem Cell Research," *Regenerative Medicine* 12, no. 7 (2017): 765–75.

47. Kalina Kamenova and Timothy Caulfield, "Stem Cell Hype: Media Portrayal of Therapy Translation," *Science Translational Medicine* 7, no. 278 (2015): 1–4.

48. Ubaka Ogbogu et al., "Chinese Newspaper Coverage of (Unproven) Stem Cell Therapies and Their Providers," *Stem Cell Reviews and Reports* 9, no. 2 (2013): 111–18.

49. Christen Rachul, John E. J. Rasko, and Timothy Caulfield, "Implicit Hype? Representations of Platelet Rich Plasma in the News Media," *PloS One* 12, no. 8 (2017): e0182496.

50. International Society for Stem Cell Research, *Guidelines for Stem Cell Research and Clinical Translation* (Skokie, IL: International Society for Stem Cell Research, 2008), 26.

51. Alan Petersen, Kate Seear, and Megan Munsie, "Therapeutic Journeys: The Hopeful Travails of Stem Cell Tourists," *Sociology of Health and Illness* 36, no. 5 (2014): 670–85, 672.

52. Sorapop Kiatpongsan and Douglas Sipp, "Offshore Stem Cell Treatments," *Nature Reports Stem Cells*, 2008. https://www.nature.com/articles/stemcells.2008.151

53. Hyun, "The Bioethics of Stem Cell Research and Therapy."

54. Charles E. Murdoch and Christopher Thomas Scott, "Stem Cell Tourism and the Power of Hope," *American Journal of Bioethics* 10, no. 5 (2010): 16–23, 19.

55. A. Blight et al., "Position Statement on the Sale of Unproven Cellular Therapies for Spinal Cord Injury The International Campaign for Cures of Spinal Cord Injury Paralysis," *Spinal Cord* 47, no. 9 (2009): 713–14.

56. Clare Dyer, "Doctor Is Found Guilty of Exploiting 'Desperate' MS Patients," *BMJ: British Medical Journal* 340 (2010). https://www.bmj.com/content/340/bmj.c2009

57. Dyer, "Doctor Is Found Guilty of Exploiting 'Desperate' MS Patients."

58. Alan Petersen, Casimir MacGregor, and Megan Munsie, "Stem Cell Tourism Exploits People by Marketing Hope," *The Conversation*, July 15, 2014, http://theconversation.com/stem-cell-tourism-exploits-people-by-marketing-hope-29146.

59. Carlos Novas, "The Political Economy of Hope: Patients' Organizations, Science and Biovalue," *BioSocieties* 1, no. 3 (2006): 289–305.

60. Jeremy Snyder et al., "'I Knew What Was Going to Happen If I Did Nothing and so I Was Going to Do Something': Faith, Hope, and Trust in the Decisions of Canadians with Multiple Sclerosis to Seek Unproven Interventions Abroad," *BMC Health Services Research* 14, no. 1 (2014): 445.

61. Petersen, Seear, and Munsie, "Therapeutic Journeys," 675.

62. Petersen, Seear, and Munsie, "Therapeutic Journeys," 675.

63. Ubaka Ogbogu, Jenny Du, and Yonida Koukio, "The Involvement of Canadian Physicians in Promoting and Providing Unproven and Unapproved Stem Cell Interventions," *BMC Medical Ethics* 19, no. 1 (2018): 32.

64. Turner and Knoepfler, "Selling Stem Cells in the USA."

65. Wayne Fu et al., "Characteristics and Scope of Training of Clinicians Participating in the US Direct-to-Consumer Marketplace for Unproven Stem Cell Interventions," *JAMA* 321, no. 24 (2019): 2463–64.

66. "Home: Stem Cell Treatments," Cell Surgical Network, accessed October 29, 2019, https://stemcellrevolution.com/.

67. "Regenexx: Stem Cell Therapy and Platelet Rich Plasma for Arthritis and Injuries," Regenexx, accessed October 29, 2019, https://regenexx.com/.

68. "Ontario Stem Cell Treatment Centre—Dr. Eric Robinson, Orthopaedic Surgeon; Dr. Barr, Plastic Surgeon," Ontario Stem Cell Treatment Centre, accessed October 29, 2019, https://stemcellrepair.ca/staff/.

69. American Medical Association Council on Ethical and Judicial Affairs, *Code of Medical Ethics: Current Opinions with Annotations* (Chicago, IL: AMA Press, 2006).

70. American Medical Association Council on Ethical and Judicial Affairs, *Code of Medical Ethics*, section 1.2.11.

71. General Medical Council, *Good Medical Practice* (Manchester, UK: General Medical Council, 2014), https://www.gmc-uk.org/-/media/documents/good-medical-practice---english-1215_pdf-51527435.pdf.

72. Canadian Medical Association, *Code of Ethics and Professionalism* (Ottawa, ON: Canadian Medical Association, 2018), https://policybase.cma.ca/documents/policypdf/PD19-03.pdf.

73. Medical Board of Australia, "Good Medical Practice: A Code of Conduct for Doctors in Australia" (Medical Board of Australia, 2014), Section 1.4, https://www.medicalboard.gov.au/Codes-Guidelines-Policies/Code-of-conduct.aspx.

74. Medical Board of Australia, "Good Medical Practice," Section 8.6.

75. Medical Board of Australia, "Good Medical Practice," Section 8.11.

76. Medical Board of Australia, "Good Medical Practice," Section 8.12.

77. European Council of Medical Orders, "Principles of European Medical Ethics" (European Council of Medical Orders, 1995), http://www.ceom-ecmo.eu/en/view/principles-of-european-medical-ethics.

78. European Council of Medical Orders, "Principles of European Medical Ethics," Article 2.

79. European Council of Medical Orders, "Principles of European Medical Ethics," Appendix B.

80. European Council of Medical Orders, "Principles of European Medical Ethics," Article 10.

81. World Medical Association, "World Medical Association International Code of Medical Ethics" (World Medical Association, 2006), https://www.wma.net/policies-post/wma-international-code-of-medical-ethics/.

82. Munsie and Hyun, "A Question of Ethics."

83. American Board of Internal Medicine, "Medical Professionalism in the New Millennium: A Physician Charter," *Annals of Internal Medicine* 136, no. 3 (2002): 243.

84. Munsie and Hyun, "A Question of Ethics," 650.

85. International Society for Stem Cell Research, *Guidelines for the Stem Cell Research and Clinical Translation*, 25.
86. Aaron D. Levine and Leslie E. Wolf, "The Roles and Responsibilities of Physicians in Patients' Decisions about Unproven Stem Cell Therapies," *Journal of Law, Medicine and Ethics* 40, no. 1 (2012): 122–34.
87. A. Caplan and B. Levine, "Hope, Hype and Help: Ethically Assessing the Growing Market in Stem Cell Therapies," *American Journal of Bioethics* 10, no. 5 (2010): 24.
88. Tamra Lysaght et al., "Ethical and Regulatory Challenges with Autologous Adult Stem Cells: A Comparative Review of International Regulations," *Journal of Bioethical Inquiry* 14, no. 2 (2017): 261–73.
89. Health Canada, "Health Canada Policy Position Paper—Autologous Cell Therapy Products."
90. I. Glenn Cohen and Shelly Simana, "Regulation of Stem Cell Therapy Travel," *Current Stem Cell Reports* 4, no. 3 (2018): 220–27.
91. Amy Zarzeczny et al., "Professional Regulation: A Potentially Valuable Tool in Responding to 'Stem Cell Tourism,'" *Stem Cell Reports* 3, no. 3 (2014): 379–84.
92. Jeremy Snyder et al., "Navigating Physicians' Ethical and Legal Duties to Patients Seeking Unproven Interventions Abroad," *Canadian Family Physician* 61, no. 7 (2015): 584–86.
93. Harold Atkins, "Stem Cell Transplantation to Treat Multiple Sclerosis," *JAMA* 321, no. 2 (2019): 153–55.
94. Richard K. Burt et al., "Effect of Nonmyeloablative Hematopoietic Stem Cell Transplantation vs Continued Disease-Modifying Therapy on Disease Progression in Patients with Relapsing-Remitting Multiple Sclerosis: A Randomized Clinical Trial," *JAMA* 321, no. 2 (2019): 165–74.
95. "HSCT México," accessed October 29, 2019, https://www.hsctmexico.com/index.php?lng=eng.
96. Paul Knoepfler, "Upbeat Burt Team Pub on Stem Cells for MS Comes with Uneasy Back Story," *The Niche* (blog), January 20, 2019, https://ipscell.com/2019/01/upbeat-burt-team-pub-on-stem-cells-for-ms-comes-with-uneasy-back-story/.
97. Sarah Chan, "Current and Emerging Global Themes in the Bioethics of Regenerative Medicine: The Tangled Web of Stem Cell Translation," *Regenerative Medicine* 12, no. 7 (2017): 839–51, 844.
98. "Vital Medical Center," accessed October 29, 2019, http://vitalmedicalcenterinc.com/.

99. Leslie Josephs, "Costa Rica Puts Brakes on Popular Stem Cell Tourism," *Reuters*, June 6, 2010, https://www.reuters.com/article/uk-costarica-stemcells-idUKTRE6560HU20100607.

100. Alan Petersen et al., "Managing Hope," in *Stem Cell Tourism and the Political Economy of Hope* (London: Springer, 2017), 59–82.

Chapter 7

1. My Right to Try Now, *Matt Bellina's Case for The Right to Try*, 2017, https://www.youtube.com/watch?v=n-t9j8mvbNE.

2. Rebecca Dresser, "'Right to Try' Laws: The Gap between Experts and Advocates," *Hastings Center Report* 45, no. 3 (2015): 9–10.

3. André Picard, "Do the Dying Have the Right to Experimental Drugs?," *Globe and Mail*, April 11, 2018, sec. Opinion, https://www.theglobeandmail.com/opinion/do-the-dying-have-the-right-to-experimental-drugs/article24377706/.

4. Diana Zuckerman, "Right to Try National Law Would Exploit False Hope," *National Center for Health Research* (blog), March 16, 2017, http://www.center4research.org/right-to-try-exploit-false-hope/.

5. Kelly Folkers, Carolyn Chapman, and Barbara Redman, "Federal Right to Try: Where Is It Going?," *Hastings Center Report* 49, no. 2 (2019): 26–36.

6. Patricia J. Zettler and Henry T. Greely, "The Strange Allure of State 'Right-to-Try' Laws," *JAMA Internal Medicine* 174, no. 12 (2014): 1885–86.

7. Thomas J. Hwang, Jonathan J. Darrow, and Aaron S. Kesselheim, "The FDA's Expedited Programs and Clinical Development Times for Novel Therapeutics, 2012–2016," *JAMA* 318, no. 21 (2017): 2137–38.

8. Zettler and Greely, "The Strange Allure of State 'Right-to-Try' Laws."

9. Alison Bateman-House et al., "Right-to-Try Laws: Hope, Hype, and Unintended Consequences," *Annals of Internal Medicine* 163, no. 10 (2015): 796–97.

10. Folkers, Chapman, and Redman, "Federal Right to Try."

11. Zettler and Greely, "The Strange Allure of State 'Right-to-Try' Laws."

12. Kenneth I. Moch, "Ethical Crossroads: Expanded Access, Patient Advocacy, and the #SaveJosh Social Media Campaign," *Medicine Access@ Point of Care* 1, no. 1 (2017): e119–30.

13. Zachary Brennan, "Who's Actually Using 'Right-To-Try' Laws? A Texas Oncologist Explains His Experience," *Regulatory Focus*, August 4, 2017, https://www.raps.org/regulatory-focus%E2%84%A2/news-articles/2017/8/who-s-actually-using-right-to-try-laws-a-texas-oncologist-explains-his-experience.

14. Arthur L. Caplan and Alison Bateman-House, "Should Patients in Need Be Given Access to Experimental Drugs?," *Expert Opinion on Pharmacotherapy* 16, no. 9 (2015): 1275–79, 1277.

15. Alison Bateman-House and Christopher T. Robertson, "The Federal Right to Try Act of 2017: A Wrong Turn for Access to Investigational Drugs and the Path Forward," *JAMA Internal Medicine* 178, no. 3 (2018): 321–22.

16. Holly Fernandez Lynch, Patricia J. Zettler, and Ameet Sarpatwari, "Promoting Patient Interests in Implementing the Federal Right to Try Act," *JAMA* 320, no. 9 (2018): 869–70.

17. Mark Flatten, *Dead on Arrival: Federal* "Compassionate Use" *Leaves Little Hope for Dying Patients* (Phoenix, AZ: Goldwater Institute, February 24, 2016), https://goldwaterinstitute.org/wp-content/uploads/2016/02/Dead-On-Arrival-Report.pdf.

18. Flatten, "Dead on Arrival," 2.

19. Flatten, "Dead on Arrival," 27.

20. Lilia Luciano, "Former Fire Captain's Fight for His 'Right to Try' and the Debate over Compassionate Use," KXTV, February 21, 2017, https://www.abc10.com/article/news/local/former-fire-captains-fight-for-his-right-to-try-and-the-debate-over-compassionate-use/103-397072418.

21. Ron Johnson, "The Terminally Ill Deserve Right-to-Try Laws," *Wall Street Journal*, September 22, 2016, https://www.wsj.com/articles/the-terminally-ill-deserve-right-to-try-laws-1474586032.

22. Nathan Nascimento et al., "Letter to the Honorable Greg Walden," January 8, 2018, https://freedompartners.org/wp-content/uploads/2018/01/RTT-Letter-to-Chairman-Walden-1.5.18-3.pdf.

23. Christina Corieri, "Everyone Deserves the Right to Try: Empowering the Terminally Ill to Take Control of Their Treatment," *Policy Report*, no. 266 (2014): 1–30, 1.

24. Corieri, "Everyone Deserves the Right to Try," 14

25. Corieri, "Everyone Deserves the Right to Try," 16, 20.

26. Erin Mershon, "'Right-to-Try' Intended to Weaken FDA, Key Senator Says in Blunt Remarks," *STAT*, May 31, 2018, https://www.statnews.com/2018/05/31/right-to-try-ron-johnson/.

27. Rebecca Dresser, "The Right to Try Investigational Drugs: Science and Stories in the Access Debate," *Texas Law Review* 93, no. 7 (2014): 1631–57.

28. Ashley F. Lanzel and James V. Lavery, "Unintended Consequences of the Right to Try Act for Palliative Care in Pediatric Oncology," *JAMA Oncology* 5, no. 5 (2019): 603–4.

29. Julie A. Jacob, "Questions of Safety and Fairness Raised as Right-to-Try Movement Gains Steam," *JAMA* 314, no. 8 (2015): 758–60.

30. Michele Munz, "Missouri's 'Right to Try' Law No Guarantee Patient Will Get Experimental Drugs," *St. Louis Post-Dispatch*, May 20, 2015, https://www.stltoday.com/news/local/metro/missouri-s-right-to-try-law-no-guarantee-patient-will/article_05c07958-5217-5c3f-9f15-1a43c8a3e740.html.

31. Jacob, "Questions of Safety and Fairness Raised as Right-to-Try Movement Gains Steam."

32. Dresser, " 'Right to Try' Laws."

33. Jonathan P. Jarow and Richard Moscicki, "Impact of Expanded Access on FDA Regulatory Action and Product Labeling," *Therapeutic Innovation and Regulatory Science* 51, no. 6 (2017): 787–89.

34. Bateman-House and Robertson, "The Federal Right to Try Act of 2017: A Wrong Turn for Access to Investigational Drugs and the Path Forward."

35. Steven Joffe and Holly Fernandez Lynch, "Federal Right-to-Try Legislation: Threatening the FDA's Public Health Mission," *New England Journal of Medicine* 378, no. 8 (2018): 695.

36. Joffe and Fernandez Lynch, "Federal Right-to-Try Legislation: Threatening the FDA's Public Health Mission."

37. Nicholas Florko, "When 'Right to Try' Isn't Enough," *STAT*, May 31, 2019, https://www.statnews.com/2019/05/31/when-right-to-try-isnt-enough/.

38. Florko, "When 'Right to Try' Isn't Enough."

39. Florko, "When 'Right to Try' Isn't Enough."

40. Florko, "When 'Right to Try' Isn't Enough."

41. Michael Carome and Sarah Sorscher, Letter to Congress Regarding S. 204, H.R. 878, and H.R. 1020, March 6, 2017, https://www.citizen.org/wp-content/uploads/migration/2362.pdf.

42. Bateman-House et al., "Right-to-Try Laws."

43. Bateman-House et al., "Right-to-Try Laws."

44. Folkers, Chapman, and Redman, "Federal Right to Try," 32.

45. Erin Mershon, "Trump Signs Right-to-Try Legislation, Widening Access to Experimental Drugs," *STAT*, May 30, 2018, https://www.statnews.com/2018/05/30/trump-signs-right-to-try/.

46. Therapeutic Solutions International Inc., "Therapeutic Solutions International Completes Phase 1 Clinical Trial in Advanced Cancer Patients for Right to Try Access of Its StemVacs Product for American Cancer Patients," *GlobeNewswire News Room*, September 4, 2018, http://www.globenewswire.com/news-release/2018/09/04/1564969/0/en/Therapeutic-Solutions-International-Completes-Phase-1-Clinical-Trial-in-Advanced-Cancer-Patients-for-Right-to-Try-Access-of-its-StemVacs-Product-for-American-Cancer-Patients.html.

47. Creative Medical Technology Holdings Inc., "Creative Medical Technology Holdings Aims to Treat Cancer Associated Wasting (Cachexia) Using AmnioStem Universal Donor Stem Cell," *PR Newswire*, July 6, 2018, https://www.prnewswire.com/news-releases/creative-medical-technology-holdings-aims-to-treat-cancer-associated-wasting-cachexia-using-amniostem-universal-donor-stem-cell-300676909.html.
48. Naomi Lopez Bauman, "Right to Try Program Offers Hope to Brain Cancer Patients," *Goldwater Institute* (blog), October 3, 2019, https://goldwaterinstitute.org/article/the-first-announced-right-to-try-program-offers-hope-to-brain-cancer-patients/.
49. Nicholas Florko, "A Year after Trump Touted Right to Try, Patients Still Aren't Getting Treatment," *STAT*, January 29, 2019, https://www.statnews.com/2019/01/29/right-to-try-patients-still-arent-getting-treatment/.
50. Kelly Folkers and Alison Bateman-House, "Glioblastoma Patient Is First to Receive Treatment under Right to Try: Our Question Is Why?," *Cancer Letter*, February 1, 2019, https://cancerletter.com/articles/20190201_6/.
51. Anna Hopkins, "Millennial Fighting Rare Bone Cancer Responds to Biden Vow: Law Supported by Trump Helped Save My Life," Fox News, June 14, 2019, https://www.foxnews.com/politics/millennial-cancer-joe-biden-trump-right-try-saved-life.
52. Zachary Brennan, "Right to Try One Year Later: Limited Patient Involvement but More FDA Clarity Coming," *Regulatory Focus*, May 30, 2019, https://www.raps.org/news-and-articles/news-articles/2019/5/right-to-try-one-year-later-limited-patient-invol.
53. Zettler and Greely, "The Strange Allure of State 'Right-to-Try' Laws," 1886.
54. D. Theodore Rave, "Politicians as Fiduciaries," *Harvard Law Review* 126, no. 3 (2013): 671–739.
55. Helen Norton, "The Government's Lies and the Constitution," *Indiana Law Journal* 91, no 1 (2015): 73–120.
56. Sissela Bok, *Lying: Moral Choice in Public and Private Life* (New York: Vintage, 1999).
57. Martin Jay, *The Virtues of Mendacity: On Lying in Politics* (Charlottesville: University of Virginia Press, 2010).
58. Goldwater Institute, *Right to Try Is All about Hope for Patients like Jordan*, 2018, https://www.youtube.com/watch?v=54bkoy7UWWw.
59. "Right to Try," Ambrose Cell Therapy, accessed October 30, 2019, https://ambrosecelltherapy.com/right-to-try/.
60. Kasper Raus, "An Analysis of Common Ethical Justifications for Compassionate Use Programs for Experimental Drugs," *BMC Medical Ethics* 17, no. 1 (2016): 60.

61. Food and Drug Administration, "Charging for Investigational Drugs under an IND: Questions and Answers," June 2016, https://www.fda.gov/media/85682/download.

62. Fernandez Lynch, Zettler, and Sarpatwari, "Promoting Patient Interests in Implementing the Federal Right to Try Act," 870.

63. Michelle Cortez, "The 'Right to Try' Could Cost Dying Patients a Fortune," *Bloomberg*, June 20, 2018, https://www.bloomberg.com/news/articles/2018-06-20/the-price-to-try-a-drug-could-be-300-000-for-dying-patients.

64. David Gorski, "As I Predicted, the Exploitation of Desperate Patients Using Right-to-Try Begins," *Respectful Insolence* (blog), June 22, 2018, https://respectfulinsolence.com/2018/06/22/as-i-predicted-the-exploitation-of-patients-under-right-to-try-begins/.

65. Tova Cohen, "BrainStorm Will Not Provide ALS Therapy under U.S. Right to Try Act," *Reuters*, June 26, 2018, https://www.reuters.com/article/us-health-brainstorm-cell-als-exclusive-idUSKBN1JM1BE.

66. Ido Efrati, "Foreign Patients to Subsidize Experimental Treatment for Israelis With ALS," *Haaretz*, February 20, 2019, https://www.haaretz.com/israel-news/.premium-foreign-patients-to-subsidize-experimental-treatment-for-israelis-with-als-1.6956407.

67. Bateman-House et al., "Right-to-Try Laws," 796.

68. Bateman-House et al., "Right-to-Try Laws," 797.

69. Folkers, Chapman, and Redman, "Federal Right to Try."

70. Raus, "An Analysis of Common Ethical Justifications for Compassionate Use Programs for Experimental Drugs," 6.

71. Bateman-House and Robertson, "The Federal Right to Try Act of 2017: A Wrong Turn for Access to Investigational Drugs and the Path Forward."

72. Eline M. Bunnik, Nikkie Aarts, and Suzanne van de Vathorst, "Little to Lose and No Other Options: Ethical Issues in Efforts to Facilitate Expanded Access to Investigational Drugs," *Health Policy* 122, no. 9 (2018): 977–83.

73. Folkers, Chapman, and Redman, "Federal Right to Try."

74. Bateman-House and Robertson, "The Federal Right to Try Act of 2017: A Wrong Turn for Access to Investigational Drugs and the Path Forward."

75. Fernandez Lynch, Zettler, and Sarpatwari, "Promoting Patient Interests in Implementing the Federal Right to Try Act."

76. Nicholas Florko, "Fed Up with FDA, ALS Advocates Consider a Take-No-Prisoners Approach," *STAT*, June 7, 2019, https://www.statnews.com/2019/06/07/als-advocates-protest-fda/.

77. Arthur Caplan, "Forget Right-to-Try Laws: Our Process Is More Effective and Ethical," *STAT*, June 3, 2019, https://www.statnews.com/2019/06/03/effective-ethical-right-to-try-process/.

78. Florko, "A Year after Trump Touted Right to Try, Patients Still Aren't Getting Treatment."

79. *Freedom and the FDA: The Matt Bellina Story*, accessed October 30, 2019, https://www.youtube.com/watch?v=IE6mzkPSVR8.

Chapter 8

1. Melanie Newman and Jim Reed, "Cancer Crowdfunding 'Couldn't Save My Daughter,'" *BBC News*, March 6, 2019, https://www.bbc.com/news/health-47442946.

2. Helen Sproates, "Gemma Nuttall Cancer Fund," GoFundMe, October 22, 2016, https://www.gofundme.com/f/teamgemma.

3. Charlotte Green, "Miracle Mum Gemma Nuttall 'Cancer-Free' after Immunotherapy Success," *Rossendale Free Press*, October 19, 2017, http://www.rossendalefreepress.co.uk/news/miracle-mum-gemma-nuttall-cancer-13780804.

4. Celena Chong, "A Group of Investors Is Buying GoFundMe," *Business Insider*, June 24, 2015, https://www.businessinsider.com/a-group-of-investors-is-buying-gofundme-2015-6.

5. Ingrid Lunden, "GoFundMe Acquires CrowdRise to Expand to Fundraising for Charities," *TechCrunch*, January 10, 2017, https://techcrunch.com/2017/01/10/gofundme-buys-crowdrise-to-expand-to-fundraising-for-charities/.

6. Ainsley Harris, "How Crowdfunding Platform GoFundMe Has Created a $3 Billion Digital Safety Net," *Fast Company*, February 13, 2017, https://www.fastcompany.com/3067472/how-crowdfunding-platform-gofundme-has-created-a-3-billion-digital.

7. Nathan Heller, "The Hidden Cost of GoFundMe Health Care," *New Yorker*, June 24, 2019, https://www.newyorker.com/magazine/2019/07/01/the-perverse-logic-of-gofundme-health-care.

8. Carolyn McClanahan, "People Are Raising $650 Million on GoFundMe Each Year to Attack Rising Healthcare Costs," *Forbes*, August 13, 2018, https://www.forbes.com/sites/carolynmcclanahan/2018/08/13/using-gofundme-to-attack-health-care-costs/.

9. "Medical Fundraising: Start a Free Fundraiser," GoFundMe, accessed October 30, 2019, https://www.gofundme.com/start/medical-fundraising.

10. Martin Lukk, Erik Schneiderhan, and Joanne Soares, "Worthy? Crowdfunding the Canadian Health Care and Education Sectors," *Canadian Review of Sociology/Revue Canadienne de Sociologie* 55, no. 3 (2018): 404–24.

11. Jeremy Snyder et al., "Appealing to the Crowd: Ethical Justifications in Canadian Medical Crowdfunding Campaigns," *Journal of Medical Ethics* 43, no. 6 (2017): 364–67.

12. Lauren S. Berliner and Nora J. Kenworthy, "Producing a Worthy Illness: Personal Crowdfunding amidst Financial Crisis," *Social Science and Medicine* 187 (2017): 233–42.

13. Lukk, Schneiderhan, and Soares, "Worthy?"

14. Varsha Palad and Jeremy Snyder, "'We Don't Want Him Worrying about How He Will Pay to Save His Life': Using Medical Crowdfunding to Explore Lived Experiences with Addiction Services in Canada," *International Journal of Drug Policy* 65 (2019): 73–77.

15. Berliner and Kenworthy, "Producing a Worthy Illness."

16. Trena M. Paulus and Katherine R. Roberts, "Crowdfunding a 'Real-Life Superhero': The Construction of Worthy Bodies in Medical Campaign Narratives," *Discourse, Context and Media* 21 (2018): 64–72.

17. Snyder et al., "Appealing to the Crowd."

18. Paulus and Roberts, "Crowdfunding a 'Real-Life Superhero.'"

19. Chris A. Barcelos, "'Bye-Bye Boobies': Normativity, Deservingness and Medicalisation in Transgender Medical Crowdfunding," *Culture, Health and Sexuality* 21, no. 12 (2019): 1–15.

20. Jeremy Snyder, "Crowdfunding for Medical Care: Ethical Issues in an Emerging Health Care Funding Practice," *Hastings Center Report* 46, no. 6 (2016): 36–42.

21. Jake Hall, "How Crowdfunding Became a Lifeline for the Trans Community," *Vice*, August 27, 2018, https://www.vice.com/en_ca/article/9km7y7/ crowdfunding-transgender-transition-healthcare-inequality-costs.

22. David U. Himmelstein et al., "Medical Bankruptcy in the United States, 2007: Results of a National Study," *American Journal of Medicine* 122, no. 8 (2009): 741–46.

23. Consumer Financial Protection Bureau, *Consumer Credit Reports: A Study of Medical and Non-Medical Collections* (Washington, DC: Consumer Financial Protection Bureau, 2014), https://files.consumerfinance.gov/ f/201412_cfpb_reports_consumer-credit-medical-and-non-medical-collections.pdf.

24. David U. Himmelstein et al., "Medical Bankruptcy: Still Common Despite the Affordable Care Act," *American Journal of Public Health* 109, no. 3 (2019): 431–33.

25. Gordon Burtch and Jason Chan, "Investigating the Relationship between Medical Crowdfunding and Personal Bankruptcy in the United States: Evidence of a Digital Divide," *MIS Quarterly* 43, no. 1 (2019): 237–62.

26. Rachel Bluth, "GoFundMe CEO: 'Gigantic Gaps' in Health System Showing Up in Crowdfunding," *Kaiser Health News*, January 16, 2019, https://khn.org/news/gofundme-ceo-gigantic-gaps-in-health-system-showing-up-in-crowdfunding/.

27. Snyder, "Crowdfunding for Medical Care."

28. Snyder et al., "Appealing to the Crowd."

29. Wesley M. Durand et al., "Medical Crowdfunding for Organ Transplantation," *Clinical Transplantation* 32, no. 6 (2018): e13267.

30. Snyder, "Crowdfunding for Medical Care."

31. Alysha van Duynhoven et al., "Spatially Exploring the Intersection of Socioeconomic Status and Canadian Cancer-Related Medical Crowdfunding Campaigns," *BMJ Open* 9, no. 6 (2019): e026365.

32. Chris A. Barcelos and Stephanie L. Budge, "Inequalities in Crowdfunding for Transgender Health Care," *Transgender Health* 4, no. 1 (2019): 81–88.

33. Barcelos, " 'Bye-Bye Boobies.' "

34. Berliner and Kenworthy, "Producing a Worthy Illness."

35. Nikki Fritz and Amy Gonzales, "Not the Normal Trans Story: Negotiating Trans Narratives While Crowdfunding at the Margins," *International Journal of Communication* 12 (2018): 1189–208.

36. Amy L. Gonzales et al., "'Better Everyone Should Know Our Business than We Lose Our House': Costs and Benefits of Medical Crowdfunding for Support, Privacy, and Identity," *New Media and Society* 20, no. 2 (2018): 641–58.

37. Snyder, "Crowdfunding for Medical Care."

38. Ford Vox et al., "Medical Crowdfunding for Scientifically Unsupported or Potentially Dangerous Treatments," *JAMA* 320, no. 16 (2018): 1705–706.

39. Jeremy Snyder and Timothy Caulfield, "Patients' Crowdfunding Campaigns for Alternative Cancer Treatments," *Lancet Oncology* 20, no. 1 (2019): 28–29.

40. Melanie Newman, "Is Cancer Fundraising Fuelling Quackery?," *BMJ* 362 (2018): k3829.

41. Vox et al., "Medical Crowdfunding for Scientifically Unsupported or Potentially Dangerous Treatments."

42. Jeremy Snyder, Leigh Turner, and Valorie A. Crooks, "Crowdfunding for Unproven Stem Cell–Based Interventions," *JAMA* 319, no. 18 (2018): 1935–36.

43. Jeremy Snyder, Leigh Turner, and Valorie A. Crooks, "Crowdfunding for Unproven Stem Cell Procedures Spreads Misinformation," *STAT*, August 6, 2018, https://www.statnews.com/2018/08/06/crowdfunding-for-unproven-stem-cell-procedures-wastes-money-and-spreads-misinformation/.

44. Michael Hiltzik, "FDA Says StemGenex Marketing of Unproven Stem Cell Treatments Is Illegal," *Los Angeles Times*, November 16, 2018, https://www.latimes.com/business/hiltzik/la-fi-hiltzik-fda-stemgenex-20181116-story.html.

45. Jeremy Snyder and Leigh Turner, "Crowdfunding for Stem Cell-Based Interventions to Treat Neurologic Diseases and Injuries," *Neurology* 93, no. 6 (2019): 252–58.

46. Snyder and Turner, "Crowdfunding for Stem Cell-Based Interventions to Treat Neurologic Diseases and Injuries."

47. Heller, "The Hidden Cost of GoFundMe Health Care."

48. Newman, "Is Cancer Fundraising Fuelling Quackery?"

49. Snyder and Caulfield, "Patients' Crowdfunding Campaigns for Alternative Cancer Treatments."

50. Snyder and Caulfield, "Patients' Crowdfunding Campaigns for Alternative Cancer Treatments."

51. Snyder, Turner, and Crooks, "Crowdfunding for Unproven Stem Cell–Based Interventions."

52. Jeremy Snyder and Leigh Turner, "Selling Stem Cell 'Treatments' as Research: Prospective Customer Perspectives from Crowdfunding Campaigns," *Regenerative Medicine* 13, no. 4 (2018): 375–84.

53. Claire Tanner et al., "The Politics of Evidence in Online Illness Narratives: An Analysis of Crowdfunding for Purported Stem Cell Treatments," *Health* 23, no. 4 (2019): 436–57.

54. Snyder, Turner, and Crooks, "Crowdfunding for Unproven Stem Cell–Based Interventions."

55. Snyder and Turner, "Crowdfunding for Stem Cell-Based Interventions to Treat Neurologic Diseases and Injuries."

56. Snyder and Caulfield, "Patients' Crowdfunding Campaigns for Alternative Cancer Treatments."

57. Kathryn Greene and Laura S. Brinn, "Messages Influencing College Women's Tanning Bed Use: Statistical versus Narrative Evidence Format and a Self-Assessment to Increase Perceived Susceptibility," *Journal of Health Communication* 8, no. 5 (2003): 443–61.

58. Leslie J. Hinyard and Matthew W. Kreuter, "Using Narrative Communication as a Tool for Health Behavior Change: A Conceptual, Theoretical, and Empirical Overview," *Health Education and Behavior* 34, no. 5 (2007): 777–92.

59. Timothy Caulfield et al., "Health Misinformation and the Power of Narrative Messaging in the Public Sphere," *Canadian Journal of Bioethics/ Revue Canadienne de Bioéthique* 2, no. 2 (2019): 52–60.

60. Guy Quenneville, "Injured Humboldt Broncos and Families of Dead 'Urgently' Need Advances from $15M GoFundMe Pool," *CBC News*, July 5, 2018, https://www.cbc.ca/news/canada/saskatoon/humboldt-broncos-gofundme-survivors-saskatchewan-1.4734347.

61. "Top Fundraising Tips," GoFundMe, accessed October 30, 2019, https://www.gofundme.com/c/fundraising-tips.

62. Blake Murdoch et al., "Media Portrayal of Illness-Related Medical Crowdfunding: A Content Analysis of Newspaper Articles in the United States and Canada," *PloS One* 14, no. 4 (2019): e0215805.

63. "Top Fundraising Tips."

64. "Medical Fundraising Tips: Financial Support When You Need It," GoFundMe, accessed October 30, 2019, https://www.gofundme.com/c/fundraising-tips/medical.

65. Paige Kutilek, "IVF Fundraising: Guide to Costs, Funding, and Treatments," GoFundMe, March 24, 2016, https://ca.gofundme.com/c/blog/ivf-fundraising.

66. GoFundMe Team, "Clinical Trials for Cancer Patients," GoFundMe, March 1, 2018, https://ca.gofundme.com/c/blog/clinical-trials-cancer-patients.

67. GoFundMe Team, "Is Stem Cell Therapy Right for You?," GoFundMe, August 22, 2018, https://web.archive.org/web/20180822211451/https:/www.gofundme.com/c/blog/stem-cell-therapy.

68. Patty Todd, "Stem Cell Therapy for Hayden Butler," GoFundMe, October 12, 2017, https://www.gofundme.com/f/2cdpj7g.

69. Cheryl Alkon, "How to Crowdfund Your Kid's Medical Expenses," March 26, 2018, https://www.todaysparent.com/kids/kids-health/how-to-crowdfund-your-kids-medical-expenses/.

70. "5 Tips For Better Medical Fundraising," DonationTo, July 23, 2012, https://www.donationto.com/blog/5-tips-for-better-medical-fundraising/.

71. Heller, "The Hidden Cost of GoFundMe Health Care."
72. Leslie Hood, "Stage IV Treatment for Sharon Mann," GoFundMe, August 8, 2018, https://www.gofundme.com/f/healing-and-community-for-sharon.
73. Amy Holmgren, "Cancer Picked the Wrong Diva," GoFundMe, August 15, 2018, https://www.gofundme.com/f/e9sy27-cancer-picked-the-wrong-diva.
74. Nadia Khomami, "Charlie Gard Parents Set up Foundation with £1.3m of Donations," *Guardian*, August 15, 2017, sec. UK news, https://www.theguardian.com/uk-news/2017/aug/15/charlie-gard-parents-set-up-foundation-with-donations.
75. Connie Yates, "Charlie Gard #charliesfight," GoFundMe, January 30, 2017, https://www.gofundme.com/f/please-help-to-save-charlies-life.
76. Paula Wolanski, "Please Help Malgosia Get Stem Cell Therapy," GoFundMe, June 6, 2019, https://www.gofundme.com/f/please-help-malgosia-get-stem-cell-therapy.
77. Neil Genzlinger, "'The God Cells' Advocates Fetal Tissue Therapy Without Debate," *New York Times*, June 2, 2016, https://www.nytimes.com/2016/06/03/movies/review-the-god-cells-advocates-fetal-tissue-therapy-without-debate.html.
78. Jessica Glenza, "How Charlie Gard Captured Trump's Attention and Animated Pro-Life Groups," *Guardian*, July 26, 2017, sec. UK news, https://www.theguardian.com/uk-news/2017/jul/26/charlie-gard-us-pro-life-rightwing-ethics.
79. Albert Anderson, *Ethics for Fundraisers* (Bloomington: Indiana University Press, 1996).
80. Bryanna Moore, "Medical Crowdfunding and the Virtuous Donor," *Bioethics* 33, no. 2 (2019): 238–44.
81. International Society for Stem Cell Research, *Patient Handbook on Stem Cell Therapies* (Skokie, IL: International Society for Stem Cell Research, 2008), http://www.isscr.org/clinical_trans/pdfs/ISSCRPatientHandbook.pdf.
82. Newman, "Is Cancer Fundraising Fuelling Quackery?"
83. Martin Coulter, "GoFundMe Blocks Cash Appeals for Controversial Cancer Clinic," *Financial Times*, March 20, 2019, https://www.ft.com/content/f2c17eaa-4afb-11e9-bbc9-6917dce3dc62.
84. Julia Arciga, "GoFundMe Bans Anti-Vaxxers Who Raise Money to Spread Misinformation," *Daily Beast*, March 22, 2019, https://www.thedailybeast.com/gofundme-bans-anti-vaxxers-who-raise-money-to-spread-misinformation.

85. "GoFundMe Terms and Conditions," GoFundMe, November 20, 2018, https://web.archive.org/web/20190401084241/https:/www.gofundme.com/terms.

86. Heller, "The Hidden Cost of GoFundMe Health Care."

87. "GoFundMe Terms of Service," GoFundMe, accessed October 30, 2019, https://www.gofundme.com/terms.

88. Sarah Hearon, "Kate Winslet, Leonardo DiCaprio Help Save the Life of a Mom With Cancer," *Us Weekly*, February 6, 2018, https://www.usmagazine.com/celebrity-news/news/kate-winslet-leonardo-dicaprio-help-save-life-of-mom-with-cancer/.

89. Newman and Reed, "Cancer Crowdfunding 'Couldn't Save My Daughter.' "

90. Jessica Gibb, "Kate Winslet Surprises Cancer Mum after Saving Her Life with Titanic Fundraiser," *Mirror*, February 5, 2018, https://www.mirror.co.uk/tv/tv-news/kate-winslet-surprises-miracle-cancer-11973038.

91. "Reviews—Testimonials of Treatment of Ovarian Cancer at Hallwang Clinic," Hallwang Clinic, May 17, 2019, https://www.hallwang-clinic.com/en/reviews/ovarian-cancer.

92. Newman and Reed, "Cancer Crowdfunding 'Couldn't Save My Daughter.' "

Conclusion

1. Adrienne M. Martin, *How We Hope: A Moral Psychology* (Princeton, NJ: Princeton University Press, 2016).

2. Alan Wertheimer, *Exploitation* (Princeton, NJ: Princeton University Press, 1999).

Bibliography

"4 File a Class-Action Suit against Sweepstakes Firm." *St. Louis Post-Dispatch*, January 31, 1998.Agrawal, Manish, and Marion Danis. "End-of-Life Care for Terminally Ill Participants in Clinical Research." *Journal of Palliative Medicine* 5, no. 5 (2002): 729–37.

Agrawal, Manish, and Ezekiel J. Emanuel. "Ethics of Phase 1 Oncology Studies: Reexamining the Arguments and Data." *JAMA* 290, no. 8 (2003): 1075–82.

Agrawal, Manish, Christine Grady, Diane L. Fairclough, Neal J. Meropol, Kim Maynard, and Ezekiel J. Emanuel. "Patients' Decision-Making Process Regarding Participation in Phase I Oncology Research." *Journal of Clinical Oncology* 24, no. 27 (2006): 4479–84.

Alkon, Cheryl. "How to Crowdfund Your Kid's Medical Expenses," March 26, 2018. https://www.todaysparent.com/kids/kids-health/how-to-crowdfund-your-kids-medical-expenses/.

Ambrose Cell Therapy. "Right to Try." Accessed October 30, 2019. https://ambrosecelltherapy.com/right-to-try/.

American Board of Internal Medicine. "Medical Professionalism in the New Millennium: A Physician Charter." *Annals of Internal Medicine* 136, no. 3 (2002): 243.

American Medical Association Council on Ethical and Judicial Affairs. *Code of Medical Ethics: Current Opinions with Annotations*. Chicago, IL: AMA Press, 2006.

Anderson, Albert. *Ethics for Fundraisers*. Bloomington: Indiana University Press, 1996.

Anele, Douglas. "Deconstructing Buharimania." *Vanguard Nigeria*, March 8, 2015. https://www.vanguardngr.com/2015/03/deconstructing-buharimania/.

Angell, Marcia. "Investigators' Responsibilities for Human Subjects in Developing Countries." *New England Journal of Medicine* 342, no. 13 (March 30, 2000): 967–69. https://doi.org/10.1056/NEJM200003303421309.

Annas, George J. "The Changing Landscape of Human Experimentation: Nuremberg, Helsinki, and Beyond." *Health Matrix* 2 (1992): 119–40.

Appelbaum, Paul S., Loren H. Roth, and Charles Lidz. "The Therapeutic Misconception: Informed Consent in Psychiatric Research." *International Journal of Law and Psychiatry* 5, no. 3–4 (1982): 319–29.

Aquinas, Saint Thomas. *Summa Theologiae.* Translated by Timothy McDermott. Allen, TX: Thomas More Press, 1991.

Arciga, Julia. "GoFundMe Bans Anti-Vaxxers Who Raise Money to Spread Misinformation." *The Daily Beast*, March 22, 2019, sec. science. https://www.thedailybeast.com/gofundme-bans-anti-vaxxers-who-raise-money-to-spread-misinformation.

Arnold, Denis G. "Exploitation and the Sweatshop Quandary." *Business Ethics Quarterly* 13, no. 2 (2003): 243–56.

Arnold, Denis G., and Norman E. Bowie. "Respect for Workers in Global Supply Chains: Advancing the Debate over Sweatshops." *Business Ethics Quarterly* 17, no. 1 (2007): 135–45.

Arnold, Denis G., and Norman E. Bowie. "Sweatshops and Respect for Persons." *Business Ethics Quarterly* 13, no. 2 (2003): 221–42.

Arnold, Denis G., and Laura P. Hartman. "Beyond Sweatshops: Positive Deviancy and Global Labour Practices." *Business Ethics* 14, no. 3 (2005): 206.

Arnold, Denis G., and Laura P. Hartman. "Moral Imagination and the Future of Sweatshops." *Business and Society Review* 108, no. 4 (2003): 425–61.

Arnold, Denis G., and Laura P. Hartman. "Worker Rights and Low Wage Industrialization: How to Avoid Sweatshops." *Human Rights Quarterly* 28 (2006): 676–700.

Atkins, Harold. "Stem Cell Transplantation to Treat Multiple Sclerosis." *JAMA* 321, no. 2 (2019): 153–55.

Bakowski, Jane. "Hazel's Star Rises in Her Bollywood Roles." *Kent and Sussex Courier*, July 10, 2009.

Ballantyne, Angela. "HIV International Clinical Research: Exploitation and Risk." *Bioethics* 19, no. 5–6 (2005): 476–91. https://doi.org/10.1111/j.1467-8519.2005.00459.x.

Barcelos, Chris A. "'Bye-Bye Boobies': Normativity, Deservingness and Medicalisation in Transgender Medical Crowdfunding." *Culture, Health & Sexuality* 21 (2019): 1–15.

Barcelos, Chris A., and Stephanie L. Budge. "Inequalities in Crowdfunding for Transgender Health Care." *Transgender Health* 4, no. 1 (2019): 81–88.

Bateman-House, Alison, Laura Kimberly, Barbara Redman, Nancy Dubler, and Arthur Caplan. "Right-to-Try Laws: Hope, Hype, and Unintended Consequences." *Annals of Internal Medicine* 163, no. 10 (2015): 796–97.

Bateman-House, Alison, and Christopher T. Robertson. "The Federal Right to Try Act of 2017: A Wrong Turn for Access to Investigational Drugs and the Path Forward." *JAMA Internal Medicine* 178, no. 3 (2018): 321–22.

Bauer, Brian. "Mine Jobs Scam." *The Cairns Sun*, July 20, 2011.

Bauer, Gerhard, Magdi Elsallab, and Mohamed Abou-El-Enein. "Concise Review: A Comprehensive Analysis of Reported Adverse Events in Patients Receiving Unproven Stem Cell-Based Interventions." *Stem Cells Translational Medicine* 7, no. 9 (2018): 676–85.

Begley, Katie. "Axed Acts Blast Twist." *Scottish Star*, October 11, 2011.

Benet, Stephen. *John Brown's Body*. Aegitas, 2015.

Berg, Carla J., Michael A. Rapoff, C. R. Snyder, and John M. Belmont. "The Relationship of Children's Hope to Pediatric Asthma Treatment Adherence." *The Journal of Positive Psychology* 2, no. 3 (2007): 176–84.

Berg, Carla J., Lorie A. Ritschel, Deanne W. Swan, Lawrence C. An, and Jasjit S. Ahluwalia. "The Role of Hope in Engaging in Healthy Behaviors among College Students." *American Journal of Health Behavior* 35, no. 4 (2011): 402–15.

Berger, Israel, Amina Ahmad, Akhil Bansal, Tanvir Kapoor, Douglas Sipp, and John E. J. Rasko. "Global Distribution of Businesses Marketing Stem Cell-Based Interventions." *Cell Stem Cell* 19, no. 2 (2016): 158–62.

Berliner, Lauren S., and Nora J. Kenworthy. "Producing a Worthy Illness: Personal Crowdfunding amidst Financial Crisis." *Social Science & Medicine* 187 (2017): 233–42.

Biessen, Diane A. van der, Peer G. van der Helm, Dennis Klein, Simone van der Burg, Ron H. Mathijssen, Martijn P. Lolkema, and Maja J. de Jonge. "Understanding How Coping Strategies and Quality of Life Maintain Hope in Patients Deliberating Phase I Trial Participation." *Psycho-Oncology* 27, no. 1 (2018): 163–70.

Blight, A., A. Curt, J. F. Ditunno, B. Dobkin, P. Ellaway, J. Fawcett, M. Fehlings, R. G. Grossman, D. P. Lammertse, and A. Privat. "Position Statement on the Sale of Unproven Cellular Therapies for Spinal Cord Injury The International Campaign for Cures of Spinal Cord Injury Paralysis." *Spinal Cord* 47, no. 9 (2009): 713.

Bluth, Rachel. "GoFundMe CEO: 'Gigantic Gaps' in Health System Showing Up in Crowdfunding." *Kaiser Health News*, January 16, 2019. https://khn. org/news/gofundme-ceo-gigantic-gaps-in-health-system-showing-up-in-crowdfunding/.

Bok, Sissela. *Lying: Moral Choice in Public and Private Life*. New York: Vintage, 1999.

Bovens, Luc. "The Value of Hope." *Philosophy and Phenomenological Research* 59, no. 3 (1999): 667–81.

Bowie, Norman E. *Business Ethics: A Kantian Perspective*. Cambridge: Cambridge University Press, 2017.

Brennan, Zachary. "Right to Try One Year Later: Limited Patient Involvement but More FDA Clarity Coming." Regulatory Focus, May 30, 2019. https://www.raps.org/news-and-articles/news-articles/2019/5/right-to-try-one-year-later-limited-patient-invol.

Brennan, Zachary. "Who's Actually Using 'Right-To-Try' Laws? A Texas Oncologist Explains His Experience." *Regulatory Focus*, August 4, 2017. https://www.raps.org/regulatory-focus™/news-articles/2017/8/whos-actually-using-right-to-try-laws-a-texas-oncologist-explains-his-experience.

Bressan, Rodrigo A., Eduardo Iacoponi, Jorge Candido de Assis, and Sukhi S. Shergill. "Hope Is a Therapeutic Tool." *BMJ* 359 (2017): j5469.

Brock, Gillian. *Global Justice: A Cosmopolitan Account*. Oxford: Oxford University Press, 2009.

Browne, Joyce L., Connie O. Rees, Johannes J. M. van Delden, Irene Agyepong, Diederick E. Grobbee, Ama Edwin, Kerstin Klipstein-Grobusch, and Rieke van der Graaf. "The Willingness to Participate in Biomedical Research Involving Human Beings in Low- and Middle-Income Countries: A Systematic Review." *Tropical Medicine & International Health* 24, no. 3 (2019): 264–79. https://doi.org/10.1111/tmi.13195.

Buchanan, Allen E. *Marx and Justice: The Radical Critique of Liberalism*. London: Methuen, 1982.

Buchanan, Allen E. "Marx, Morality, and History: An Assessment of Recent Analytical Work on Marx." *Ethics* 98, no. 1 (1987): 104–36.

Bull, Arla. "Supporters Rally to Raise Cancer Treatment Funds for Teacher." *Kitsap Sun*, September 25, 2105. http://www.kitsapsun.com/news/local/mason/supporters-rally-to-raise-cancer-treatment-funds-for-teacher-ep-1288128229-354418171.html.

Bunnik, Eline M., Nikkie Aarts, and Suzanne van de Vathorst. "Little to Lose and No Other Options: Ethical Issues in Efforts to Facilitate Expanded Access to Investigational Drugs." *Health Policy* 122, no. 9 (2018): 977–83.

Burt, Richard K., Roumen Balabanov, Joachim Burman, Basil Sharrack, John A. Snowden, Maria Carolina Oliveira, Jan Fagius, John Rose, Flavia Nelson, and Amilton Antunes Barreira. "Effect of Nonmyeloablative Hematopoietic Stem Cell Transplantation vs Continued Disease-Modifying Therapy on Disease Progression in Patients with Relapsing-Remitting Multiple Sclerosis: A Randomized Clinical Trial." *JAMA* 321, no. 2 (2019): 165–74.

Burtch, Gordon, and Jason Chan. "Investigating the Relationship between Medical Crowdfunding and Personal Bankruptcy in the United States: Evidence of a Digital Divide." *MIS Quarterly* 43, no. 1 (2019): 237–62.

"California Man Arrested, Charged for Adult Adoption Scheme to Defraud Undocumented Immigrants." February 11, 2016. https://www.justice.gov/opa/pr/california-man-arrested-charged-adult-adoption-scheme-defraud-undocumented-immigrants.

Campana, Paolo. "Out of Africa: The Organization of Migrant Smuggling across the Mediterranean." *European Journal of Criminology* 15, no. 4 (2018): 481–502.

Canadian Medical Association. "Code of Ethics and Professionalism." *Canadian Medical Association*, 2018. https://policybase.cma.ca/documents/policypdf/PD19-03.pdf

Caney, Simon. "International Distributive Justice." *Political Studies* 49, no. 5 (2001): 974–97.

Caplan, A., and B. Levine. "Hope, Hype and Help: Ethically Assessing the Growing Market in Stem Cell Therapies." *The American Journal of Bioethics* 10, no. 5 (2010): 24.

Caplan, Arthur. "Forget Right-to-Try Laws: Our Process Is More Effective and Ethical." *STAT*, June 3, 2019. https://www.statnews.com/2019/06/03/effective-ethical-right-to-try-process/.

Caplan, Arthur L., and Alison Bateman-House. "Should Patients in Need Be Given Access to Experimental Drugs?" *Expert Opinion on Pharmacotherapy* 16, no. 9 (2015): 1275–79.

Carome, Michael, and Sarah Sorscher. Letter in Opposition to S.204, H.R. 878 and H.R. 1020. March 6, 2017. https://www.citizen.org/wp-content/uploads/migration/2362.pdf.

Catt, S., C. Langridge, L. Fallowfield, D. C. Talbot, and V. Jenkins. "Reasons Given by Patients for Participating, or Not, in Phase 1 Cancer Trials." *European Journal of Cancer* 47, no. 10 (2011): 1490–97.

Caulfield, Timothy, Alessandro R. Marcon, Blake Murdoch, Jasmine M. Brown, Sarah Tinker Perrault, Jonathan Jarry, Jeremy Snyder, Samantha J. Anthony, Stephanie Brooks, and Zubin Master. "Health Misinformation and the Power of Narrative Messaging in the Public Sphere." *Canadian Journal of Bioethics/Revue Canadienne de Bioéthique* 2, no. 2 (2019): 52–60.

Cell Surgical Network. "Home : Stem Cell Treatments." Accessed October 29, 2019. https://stemcellrevolution.com/.

Chan, Sarah. "Current and Emerging Global Themes in the Bioethics of Regenerative Medicine: The Tangled Web of Stem Cell Translation." *Regenerative Medicine* 12, no. 7 (2017): 839–51.

Chez, Michael, Christopher Lepage, Carol Parise, Ashley Dang-Chu, Andrea Hankins, and Michael Carroll. "Safety and Observations from a Placebo-Controlled, Crossover Study to Assess Use of Autologous Umbilical Cord Blood Stem Cells to Improve Symptoms in Children with Autism." *Stem Cells Translational Medicine* 7, no. 4 (2018): 333–41.

Chong, Celena. "A Group of Investors Is Buying GoFundMe." *Business Insider*, June 24, 2015. https://www.businessinsider.com/a-group-of-investors-is-buying-gofundme-2015-6.

Clark, Luke, Bruno Averbeck, Doris Payer, Guillaume Sescousse, Catharine A. Winstanley, and Gui Xue. "Pathological Choice: The Neuroscience of Gambling and Gambling Addiction." *Journal of Neuroscience* 33, no. 45 (2013): 17617–23.

Cohen, Gerald A. "The Labor Theory of Value and the Concept of Exploitation." *Philosophy & Public Affairs* 8, no. 4 (1979): 338–360.

Cohen, I. Glenn. *Patients with Passports: Medical Tourism, Law, and Ethics.* Oxford: Oxford University Press, 2014.

Cohen, I. Glenn, and Shelly Simana. "Regulation of Stem Cell Therapy Travel." *Current Stem Cell Reports* 4, no. 3 (2018): 220–27.

Cohen, Tova. "BrainStorm Will Not Provide ALS Therapy under U.S. Right to Try Act." *Reuters*, June 26, 2018. https://www.reuters.com/article/us-health-brainstorm-cell-als-exclusive-idUSKBN1JM1BE.

Commissioner, Office of the. "FDA Seeks Permanent Injunctions against Two Stem Cell Clinics." FDA, September 10, 2019. http://www.fda.gov/news-events/press-announcements/fda-seeks-permanent-injunctions-against-two-stem-cell-clinics.

Connolly, Ruairi, Timothy O'Brien, and Gerard Flaherty. "Stem Cell Tourism: A Web-Based Analysis of Clinical Services Available to International Travellers." *Travel Medicine and Infectious Disease* 12, no. 6 (2014): 695–701.

Consumer Financial Protection Bureau. "Consumer Credit Reports: A Study of Medical and Non-Medical Collections," December 2014. https://files.consumerfinance.gov/f/201412_cfpb_reports_consumer-credit-medical-and-non-medical-collections.pdf.

Corieri, Christina. "Everyone Deserves the Right to Try: Empowering the Terminally Ill to Take Control of Their Treatment." *Policy Report*, no. 266 (2014): 1–30.

Cortez, Michelle. "The 'Right to Try' Could Cost Dying Patients a Fortune." *Bloomberg*, June 20, 2018. https://www.bloomberg.com/news/articles/2018-06-20/the-price-to-try-a-drug-could-be-300-000-for-dying-patients.

Coulter, Martin. "GoFundMe Blocks Cash Appeals for Controversial Cancer Clinic." *Financial Times*, March 20, 2019. https://www.ft.com/content/f2c17eaa-4afb-11e9-bbc9-6917dce3dc62.

Crane, Andrew, and Dirk Matten. "Incorporating the Corporation in Citizenship: A Response to Néron and Norman." *Business Ethics Quarterly* 18, no. 1 (2008): 27–33.

Creative Medical Technology Holdings Inc. "Creative Medical Technology Holdings Aims to Treat Cancer Associated Wasting (Cachexia) Using AmnioStem Universal Donor Stem Cell." *PR Newswire*, July 6, 2018. https://www.prnewswire.com/news-releases/creative-medical-technology-holdings-aims-to-treat-cancer-associated-wasting-cachexia-using-amniostem-universal-donor-stem-cell-300676909.html.

Crites, Joshua, and Eric Kodish. "Unrealistic Optimism and the Ethics of Phase I Cancer Research." *Journal of Medical Ethics* 39, no. 6 (2013): 403–6.

Daugherty, Christopher, Mark J. Ratain, Eugene Grochowski, Carol Stocking, Eric Kodish, Rosemarie Mick, and Mark Siegler. "Perceptions of Cancer

Patients and Their Physicians Involved in Phase I Trials." *Journal of Clinical Oncology* 13, no. 5 (1995): 1062–72.

Davies, Lizzy. "Italy Boat Wreck: Scores of Migrants Die as Boat Sinks off Lampedusa." *The Guardian*, October 3, 2013, sec. World news. https://www.theguardian.com/world/2013/oct/03/lampedusa-migrants-killed-boat-sinks-italy.

Dawson, Geraldine, Jessica M. Sun, Katherine S. Davlantis, Michael Murias, Lauren Franz, Jesse Troy, Ryan Simmons, Maura Sabatos-DeVito, Rebecca Durham, and Joanne Kurtzberg. "Autologous Cord Blood Infusions Are Safe and Feasible in Young Children with Autism Spectrum Disorder: Results of a Single-Center Phase I Open-Label Trial." *Stem Cells Translational Medicine* 6, no. 5 (2017): 1332–39.

"Debate on Stem-Cell Research." *The Irish Times*, December 3, 2003.

Dellson, Pia, Kerstin Nilsson, Helena Jernström, and Christina Carlsson. "Patients' Reasoning Regarding the Decision to Participate in Clinical Cancer Trials: An Interview Study." *Trials* 19, no. 1 (2018): 528.

Demir, Oguzhan Omer, Murat Sever, and Yavuz Kahya. "The Social Organisation of Migrant Smugglers in Turkey: Roles and Functions." *European Journal on Criminal Policy and Research* 23, no. 3 (2017): 371–91.

Dhanapala, Jayantha, and Savitri Goonesekere. "'Torch of Awareness' for Voters." *Daily Mirror*, September 5, 2013. http://www.dailymirror.lk/opinion/torch-of-awareness-for-voters/172-34912.

Dickinson, Emily. *The Complete Poems of Emily Dickinson*. Boston: Back Bay Books, 1976.

Dolly, Saoirse O., Eleftheria Kalaitzaki, Martina Puglisi, Sarah Stimpson, Janet Hanwell, Sonia Serrano Fandos, Sarah Stapleton, Thushara Ansari, Clare Peckitt, and Stan Kaye. "A Study of Motivations and Expectations of Patients Seen in Phase 1 Oncology Clinics." *Cancer* 122, no. 22 (2016): 3501–8.

DonationTo. "5 Tips For Better Medical Fundraising," July 23, 2012. https://www.donationto.com/blog/5-tips-for-better-medical-fundraising/.

Dresser, Rebecca. "First-in-Human Trial Participants: Not a Vulnerable Population, but Vulnerable Nonetheless." *The Journal of Law, Medicine & Ethics* 37, no. 1 (2009): 38–50.

Dresser, Rebecca. "'Right to Try' Laws: The Gap between Experts and Advocates." *Hastings Center Report* 45, no. 3 (2015): 9–10.

Dresser, Rebecca. "The Right to Try Investigational Drugs: Science and Stories in the Access Debate." *Texas Law Review* 93, no. 7 (2014): 1631–57.

Drews, Maria Francesca. "The Evolution of Hope in Patients with Terminal Illness." *Nursing* 47, no. 1 (2017): 13–14.

Dubov, Alex. "Moral Justification of Phase 1 Oncology Trials." *Journal of Pain & Palliative Care Pharmacotherapy* 28, no. 2 (June 1, 2014): 138–51. https://doi.org/10.3109/15360288.2014.908994.

Durand, Wesley M., Jillian L. Peters, Adam E. M. Eltorai, Saisanjana Kalagara, Adena J. Osband, and Alan H. Daniels. "Medical Crowdfunding for Organ Transplantation." *Clinical Transplantation* 32, no. 6 (2018): e13267.

Duynhoven, Alysha van, Anthony Lee, Ross Michel, Jeremy Snyder, Valorie Crooks, Peter Chow-White, and Nadine Schuurman. "Spatially Exploring the Intersection of Socioeconomic Status and Canadian Cancer-Related Medical Crowdfunding Campaigns." *BMJ Open* 9, no. 6 (2019): e026365.

Dwyer, James. "What's Wrong with the Global Migration of Health Care Professionals? Individual Rights and International Justice." *Hastings Center Report* 37, no. 5 (2007): 36–43.

Dyer, Clare. "Doctor Is Found Guilty of Exploiting 'Desperate' MS Patients." *BMJ: British Medical Journal* 340 (2010): C2009.

Efrati, Ido. "Foreign Patients to Subsidize Experimental Treatment for Israelis with ALS." *Haaretz*, February 20, 2019. https://www.haaretz.com/israel-news/.premium-foreign-patients-to-subsidize-experimental-treatment-for-israelis-with-als-1.6956407.

Eisenhauer, E. A., P. J. O'Dwyer, M. Christian, and J. S. Humphrey. "Phase I Clinical Trial Design in Cancer Drug Development." *Journal of Clinical Oncology: Official Journal of the American Society of Clinical Oncology* 18, no. 3 (2000): 684–92.

El Setouhy, Maged, Tsiri Agbenyega, Francis Anto, Christine Alexandra Clerk, Kwadwo A. Koram, Michael English, Rashid Juma, et al. "Moral Standards for Research in Developing Countries from 'Reasonable Availability' to 'Fair Benefits.'" *The Hastings Center Report* 34, no. 3 (2004): 17–27. https://doi.org/10.2307/3528416.

Eliott, Jaklin A., and Ian N. Olver. "Hope and Hoping in the Talk of Dying Cancer Patients." *Social Science & Medicine* 64, no. 1 (2007): 138–49.

Elster, Jon. "Exploring Exploitation." *Journal of Peace Research* 15, no. 1 (1978): 3–17.

European Council of Medical Orders. "Principles of European Medical Ethics." European Council of Medical Orders, 1995. http://www.ceom-ecmo.eu/en/view/principles-of-european-medical-ethics.

"Fake Mining Ads Trick Eager Job-Seekers." *Central Telegraph and Rural Weekly*, July 8, 2011.

Flatten, Mark. "Dead on Arrival: Federal 'Compassionate Use' Leaves Little Hope for Dying Patients." Goldwater Institute, February 24, 2016. https://goldwaterinstitute.org/wp-content/uploads/2016/02/Dead-On-Arrival-Report.pdf.

Florko, Nicholas. "A Year after Trump Touted Right to Try, Patients Still Aren't Getting Treatment." *STAT*, January 29, 2019. https://www.statnews.com/2019/01/29/right-to-try-patients-still-arent-getting-treatment/.

Florko, Nicholas. "Fed up with FDA, ALS Advocates Consider a Take-No-Prisoners Approach." *STAT*, June 7, 2019. https://www.statnews.com/2019/06/07/als-advocates-protest-fda/.

Florko, Nicholas. "When 'Right to Try' Isn't Enough." *STAT*, May 31, 2019. https://www.statnews.com/2019/05/31/when-right-to-try-isnt-enough/.

Folkers, Kelly, and Alison Bateman-House. "Glioblastoma Patient Is First to Receive Treatment under Right to Try. Our Question Is Why?" *The Cancer Letter*, February 1, 2019. https://cancerletter.com/articles/20190201_6/.

Folkers, Kelly, Carolyn Chapman, and Barbara Redman. "Federal Right to Try: Where Is It Going?" *Hastings Center Report* 49, no. 2 (2019): 26–36.

Food and Drug Administration. "Charging for Investigational Drugs under an IND: Questions and Answers," June 2016. https://www.fda.gov/media/85682/download.

Freedman, Benjamin. "Equipoise and the Ethics of Clinical Research." *The New England Journal of Medicine* 317, no. 3 (July 16, 1987): 141–45. https://doi.org/10.1056/NEJM198707163170304.

Freedom and the FDA: The Matt Bellina Story. Accessed October 30, 2019. https://www.youtube.com/watch?v=IE6mzkPSVR8.

Fritz, Nikki, and Amy Gonzales. "Not the Normal Trans Story: Negotiating Trans Narratives While Crowdfunding at the Margins." *International Journal of Communication* 12 (2018): 1189–1208.

Frketich, Joanna. "Family Raising $100,000 for Experimental Treatment for Teen's Lyme Disease." *The Hamilton Spectator*, April 16, 2015. https://www.therecord.com/news-story/5562614-family-raising-100-000-for-experimental-treatment-for-teen-s-lyme-disease/.

Fu, Wayne, Cambray Smith, Leigh Turner, Joseph Fojtik, Joel E. Pacyna, and Zubin Master. "Characteristics and Scope of Training of Clinicians Participating in the US Direct-to-Consumer Marketplace for Unproven Stem Cell Interventions." *JAMA* 321, no. 24 (2019): 2463–64.

Gbadegesin, Segun, and David Wendler. "Protecting Communities in Health Research from Exploitation." *Bioethics* 20, no. 5 (2006): 248–53. https://doi.org/10.1111/j.1467-8519.2006.00501.x.

General Medical Council. "Good Medical Practice." General Medical Council, 2014. https://www.gmc-uk.org/-/media/documents/good-medical-practice--english-1215_pdf-51527435.pdf.

Genzlinger, Neil. "'The God Cells' Advocates Fetal Tissue Therapy Without Debate." *New York Times*, June 2, 2016, sec. Movies. https://www.nytimes.com/2016/06/03/movies/review-the-god-cells-advocates-fetal-tissue-therapy-without-debate.html.

Gibb, Jessica. "Kate Winslet Surprises Cancer Mum after Saving Her Life with Titanic Fundraiser." *Mirror*, February 5, 2018. https://www.mirror.co.uk/tv/tv-news/kate-winslet-surprises-miracle-cancer-11973038.

Gibson, Gordon. "Gaming or Gambling: By Any Name It Exploits the Hopes and Dreams of Losers." *Calgary Herald*, February 14, 1998.

Glantz, Leonard H., George J. Annas, Michael A. Grodin, and Wendy K. Mariner. "Research in Developing Countries: Taking 'Benefit' Seriously." *The Hastings Center Report* 28, no. 6 (November 1, 1998): 38.

Glenza, Jessica. "How Charlie Gard Captured Trump's Attention and Animated Pro-Life Groups." *The Guardian*, July 26, 2017, sec. UK news. https://www.theguardian.com/uk-news/2017/jul/26/charlie-gard-us-pro-life-rightwing-ethics.

GoFundMe. "GoFundMe Terms & Conditions," November 20, 2018. https://web.archive.org/web/20190401084241/https:/www.gofundme.com/terms.

GoFundMe. "GoFundMe Terms of Service." Accessed October 30, 2019. https://www.gofundme.com/terms.

GoFundMe. "Medical Fundraising—Start a Free Fundraiser." Accessed October 30, 2019. https://www.gofundme.com/start/medical-fundraising.

GoFundMe. "Medical Fundraising Tips: Financial Support When You Need It." Accessed October 30, 2019. https://www.gofundme.com/c/fundraising-tips/medical.

GoFundMe. "Top Fundraising Tips." Accessed October 30, 2019. https://www.gofundme.com/c/fundraising-tips.

GoFundMe Team. "Clinical Trials for Cancer Patients." GoFundMe, March 1, 2018. https://ca.gofundme.com/c/blog/clinical-trials-cancer-patients.

GoFundMe Team. "Is Stem Cell Therapy Right for You?" GoFundMe, August 22, 2018. https://web.archive.org/web/20180822211451/https:/www.gofundme.com/c/blog/stem-cell-therapy. Goldwater Institute. *Right to Try Is All about Hope for Patients like Jordan*, 2018. https://www.youtube.com/watch?v=54bkoy7UWWw.

Gonzales, Amy L., Elizabeth Y. Kwon, Teresa Lynch, and Nicole Fritz. "'Better Everyone Should Know Our Business than We Lose Our House': Costs and Benefits of Medical Crowdfunding for Support, Privacy, and Identity." *New Media & Society* 20, no. 2 (2018): 641–58.

Gorski, David. "As I Predicted, the Exploitation of Desperate Patients Using Right-to-Try Begins." *Respectful Insolence* (blog), June 22, 2018. https://respectfulinsolence.com/2018/06/22/as-i-predicted-the-exploitation-of-patients-under-right-to-try-begins/.

Green, Charlotte. "Miracle Mum Gemma Nuttall 'Cancer-Free' after Immunotherapy Success." *Rossendale Free Press*, October 19, 2017. http://www.rossendalefreepress.co.uk/news/miracle-mum-gemma-nuttall-cancer-13780804.

Greene, Kathryn, and Laura S. Brinn. "Messages Influencing College Women's Tanning Bed Use: Statistical versus Narrative Evidence Format and a Self-Assessment to Increase Perceived Susceptibility." *Journal of Health Communication* 8, no. 5 (2003): 443–61.

Hall, Jake. "How Crowdfunding Became a Lifeline for the Trans Community." *Vice*, August 27, 2018. https://www.vice.com/en_ca/article/9km7y7/crowdfunding-transgender-transition-healthcare-inequality-costs.

Hallwang Clinic. "Reviews—Testimonials of Treatment of Ovarian Cancer at Hallwang Clinic," May 17, 2019. https://www.hallwang-clinic.com/en/reviews/ovarian-cancer.

Hanlon, Gerard. "Rethinking Corporate Social Responsibility and the Role of the Firm: On the Denial of Politics." *The Oxford Handbook of Corporate Social Responsibility*, edited by Andrew Crane, Dirk Matten, Abagail McWilliams, Jeremy Moon, and Donald S. Siegel. New York, NY: Oxford University Press, 2008: 156–72.

Harris, Ainsley. "How Crowdfunding Platform GoFundMe Has Created a $3 Billion Digital Safety Net." *Fast Company*, February 13, 2017. https://www.fastcompany.com/3067472/how-crowdfunding-platform-gofundme-has-created-a-3-billion-digital.

Harris Interactive. "Participation in Clinical Trials Lower in Europe and India than in the United States." *Healthcare News*, 5 (2005): 7.

Hawkins, Jennifer S., and Ezekiel J. Emanuel. *Exploitation and Developing Countries: The Ethics of Clinical Research*. Princeton, NJ: Princeton University Press, 2008.

Health Canada. "Health Canada Policy Position Paper: Autologous Cell Therapy Products," May 15, 2019. https://www.canada.ca/en/health-canada/services/drugs-health-products/biologics-radiopharmaceuticals-genetic-therapies/applications-submissions/guidance-documents/cell-therapy-policy.html.

Hearon, Sarah. "Kate Winslet, Leonardo DiCaprio Help Save the Life of a Mom with Cancer." *Us Weekly*, February 6, 2018. https://www.usmagazine.com/celebrity-news/news/kate-winslet-leonardo-dicaprio-help-save-life-of-mom-with-cancer/.

Heller, Nathan. "The Hidden Cost of GoFundMe Health Care," June 24, 2019. https://www.newyorker.com/magazine/2019/07/01/the-perverse-logic-of-gofundme-health-care.

Henderson, Gail E., Michele M. Easter, Catherine Zimmer, Nancy M. P. King, Arlene M. Davis, Barbra Bluestone Rothschild, Larry R. Churchill, Benjamin S. Wilfond, and Daniel K. Nelson. "Therapeutic Misconception in Early Phase Gene Transfer Trials." *Social Science & Medicine* 62, no. 1 (2006): 239–253.

Herman, Barbara. *Moral Literacy*. Cambridge, MA: Harvard University Press, 2007.

Hesiod. *Works of Hesiod and the Homeric Hymns*. Translated by Daryl Hine. Chicago: University of Chicago Press, 2008.

Hill, Douglas L., and Chris Feudtner. "Hope in the Midst of Terminal Illness." In *The Oxford Handbook of Hope*, edited by Matthew W. Gallagher and Shane J. Lopez. Oxford: Oxford University Press, 2017: 191–206.

Hill, Thomas. *Dignity and Practical Reason in Kant's Moral Theory*. Ithaca, NY: Cornell University Press, 1992.

Hill, Thomas E. *Human Welfare and Moral Worth: Kantian Perspectives*. Oxford: Oxford University Press, 2002.

Hiltzik, Michael. "FDA Says StemGenex Marketing of Unproven Stem Cell Treatments Is Illegal." *Los Angeles Times*, November 16, 2018. https://www.latimes.com/business/hiltzik/la-fi-hiltzik-fda-stemgenex-20181116-story.html.

Himmelstein, David U., Robert M. Lawless, Deborah Thorne, Pamela Foohey, and Steffie Woolhandler. "Medical Bankruptcy: Still Common Despite the Affordable Care Act." *American Journal of Public Health* 109, no. 3 (2019): 431–33.

Himmelstein, David U., Deborah Thorne, Elizabeth Warren, and Steffie Woolhandler. "Medical Bankruptcy in the United States, 2007: Results of a National Study." *The American Journal of Medicine* 122, no. 8 (2009): 741–46.

Hinyard, Leslie J., and Matthew W. Kreuter. "Using Narrative Communication as a Tool for Health Behavior Change: A Conceptual, Theoretical, and Empirical Overview." *Health Education & Behavior* 34, no. 5 (2007): 777–92.

Hobbes, Thomas. *Leviathan: Or The Matter, Forme, & Power of a Common-Wealth Ecclesiasticall and Civill*. New Haven, CT: Yale University Press, 2010.

Holmgren, Amy. "Cancer Picked the Wrong Diva." GoFundMe, August 15, 2018. https://www.gofundme.com/f/e9sy27-cancer-picked-the-wrong-diva.Hood, Leslie. "Stage IV Treatment for Sharon Mann." GoFundMe, August 8, 2018. https://www.gofundme.com/f/healing-and-community-for-sharon.

Hopkins, Anna. "Millennial Fighting Rare Bone Cancer Responds to Biden Vow: Law Supported by Trump Helped Save My Life." *Fox News*, June 14, 2019. https://www.foxnews.com/politics/millennial-cancer-joe-biden-trump-right-try-saved-life.

Horng, Sam, and Christine Grady. "Misunderstanding in Clinical Research: Distinguishing Therapeutic Misconception, Therapeutic Misestimation, & Therapeutic Optimism." *IRB: Ethics & Human Research* 25, no. 1 (2003): 11–16.

Horng, Sam, and Christine Grady. "Misunderstanding in Clinical Research: Distinguishing Therapeutic Misconception, Therapeutic Misestimation, & Therapeutic Optimism." *IRB: Ethics & Human Research* 25, no. 1 (2003): 11–16.

Horstmann, Elizabeth, Mary S. McCabe, Louise Grochow, Seiichiro Yamamoto, Larry Rubinstein, Troy Budd, Dale Shoemaker, Ezekiel J. Emanuel, and Christine Grady. "Risks and Benefits of Phase 1 Oncology Trials, 1991 through 2002." *New England Journal of Medicine* 352, no. 9 (2005): 895–904.

Hosking, Patrick. "Publishing Outfit That Is Aiming to Make Vanity Fair." *The Evening Standard*, February 18, 1999.

Howell, Andrew J., Ryan M. Jacobson, and Denise J. Larsen. "Enhanced Psychological Health among Chronic Pain Clients Engaged in Hope-Focused Group Counseling." *The Counseling Psychologist* 43, no. 4 (2015): 586–613.

"HSCT México." Accessed October 29, 2019. https://www.hsctmexico.com/index.php?lng=eng.

Hume, David. *A Treatise of Human Nature: Being an Attempt to Introduce the Experimental Method of Reasoning into Moral Subjects*. Aukland, NZ: The Floating Press, 2009.

Hwang, Thomas J., Jonathan J. Darrow, and Aaron S. Kesselheim. "The FDA's Expedited Programs and Clinical Development Times for Novel Therapeutics, 2012–2016." *JAMA* 318, no. 21 (2017): 2137–38.

Hyun, Insoo. "The Bioethics of Stem Cell Research and Therapy." *The Journal of Clinical Investigation* 120, no. 1 (2010): 71–75.

Illes, Judy, and Fabio Rossi. "Opinion: No Miracle Therapy for Stroke." *Vancouver Sun*, February 12, 2015. http://www.vancouversun.com/health/Opinion+miracle+therapy+stroke/10787468/story.html.

International Society for Stem Cell Research. "Guidelines for the Clinical Translation of Stem Cells." International Society for Stem Cell Research, 2008. https://www.isscr.org/docs/default-source/all-isscr-guidelines/guidelines-2016/isscr-guidelines-for-stem-cell-research-and-clinical-translationd67119731dff6ddbb37cff0000940c19.pdf?sfvrsn=4

International Society for Stem Cell Research. "Patient Handbook on Stem Cell Therapies." International Society for Stem Cell Research, 2008. http://www.isscr.org/clinical_trans/pdfs/ISSCRPatientHandbook.pdf.

Italiano, A., C. Massard, R. Bahleda, A.-L. Vataire, E. Deutsch, N. Magne, J.-P. Pignon, G. Vassal, J.-P. Armand, and J.-C. Soria. "Treatment Outcome and Survival in Participants of Phase I Oncology Trials Carried out from 2003 to 2006 at Institut Gustave Roussy." *Annals of Oncology* 19, no. 4 (2007): 787–92.

Jacob, Julie A. "Questions of Safety and Fairness Raised as Right-to-Try Movement Gains Steam." *JAMA* 314, no. 8 (2015): 758–60.

Jansen, Lynn A. "Two Concepts of Therapeutic Optimism." *Journal of Medical Ethics* 37, no. 9 (2011): 563–66.

Jansen, Lynn A., Daruka Mahadevan, Paul S. Appelbaum, William MP Klein, Neil D. Weinstein, Motomi Mori, Catherine Degnin, and Daniel P. Sulmasy. "Perceptions of Control and Unrealistic Optimism in Early-Phase Cancer Trials." *Journal of Medical Ethics* 44, no. 2 (2018): 121–27.

Jarow, Jonathan P., and Richard Moscicki. "Impact of Expanded Access on FDA Regulatory Action and Product Labeling." *Therapeutic Innovation & Regulatory Science* 51, no. 6 (2017): 787–89.

Jay, Martin. *The Virtues of Mendacity: On Lying in Politics*. Charlottesville: University of Virginia Press, 2010.

Jecker, Nancy S. "Exploiting Subjects in Placebo-Controlled Trials." *The American Journal of Bioethics* 2, no. 2 (June 1, 2002): 19–20.

Jenkins, Valerie, Ivonne Solis-Trapala, Carolyn Langridge, Susan Catt, Denis C. Talbot, and Lesley J. Fallowfield. "What Oncologists Believe They Said and What Patients Believe They Heard: An Analysis of Phase I Trial Discussions." *Journal of Clinical Oncology* 29, no. 1 (2011): 61–68.

"Jobhunters Exploited in Mining." *The Cairns Sun*, June 26, 2008.

Joffe, Steven, E. Francis Cook, Paul D. Cleary, Jeffrey W. Clark, and Jane C. Weeks. "Quality of Informed Consent in Cancer Clinical Trials: A Cross-Sectional Survey." *The Lancet* 358, no. 9295 (2001): 1772–77.

Joffe, Steven, and Holly Fernandez Lynch. "Federal Right-to-Try Legislation-Threatening the FDA's Public Health Mission." *The New England Journal of Medicine* 378, no. 8 (2018): 695.

Joffe, Steven, and Franklin G. Miller. "Bench to Bedside: Mapping the Moral Terrain of Clinical Research." *The Hastings Center Report* 38, no. 2 (April 2008): 30–42.

Johnson, Ron. "The Terminally Ill Deserve Right-to-Try Laws." *Wall Street Journal*, September 22, 2016, sec. Opinion. https://www.wsj.com/articles/the-terminally-ill-deserve-right-to-try-laws-1474586032.

Johnstone, Kari. "The Power of Local Communities in the Fight Against Human Trafficking." *DipNote*, June 28, 2018. https://blogs.state.gov/stories/2018/06/28/en/power-local-communities-fight-against-human-trafficking.

Josephs, Leslie. "Costa Rica Puts Brakes on Popular Stem Cell Tourism." *Reuters*, June 6, 2010. https://www.reuters.com/article/uk-costarica-stemcells-idUKTRE6560HU20100607.

Kamenova, Kalina, and Timothy Caulfield. "Stem Cell Hype: Media Portrayal of Therapy Translation." *Science Translational Medicine* 7, no. 278 (2015): 1–4.

Kant, Immanuel. *Groundwork of the Metaphysics of Morals*. Edited by Christine M. Korsgaard. 2nd edition. Cambridge: Cambridge University Press, 2012.

Kant, Immanuel. *The Metaphysics of Morals*. Edited by Mary J. Gregor. 2nd edition. Cambridge; New York: Cambridge University Press, 1996.

Kaplan, Tracey. "DA Launches Effort Warning Obama-Plan Applicants of Scams." *Contra Costa Times*, February 9, 2015. https://www.mercurynews.com/2015/02/09/da-launches-effort-warning-obama-plan-applicants-of-scams/.

Kates, Michael. "The Ethics of Sweatshops and the Limits of Choice." *Business Ethics Quarterly* 25, no. 2 (2015): 191–212.

Kerry, John. "Remarks at the 2015 Trafficking in Persons Report Ceremony." U.S. Embassy in the Dominican Republic, July 27, 2015. https://do.usembassy.gov/remarks-2015-trafficking-persons-report-ceremony/.

Khomami, Nadia. "Charlie Gard Parents Set up Foundation with £1.3m of Donations." *The Guardian*, August 15, 2017, sec. UK news.

https://www.theguardian.com/uk-news/2017/aug/15/charlie-gard-parents-set-up-foundation-with-donations.

Kiatpongsan, Sorapop, and Douglas Sipp. "Offshore Stem Cell Treatments." *Nature Reports Stem Cells*, 3 December 2008. doi:10.1038/stemcells.2008.151

Kipnis, Kenneth. "Vulnerability in Research Subjects: A Bioethical Taxonomy." In *Ethical and Policy Issues in Research Involving Human* Participants, Vol. 2, 2001. Rockville, MD: National Bioethics Advisory Commission [NBAC]; 2001: G1–G13.

Kline, Donna S. "Push and Pull Factors in International Nurse Migration." *Journal of Nursing Scholarship* 35, no. 2 (2003): 107–11.

Knoepfler, Paul. "Upbeat Burt Team Pub on Stem Cells for MS Comes with Uneasy Back Story." *The Niche* (blog), January 20, 2019. https://ipscell.com/2019/01/upbeat-burt-team-pub-on-stem-cells-for-ms-comes-with-uneasy-back-story/.

Knoepfler, Paul S. "The Stem Cell Hard Sell: Report from a Clinic's Patient Recruitment Seminar." *Stem Cells Translational Medicine* 6, no. 1 (2017): 14–16.

Knoepfler, Paul S., and Leigh G Turner. "The FDA and the US Direct-to-Consumer Marketplace for Stem Cell Interventions: A Temporal Analysis." *Regenerative Medicine* 13, no. 1 (2018): 19–27.

Krieg, Norbert. "Perils of Illegal Entry into the United States." *The Independent*, September 20, 1990.

Kristof, Nicholas. "Opinion | Where Sweatshops Are a Dream." *New York Times*, January 14, 2009, sec. Opinion. https://www.nytimes.com/2009/01/15/opinion/15kristof.html.

Kristof, Nicholas D., and Sheryl Wudunn. "Two Cheers for Sweatshops." *New York Times*, September 24, 2000, sec. Magazine. https://www.nytimes.com/2000/09/24/magazine/two-cheers-for-sweatshops.html.

Kuriyan, Ajay E., Thomas A. Albini, Justin H. Townsend, Marianeli Rodriguez, Hemang K. Pandya, Robert E. Leonard, M. Brandon Parrott, Philip J. Rosenfeld, Harry W. Flynn Jr, and Jeffrey L. Goldberg. "Vision Loss after Intravitreal Injection of Autologous 'Stem Cells' for AMD." *New England Journal of Medicine* 376, no. 11 (2017): 1047–53.

Kutilek, Paige. "IVF Fundraising: Guide to Costs, Funding, and Treatments." GoFundMe, March 24, 2016. https://ca.gofundme.com/c/blog/ivf-fundraising.

Lanzel, Ashley F., and James V. Lavery. "Unintended Consequences of the Right to Try Act for Palliative Care in Pediatric Oncology." *JAMA Oncology* 5, no. 5 (2019): 603–4.

Lau, Darren, Ubaka Ogbogu, Benjamin Taylor, Tania Stafinski, Devidas Menon, and Timothy Caulfield. "Stem Cell Clinics Online: The Direct-to-Consumer Portrayal of Stem Cell Medicine." *Cell Stem Cell* 3, no. 6 (2008): 591–94.

Lavigne, Yves. "Groups Demand Tobacco Licencing." *Globe & Mail*, September 23, 1987.

Lee, Jenny Y., and Matthew W. Gallagher. "Hope and Well-Being." In *The Oxford Handbook of Hope*, edited by Matthew W. Gallagher and Shane J. Lopez. Oxford: Oxford University Press, 2018: 287–98.

Lerner, Barron H. *The Breast Cancer Wars: Hope, Fear, and the Pursuit of a Cure in Twentieth-Century America*. Oxford: Oxford University Press, 2003.

Levine, Aaron D., and Leslie E. Wolf. "The Roles and Responsibilities of Physicians in Patients' Decisions about Unproven Stem Cell Therapies." *The Journal of Law, Medicine & Ethics* 40, no. 1 (2012): 122–34.

Livingstone, David. "Beyond Hats and Bags: How Clothes Look and What They May (or May Not) Mean." *Globe & Mail*, February 13, 1982.

Lopez Bauman, Naomi. "Right to Try Program Offers Hope to Brain Cancer Patients." *Goldwater Institute* (blog), October 3, 2019. https://goldwaterinstitute.org/article/the-first-announced-right-to-try-program-offers-hope-to-brain-cancer-patients/.

Luciano, Lilia. "Former Fire Captain's Fight for His 'Right to Try' and the Debate over Compassionate Use." KXTV, February 21, 2017. https://www.abc10.com/article/news/local/former-fire-captains-fight-for-his-right-to-try-and-the-debate-over-compassionate-use/103-397072418.

Lukk, Martin, Erik Schneiderhan, and Joanne Soares. "Worthy? Crowdfunding the Canadian Health Care and Education Sectors." *Canadian Review of Sociology/Revue Canadienne de Sociologie* 55, no. 3 (2018): 404–24.

Luna, David. "Ending Human Trafficking: Building a Better World and Partnerships for Sustainable Security and Human Dignity." OECD-APEC Roundtable on Combating Corruption Related to Human Trafficking, August 27, 2015. https://www.oecd.org/gov/risk/HumanTraffickingStatement-D.M.Luna-27August2015.pdf.

Lunden, Ingrid. "GoFundMe Acquires CrowdRise to Expand to Fundraising for Charities." *TechCrunch*, January 10, 2017. http://social.techcrunch.com/2017/01/10/gofundme-buys-crowdrise-to-expand-to-fundraising-for-charities/.

Lurie, Peter, and Sidney Wolfe. "The Developing World as the 'Answer' to the Dreams of Pharmaceutical Companies: The Surfaxin Story." In *Ethical Issues in International Biomedical Research: A Casebook*, edited by Ezekiel J. Emanuel, Christine Grady, and Elizabeth Wahl. Oxford: Oxford University Press, 2007: 159–170.

Lynch, Holly Fernandez, Patricia J. Zettler, and Ameet Sarpatwari. "Promoting Patient Interests in Implementing the Federal Right to Try Act." *JAMA* 320, no. 9 (2018): 869–870.

Lynn, Barry C. "Breaking the Chain." *Harper's Magazine*, July 2006. https://harpers.org/archive/2006/07/breaking-the-chain/.

Lysaght, Tamra, Ian H. Kerridge, Douglas Sipp, Gerard Porter, and Benjamin J. Capps. "Ethical and Regulatory Challenges with Autologous Adult Stem Cells: A Comparative Review of International Regulations." *Journal of Bioethical Inquiry* 14, no. 2 (2017): 261–73.

Madan, Sindia, and Kenneth I. Pakenham. "The Stress-Buffering Effects of Hope on Adjustment to Multiple Sclerosis." *International Journal of Behavioral Medicine* 21, no. 6 (2014): 877–90.

Maikranz, Julie M., Ric G. Steele, Meredith L. Dreyer, Aaron C. Stratman, and James A. Bovaird. "The Relationship of Hope and Illness-Related Uncertainty to Emotional Adjustment and Adherence among Pediatric Renal and Liver Transplant Recipients." *Journal of Pediatric Psychology* 32, no. 5 (2006): 571–81.

Maitland, Ian. "The Great Non-Debate over International Sweatshops." In *Ethical Theory and Business*, edited by Tom L. Beauchamp and Norman E. Bowie. 7th edition. New York: Pearson Education, 2004: 579–90.

Marcon, Alessandro R., Blake Murdoch, and Timothy Caulfield. "Fake News Portrayals of Stem Cells and Stem Cell Research." *Regenerative Medicine* 12, no. 7 (2017): 765–75.

Martin, Adrienne. *How We Hope: A Moral Psychology*. Princeton, NJ: Princeton University Press, 2016.

Martin, Adrienne M. "Hope and Exploitation." *Hastings Center Report* 38, no. 5 (2008): 49–55.

Martin, Adrienne M. "Hopes and Dreams." *Philosophy and Phenomenological Research* 83, no. 1 (2011): 148–73.

Martin, Melissa, and Mary Agnes Welch. "City Man Who Ran Stem-Cell Trial for MS Patients Fabricated Credentials, Overstated Results." *Winnipeg Free Press*, January 13, 2015, sec. News. https://www.winnipegfreepress.com/breakingnews/Sufferers-feel-swindled-288496041.html.

Martinich, Rex. "Broad Wants Exemptions for Asylum Seeker Ban." *Wimmera Mail-Times*, November 9, 2016.

Marx, Karl. *Karl Marx: Selected Writings*. Edited by David McLellan. New York: Oxford University Press, 2000.

Mayer, Robert. "Sweatshops, Exploitation, and Moral Responsibility." *Journal of Social Philosophy* 38, no. 4 (2007): 605–19.

Mayer, Robert. "What's Wrong with Exploitation?" *Journal of Applied Philosophy* 24, no. 2 (2007): 137–50.

McBride, Gail. "Phase One Trials Can Exploit Terminally Ill Patients." *British Medical Journal* 308, no. 6930 (1994): 679–80.

McClanahan, Carolyn. "People Are Raising $650 Million on GoFundMe Each Year to Attack Rising Healthcare Costs." *Forbes*, August 13, 2018. https://www.forbes.com/sites/carolynmcclanahan/2018/08/13/using-gofundme-to-attack-health-care-costs/.

Mcfarland, Sheena. "Victims Face Deportation." *Salt Lake Tribune*, May 10, 2009. https://archive.sltrib.com/article.php?id=&itype=ngpsid.

Medical Board of Australia. "Good Medical Practice: A Code of Conduct for Doctors in Australia." Medical Board of Australia, 2014. https://www. medicalboard.gov.au/Codes-Guidelines-Policies/Code-of-conduct. aspx.Mershon, Erin. "'Right-to-Try' Intended to Weaken FDA, Key Senator Says in Blunt Remarks." *STAT*, May 31, 2018. https://www.statnews.com/ 2018/05/31/right-to-try-ron-johnson/.

Mershon, Erin. "Trump Signs Right-to-Try Legislation, Widening Access to Experimental Drugs." *STAT*, May 30, 2018. https://www.statnews.com/ 2018/05/30/trump-signs-right-to-try/.

Meyers, C. D. "Moral Duty, Individual Responsibility, and Sweatshop Exploitation." *Journal of Social Philosophy* 38, no. 4 (2007): 620–26.

Meyers, Chris. "Wrongful Beneficence: Exploitation and Third World Sweatshops." *Journal of Social Philosophy* 35, no. 3 (2004): 319–33.

Miller, Franklin G., and Howard Brody. "Clinical Equipoise and the Incoherence of Research Ethics." *The Journal of Medicine and Philosophy: A Forum for Bioethics and Philosophy of Medicine* 32, no. 2 (January 1, 2007): 151–65. https://doi.org/10.1080/03605310701255750.

Miller, Franklin G., and Steven Joffe. "Phase 1 Oncology Trials and Informed Consent." *Journal of Medical Ethics* 39, no. 12 (2013): 761–64.

Miller, Matthew. "Phase I Cancer Trials: A Collusion of Misunderstanding." *Hastings Center Report* 30, no. 4 (2000): 34–43.

Milona, Michael, and Katie Stockdale. "A Perceptual Theory of Hope." *Ergo: An Open Access Journal of Philosophy* 5, no. 8 (2018): 203–22.

Moch, Kenneth I. "Ethical Crossroads: Expanded Access, Patient Advocacy, and The #SaveJosh Social Media Campaign." *Medicine Access@ Point of Care* 1, no. 1 (2017): e119–30.

"Model Dreams." *South China Morning Post*, August 11, 1998.

Moore, Bryanna. "Medical Crowdfunding and the Virtuous Donor." *Bioethics* 33, no. 2 (2019): 238–44.

Morley, Jefferson. "Why Slam Kids' Dreams?" *San Jose Mercury News*, March 28, 1995.

Munsie, Megan, and Insoo Hyun. "A Question of Ethics: Selling Autologous Stem Cell Therapies Flaunts Professional Standards." *Stem Cell Research* 13, no. 3 (2014): 647–53.

Munz, Michele. "Missouri's 'Right to Try' Law No Guarantee Patient Will Get Experimental Drugs." *St. Louis Post-Dispatch*, May 20, 2015. https:// www.stltoday.com/news/local/metro/missouri-s-right-to-try-law-no-guarantee-patient-will/article_05c07958-5217-5c3f-9f15-1a43c8a3e740. html.

Murdoch, Blake, Alessandro R. Marcon, Daniel Downie, and Timothy Caulfield. "Media Portrayal of Illness-Related Medical Crowdfunding:

A Content Analysis of Newspaper Articles in the United States and Canada." *PloS One* 14, no. 4 (2019): e0215805.

Murdoch, Blake, Amy Zarzeczny, and Timothy Caulfield. "Exploiting Science? A Systematic Analysis of Complementary and Alternative Medicine Clinic Websites' Marketing of Stem Cell Therapies." *BMJ Open* 8, no. 2 (2018): e019414.

Murdoch, Charles E., and Christopher Thomas Scott. "Stem Cell Tourism and the Power of Hope." *The American Journal of Bioethics* 10, no. 5 (2010): 16–23.

Murphy, Wendy. "When We Exploit Hope, Feed Greed." *The Patriot Ledger*, December 3, 2011.

My Right to Try Now. *Matt Bellina's Case for The Right to Try*, 2017. https://www.youtube.com/watch?v=n-t9j8mvbNE.

Myerson, Allen R. "In Principle, a Case For More 'Sweatshops.'" *New York Times*, June 22, 1997, sec. Week in Review. https://www.nytimes.com/1997/06/22/weekinreview/in-principle-a-case-for-more-sweatshops.html.

"Mystery Call Offers Prize." *Wiltshire Gazette and Herald*, June 19, 2002. https://www.gazetteandherald.co.uk/news/7347542.mystery-call-offers-prize/.

Nascimento, Nathan, Brent Gardner, David Barnes, and Daniel Garza. "Letter to the Honorable Greg Walden," January 8, 2018. https://freedompartners.org/wp-content/uploads/2018/01/RTT-Letter-to-Chairman-Walden-1.5.18-3.pdf.

Natta, Don van. "Sweatshop Job Abuse Worsening, Workers Say." *New York Times*, September 13, 1995, sec. New York. https://www.nytimes.com/1995/09/13/nyregion/sweatshop-job-abuse-worsening-workers-say.html.

Néron, Pierre-Yves, and Wayne Norman. "Citizenship, Inc.: Do We Really Want Businesses to Be Good Corporate Citizens?" *Business Ethics Quarterly* 18, no. 1 (2008): 1–26.

Newman, Melanie. "Is Cancer Fundraising Fuelling Quackery?" *BMJ: British Medical Journal* 362 (2018): k3829.

Newman, Melanie, and Jim Reed. "Cancer Crowdfunding 'Couldn't Save My Daughter.'" *BBC News*, March 6, 2019. https://www.bbc.com/news/health-47442946.

Nierop-van Baalen, Carine, Maria Grypdonck, Ann Van Hecke, and Sofie Verhaeghe. "Hope Dies Last . . . A Qualitative Study into the Meaning of Hope for People with Cancer in the Palliative Phase." *European Journal of Cancer Care* 25, no. 4 (2016): 570–79.

Nietzsche, Friedrich. *Human, All Too Human: A Book for Free Spirits*. Cambridge: Cambridge University Press, 1996.

Noell, Edd S. "Bargaining, Consent and the Just Wage in the Sources of Scholastic Economic Thought." *Journal of the History of Economic Thought* 20, no. 4 (1998): 467–78.

Norris, Andrew. "Becoming Who We Are: Democracy and the Political Problem of Hope." *Critical Horizons* 9, no. 1 (2008): 77–89.

Norton, Helen. "The Government's Lies and the Constitution." *Indiana Law Journal* 91 (2015): 73–120.

Novas, Carlos. "The Political Economy of Hope: Patients' Organizations, Science and Biovalue." *BioSocieties* 1, no. 3 (2006): 289–305.

Nyamathi, Adeline M., Mohanarani Suhadev, Soumya Swaminathan, and John L. Fahey. "Perceptions of a Community Sample about Participation in Future HIV Vaccine Trials in South India." *AIDS and Behavior* 11, no. 4 (July 1, 2007): 619–27. https://doi.org/10.1007/s10461-006-9173-8.

Nycum, Gillian, and Lynette Reid. "The Harm-Benefit Tradeoff in 'Bad Deal' Trials." *Kennedy Institute of Ethics Journal* 17, no. 4 (2007): 321–50. https://doi.org/10.1353/ken.2008.0004.

O'Brien, Ciara, Louise Carter, Natalie Cook, and Emma Dean. "Novel Early Phase Clinical Trial Design in Oncology." *Pharmaceutical Medicine* 31, no. 5 (2017): 297–307.

O'Cleirigh, Fiona. "It's Time to Pay Interns What They Are Worth." *The Guardian*, October 11, 2010.

Ogbogu, Ubaka, Jenny Du, and Yonida Koukio. "The Involvement of Canadian Physicians in Promoting and Providing Unproven and Unapproved Stem Cell Interventions." *BMC Medical Ethics* 19, no. 1 (2018): 32.

Ogbogu, Ubaka, Li Du, Christen Rachul, Lisa Bélanger, and Timothy Caulfield. "Chinese Newspaper Coverage of (Unproven) Stem Cell Therapies and Their Providers." *Stem Cell Reviews and Reports* 9, no. 2 (2013): 111–118.

O'Neill, Onora. *Constructions of Reason: Explorations of Kant's Practical Philosophy.* Cambridge; New York: Cambridge University Press, 1990.

Ontario Stem Cell Treatment Centre. "Ontario Stem Cell Treatment Centre: Dr. Eric Robinson Orthopaedic Surgeon, Dr. Barr Plastic Surgeon." Accessed October 29, 2019. https://stemcellrepair.ca/staff/.

Oosterhout, J. (Hans) van. "Corporate Citizenship: An Idea Whose Time Has Not Yet Come." *The Academy of Management Review* 30, no. 4 (2005): 677–81.

Orentlicher, David. "Universality and Its Limits: When Research Ethics Can Reflect Local Circumstances." *The Journal of Law, Medicine & Ethics* 30, no. 3 (2002): 403–10. https://doi.org/10.1111/j.1748-720X.2002.tb00409.x.

Palad, Varsha, and Jeremy Snyder. "'We Don't Want Him Worrying about How He Will Pay to Save His Life': Using Medical Crowdfunding to Explore Lived Experiences with Addiction Services in Canada." *International Journal of Drug Policy* 65 (2019): 73–77.

Paulus, Trena M., and Katherine R. Roberts. "Crowdfunding a 'Real-Life Superhero': The Construction of Worthy Bodies in Medical Campaign Narratives." *Discourse, Context & Media* 21 (2018): 64–72.

Penman, Andrew, and Nick Sommerlad. "Visas Scam Rides Again." *The Mirror*, February 19, 2009.

Global News. "Penticton Teen Hopes to Have Experimental Cancer Treatment in Texas." March 5, 2015. https://globalnews.ca/news/1867313/penticton-teen-hopes-to-have-experimental-cancer-treatment-in-texas/.

Pentz, Rebecca D., Margaret White, R. Donald Harvey, Zachary Luke Farmer, Yuan Liu, Colleen Lewis, Olga Dashevskaya, Taofeek Owonikoko, and Fadlo R. Khuri. "Therapeutic Misconception, Misestimation, and Optimism in Participants Enrolled in Phase 1 Trials." *Cancer* 118, no. 18 (2012): 4571–78.

Petersen, Alan, Casimir MacGregor, and Megan Munsie. "Stem Cell Tourism Exploits People by Marketing Hope." *The Conversation*, July 15, 2014. http://theconversation.com/stem-cell-tourism-exploits-people-by-marketing-hope-29146.

Petersen, Alan, Casimir MacGregor, and Megan Munsie. "Stem Cell Tourism Exploits People by Marketing Hope." *The Conversation*. Accessed October 23, 2019. http://theconversation.com/stem-cell-tourism-exploits-people-by-marketing-hope-29146.

Petersen, Alan, Megan Munsie, Claire Tanner, Casimir MacGregor, and Jane Brophy. "Managing Hope." In *Stem Cell Tourism and the Political Economy of Hope*, edited by Alan Petersen, Megan Munsie, Claire Tanner, Casimir MacGregor, Jane Brophy. London, UK: Springer, 2017: 59–82.

Petersen, Alan, Megan Munsie, Claire Tanner, Casimir MacGregor, and Jane Brophy. "Selling Hope in China." In *Stem Cell Tourism and the Political Economy of Hope*, 121–154. Springer, 2017.

Petersen, Alan, and Kate Seear. "Technologies of Hope: Techniques of the Online Advertising of Stem Cell Treatments." *New Genetics and Society* 30, no. 4 (2011): 329–46.

Petersen, Alan, Kate Seear, and Megan Munsie. "Therapeutic Journeys: The Hopeful Travails of Stem Cell Tourists." *Sociology of Health & Illness* 36, no. 5 (2014): 670–685.

Petersen, Alan, Kate Seear, and Megan Munsie. "Therapeutic Journeys: The Hopeful Travails of Stem Cell Tourists." *Sociology of Health & Illness* 36, no. 5 (2014): 670–685.

Pettit, Philip. "Hope and Its Place in Mind." *The Annals of the American Academy of Political and Social Science* 592, no. 1 (2004): 152–165.

Picard, André. "Do the Dying Have the Right to Experimental Drugs?" *Globe & Mail*, April 11, 2018, sec. Opinion. https://www.theglobeandmail.com/opinion/do-the-dying-have-the-right-to-experimental-drugs/article24377706/.

Pimentel, Benjamin. "Temporary Workers Sue HP over Overtime Pay." *SFGate*, January 22, 2003. https://www.sfgate.com/business/article/Temporary-workers-sue-HP-over-overtime-pay-2639704.php.

Pogge, Thomas. "Access to Medicines." *Public Health Ethics* 1, no. 2 (2008): 73–82.

Pogge, Thomas. "Testing Our Drugs on the Poor Abroad." In *Exploitation and Developing Countries: The Ethics of Clinical Research*, edited by Jennifer S. Hawkins and Ezekiel Emanuel. Princeton, NJ: Princeton University Press, 2008: 105–41.

Pogge, Thomas. "World Poverty and Human Rights." *Ethics & International Affairs* 19, no. 1 (March 2005): 1–7. https://doi.org/10.1111/j.1747-7093.2005.tb00484.x.

Pogge, Thomas W. *World Poverty and Human Rights*. 2nd edition. Cambridge: Polity, 2008.

Popper, Helen. "Bolivians See Dreams Fade In Argentina." *Washington Post*, May 21, 2006. https://www.washingtonpost.com/archive/politics/2006/05/21/bolivians-see-dreams-fade-in-argentina-spanclassbankheadexploitation-widespread-in-clothing-sweatshopsspan/de589d80-98f9-4b63-a809-8a38afc7e56a/.

Porter, Henry. "Crowd Control." *The Guardian*, October 12, 1995.

Preiss, Joshua. "Global Labor Justice and the Limits of Economic Analysis." *Business Ethics Quarterly* 24, no. 1 (2014): 55–83.

Pugh, Tony. "Supplements Stuff of Fraud, Senators Told." *Philadelphia Inquirer*, September 11, 2001.

Pullman, Daryl, Amy Zarzeczny, and André Picard. "Media, Politics and Science Policy: MS and Evidence from the CCSVI Trenches." *BMC Medical Ethics* 14, no. 1 (2013): 6.

Quenneville, Guy. "Injured Humboldt Broncos and Families of Dead 'Urgently' Need Advances from $15M GoFundMe Pool." *CBC News*, July 5, 2018. https://www.cbc.ca/news/canada/saskatoon/humboldt-broncos-gofundme-survivors-saskatchewan-1.4734347.

Rachul, Christen M., Ivona Percec, and Timothy Caulfield. "The Fountain of Stem Cell-Based Youth? Online Portrayals of Anti-Aging Stem Cell Technologies." *Aesthetic Surgery Journal* 35, no. 6 (2015): 730–36.

Rachul, Christen, John EJ Rasko, and Timothy Caulfield. "Implicit Hype? Representations of Platelet Rich Plasma in the News Media." *PloS One* 12, no. 8 (2017): e0182496.

Radin, Tara J., and Martin Calkins. "The Struggle against Sweatshops: Moving Toward Responsible Global Business." *Journal of Business Ethics* 66, no. 2 (2006): 261–72.

Rasmussen, Heather N., Kristin Koetting O'Byrne, Marcy Vandamente, and Brian P. Cole. "Hope and Physical Health." In *The Oxford Handbook of Hope*, edited by Matthew W. Gallagher and Shane J. Lopez. Oxford: Oxford University Press, 2017: 159–68.

Raus, Kasper. "An Analysis of Common Ethical Justifications for Compassionate Use Programs for Experimental Drugs." *BMC Medical*

Ethics 17, no. 1 (2016): 60.Rave, D. Theodore. "Politicians as Fiduciaries." *Harvard Law Review* 126, no. 3 (2013): 671–739.

"Refugees Wait as Camp's Future Is Decided." *Birmingham Post,* July 13, 2002.

Regenberg, Alan C., Lauren A. Hutchinson, Benjamin Schanker, and Debra J. H. Mathews. "Medicine on the Fringe: Stem Cell-Based Interventions in Advance of Evidence." *Stem Cells* 27, no. 9 (2009): 2312–19.

Regenexx. "Regenexx: Stem Cell Therapy & Platelet Rich Plasma for Arthritis & Injuries." Accessed October 29, 2019. https://regenexx.com/.

Resnik, David B. "Exploitation in Biomedical Research." *Theoretical Medicine and Bioethics* 24, no. 3 (May 1, 2003): 233–59. https://doi.org/10.1023/A:1024811830049.

Resnik, David B. "The Clinical Investigator-Subject Relationship: A Contextual Approach." *Philosophy, Ethics, and Humanities in Medicine* 4, no. 1 (December 3, 2009): 16. https://doi.org/10.1186/1747-5341-4-16.

Resnik, David B. "Therapeutic Misconception, Unrealistic Optimism, and Hope in Phase I Oncology Trials." *Journal of Clinical Research Best Practices* 14, no. 8 (2018): 1–6.

Revello, Lidia. "Shows 'Exploit' People Says Star." *Aberdeen Evening Express,* May 6, 2014.Richardson, Henry S. *Moral Entanglements: The Ancillary-Care Obligations of Medical Researchers.* Oxford: Oxford University Press, 2012.

Richardson, Henry S., and Leah Belsky. "The Ancillary-Care Responsibilities of Medical Researchers: An Ethical Framework for Thinking about the Clinical Care That Researchers Owe Their Subjects." *Hastings Center Report* 34, no. 1 (2004): 25–33. https://doi.org/10.2307/3528248.Roberts, Mike. "'A Wedding Party Hijack': Left Behind in India with a Son, A Mother Demands Financial Support." *The Province,* October 17, 2005.

Rolfe, John, and Rosemarie Lentini. "Bond Was Her Word: Subletting Opportunity That Proved Too Good to Be True." *Daily Telegraph,* April 26, 2012.

Rosenberg, Tina. "Globalization." *New York Times,* August 18, 2002, sec. Magazine. https://www.nytimes.com/2002/08/18/magazine/globalization.html.

Sample, Ruth J. *Exploitation: What It Is and Why It's Wrong.* Lanham, MD: Rowman & Littlefield, 2003.

Scherer, Andreas Georg, and Guido Palazzo. "Toward a Political Conception of Corporate Responsibility: Business and Society Seen from a Habermasian Perspective." *Academy of Management Review* 32, no. 4 (2007): 1096–120.

Scherer, Andreas Georg, Guido Palazzo, and Dorothée Baumann. "Global Rules and Private Actors: Toward a New Role of the Transnational Corporation in Global Governance." *Business Ethics Quarterly* 16, no. 4 (2006): 505–32.

Scott, Christopher Thomas, Mindy C. DeRouen, and LaVera M. Crawley. "The Language of Hope: Therapeutic Intent in Stem-Cell Clinical Trials." *AJOB Primary Research* 1, no. 3 (2010): 4–11.

Seidenfeld, Justine, Elizabeth Horstmann, Ezekiel J. Emanuel, and Christine Grady. "Participants in Phase 1 Oncology Research Trials: Are They Vulnerable?" *Archives of Internal Medicine* 168, no. 1 (January 14, 2008): 16–20. https://doi.org/10.1001/archinternmed.2007.6.

"Sex Ring Smashed." *Sunday Tasmanian*, July 3, 2005.

Shah, Jatin Y., Amruta Phadtare, Dimple Rajgor, Meenakshi Vaghasia, Shreyasee Pradhan, Hilary Zelko, and Ricardo Pietrobon. "What Leads Indians to Participate in Clinical Trials? A Meta-Analysis of Qualitative Studies." *PLOS One* 5, no. 5 (May 20, 2010): e10730. https://doi.org/10.1371/journal.pone.0010730.

Shakespeare, William. *Richard II: The Oxford Shakespeare*. Oxford: Oxford University Press, 2011.

Shamoo, Adil E., and David B. Resnik. "Strategies to Minimize Risks and Exploitation in Phase One Trials on Healthy Subjects." *The American Journal of Bioethics* 6, no. 3 (2006): W1–W13.

Shepperd, James A., Erika A. Waters, Neil D. Weinstein, and William MP Klein. "A Primer on Unrealistic Optimism." *Current Directions in Psychological Science* 24, no. 3 (2015): 232–37.

Simpson, Christy. "When Hope Makes Us Vulnerable: A Discussion of Patient–Healthcare Provider Interactions in the Context of Hope." *Bioethics* 18, no. 5 (2004): 428–47.

Sipp, Douglas. "The Malignant Niche: Safe Spaces for Toxic Stem Cell Marketing." *NPJ Regenerative Medicine* 2, no. 1 (2017): 33.

Sipp, Douglas, Pamela G. Robey, and Leigh Turner. "Clear up This Stem-Cell Mess." *Nature* 561, no. 7724 (2018): 455–57.

Snyder, C. R., Carla Berg, Julia T. Woodward, Amber Gum, Kevin L. Rand, Kristin K. Wrobleski, Jill Brown, and Ashley Hackman. "Hope against the Cold: Individual Differences in Trait Hope and Acute Pain Tolerance on the Cold Pressor Task." *Journal of Personality* 73, no. 2 (2005): 287–312.

Snyder, Charles R., Cheri Harris, John R. Anderson, Sharon A. Holleran, Lori M. Irving, Sandra T. Sigmon, Lauren Yoshinobu, June Gibb, Charyle Langelle, and Pat Harney. "The Will and the Ways: Development and Validation of an Individual-Differences Measure of Hope." *Journal of Personality and Social Psychology* 60, no. 4 (1991): 570.

Snyder, Jeremy. "Crowdfunding for Medical Care: Ethical Issues in an Emerging Health Care Funding Practice." *Hastings Center Report* 46, no. 6 (2016): 36–42.

Snyder, Jeremy. "Exploitation and Demeaning Choices." *Politics, Philosophy & Economics* 12, no. 4 (2013): 345–60.

Snyder, Jeremy. "What's the Matter with Price Gouging?" *Business Ethics Quarterly* 19, no. 2 (2009): 275–93.

Snyder, Jeremy C. "Needs Exploitation." *Ethical Theory and Moral Practice* 11, no. 4 (2008): 389–405.

Snyder, Jeremy, Krystyna Adams, Y. Y. Chen, Daniel Birch, Timothy Caulfield, I. Glenn Cohen, Valorie A. Crooks, Judy Illes, and Amy Zarzeczny. "Navigating Physicians' Ethical and Legal Duties to Patients Seeking Unproven Interventions Abroad." *Canadian Family Physician* 61, no. 7 (2015): 584–86.

Snyder, Jeremy, Krystyna Adams, Valorie A. Crooks, David Whitehurst, and Jennifer Vallee. "'I Knew What Was Going to Happen If I Did Nothing and so I Was Going to Do Something': Faith, Hope, and Trust in the Decisions of Canadians with Multiple Sclerosis to Seek Unproven Interventions Abroad." *BMC Health Services Research* 14, no. 1 (2014): 445.Snyder, Jeremy, and Timothy Caulfield. "Patients' Crowdfunding Campaigns for Alternative Cancer Treatments." *The Lancet Oncology* 20, no. 1 (2019): 28–29.

Snyder, Jeremy, Valorie A. Crooks, Annalise Mathers, and Peter Chow-White. "Appealing to the Crowd: Ethical Justifications in Canadian Medical Crowdfunding Campaigns." *Journal of Medical Ethics* 43, no. 6 (2017): 364–67.

Snyder, Jeremy, and Leigh Turner. "Crowdfunding for Stem Cell-Based Interventions to Treat Neurologic Diseases and Injuries." *Neurology* 93, no. 6 (2019): 252–58.

Snyder, Jeremy, and Leigh Turner. "Selling Stem Cell 'Treatments' as Research: Prospective Customer Perspectives from Crowdfunding Campaigns." *Regenerative Medicine* 13, no. 4 (2018): 375–84.

Snyder, Jeremy, Leigh Turner, and Valorie A. Crooks. "Crowdfunding for Unproven Stem Cell Procedures Spreads Misinformation." *STAT*, August 6, 2018. https://www.statnews.com/2018/08/06/crowdfunding-for-unproven-stem-cell-procedures-wastes-money-and-spreads-misinformation/.

Snyder, Jeremy, Leigh Turner, and Valorie A. Crooks. "Crowdfunding for Unproven Stem Cell–Based Interventions." *JAMA* 319, no. 18 (2018): 1935–36.

Sollars, Gordon G., and Fred Englander. "Sweatshops: Kant and Consequences." *Business Ethics Quarterly* 17, no. 1 (2007): 115–33.

Sproates, Helen. "Gemma Nuttall Cancer Fund." gofundme.com, October 22, 2016. https://www.gofundme.com/f/teamgemma.

Stanton, Annette L., Sharon Danoff-burg, and Melissa E. Huggins. "The First Year after Breast Cancer Diagnosis: Hope and Coping Strategies as Predictors of Adjustment." *Psycho-Oncology: Journal of the Psychological, Social and Behavioral Dimensions of Cancer* 11, no. 2 (2002): 93–102.

Steinbeck, John. *The Grapes of Wrath*. New York: Penguin, 2006.

Steiner, Hillel. "A Liberal Theory of Exploitation." *Ethics* 94, no. 2 (1984): 225–41.

Subbaraman, Nidhi. "Experts Balk at Large Trial of Stem Cells for Autism." *Spectrum* (blog), July 14, 2014. https://www.spectrumnews.org/news/experts-balk-at-large-trial-of-stem-cells-for-autism/.

Sulmasy, Daniel P., Alan B. Astrow, M. Kai He, Damon M. Seils, Neal J. Meropol, Ellyn Micco, and Kevin P. Weinfurt. "The Culture of Faith and Hope: Patients' Justifications for Their High Estimations of Expected Therapeutic Benefit When Enrolling in Early Phase Oncology Trials." *Cancer* 116, no. 15 (2010): 3702–11.

Sweetman, Terry. "After 13 Years, the Australian Writers-Authors Group Has Packed up Its Quills and Closed Its Doors." *Sunday Mail*, March 1, 1998.

Szabo, Liz. "Doctor Accused of Selling False Hope to Families." *USA Today*, November 15, 2013. https://www.usatoday.com/story/news/nation/2013/11/15/stanislaw-burzynski-cancer-controversy/2994561/.

Szklarski, Cassandra. "Plan to End Immigrant Backlog Gets $700 Million." *Vancouver Sun*, November 25, 2005.

Tanner, Claire, Megan Munsie, Doug Sipp, Leigh Turner, and Chloe Wheatland. "The Politics of Evidence in Online Illness Narratives: An Analysis of Crowdfunding for Purported Stem Cell Treatments." *Health* 23, no. 4 (2019): 436–57.

Temple, Robert, and Susan S. Ellenberg. "Placebo-Controlled Trials and Active-Control Trials in the Evaluation of New Treatments. Part 1: Ethical and Scientific Issues." *Annals of Internal Medicine* 133, no. 6 (2000): 455–63.

"The Government as Bookie." *The Globe and Mail*, May 23, 1995.

Therapeutic Solutions International Inc. "Therapeutic Solutions International Completes Phase 1 Clinical Trial in Advanced Cancer Patients for Right to Try Access of Its StemVacs Product for American Cancer Patients." *GlobeNewswire News Room*, September 4, 2018. http://www.globenewswire.com/news-release/2018/09/04/1564969/0/en/Therapeutic-Solutions-International-Completes-Phase-1-Clinical-Trial-in-Advanced-Cancer-Patients-for-Right-to-Try-Access-of-its-StemVacs-Product-for-American-Cancer-Patients.html.

Thompson, Alexandra. "Parents of an Autistic Boy, 11, Claim He Spoke His First Full Sentence." *Daily Mail*, April 11, 2019. https://www.dailymail.co.uk/health/article-6912381/Parents-non-verbal-autistic-schoolboy-11-claim-spoke-sentence.html.

Thompson, Alexandra. "Parents of Autistic Boy Hope to Raise £26,500 for Stem Cell Treatment." *Daily Mail*, January 23, 2019. https://www.dailymail.co.uk/health/article-6623311/Parents-non-verbal-autistic-boy-hope-raise-26-500-pay-stem-cell-treatment-Miami.html.

Thorsell, Thorsell. "Games Governments Play." *Globe & Mail*, January 15, 1994.

Todd, Patty. "Stem Cell Therapy for Hayden Butler." GoFundMe, October 12, 2017. https://www.gofundme.com/f/2cdpj7g.

Turner, Leigh. "Direct-to-Consumer Marketing of Stem Cell Interventions by Canadian Businesses." *Regenerative Medicine* 13, no. 06 (2018): 643–58.

Turner, Leigh. "The US Direct-to-Consumer Marketplace for Autologous Stem Cell Interventions." *Perspectives in Biology and Medicine* 61, no. 1 (2018): 7–24.

Turner, Leigh, and Paul Knoepfler. "Selling Stem Cells in the USA: Assessing the Direct-to-Consumer Industry." *Cell Stem Cell* 19, no. 2 (2016): 154–57.

"Utterly Wrong to Exploit the Hope of Those Wanting a Baby." *Bath Chronicle*, July 20, 2016.

Valdman, Mikhail. "A Theory of Wrongful Exploitation." *Philosopher's Imprint* 9, no. 6 (2009): 1–14.

Valdman, Mikhail. "Exploitation and Injustice." *Social Theory and Practice* 34, no. 4 (2008): 551–72.

"Vital Medical Center." Accessed October 29, 2019. http://vitalmedicalcenterinc.com/.

Vox, Ford, Kelly McBride Folkers, Angela Turi, and Arthur L. Caplan. "Medical Crowdfunding for Scientifically Unsupported or Potentially Dangerous Treatments." *JAMA* 320, no. 16 (2018): 1705–6.

"Waging War against a Deadly Disorder." *New Zealand Herald*, February 4, 2006.

Weber, Caroline. "Holiday Books: Fashion." *New York Times*, December 3, 2006.

Weber, Jeffrey S., Laura A. Levit, Peter C. Adamson, Suanna Bruinooge, and Howard A. Burris. "American Society of Clinical Oncology Policy Statement Update: The Critical Role of Phase I Trials in Cancer Research and Treatment." *Journal of Clinical Oncology* 33, no. 3 (2015): 278.

Weinstein, Neil D. "Unrealistic Optimism about Future Life Events." *Journal of Personality and Social Psychology* 39, no. 5 (1980): 806.

Wendler, David, Benjamin Krohmal, Ezekiel J. Emanuel, and Christine Grady. "Why Patients Continue to Participate in Clinical Research." *Archives of Internal Medicine* 168, no. 12 (June 23, 2008): 1294–99. https://doi.org/10.1001/archinte.168.12.1294.

Wertheimer, Alan. *Exploitation*. Princeton, NJ: Princeton University Press, 1999.

Wertheimer, Alan. *Rethinking the Ethics of Clinical Research: Widening the Lens*. Oxford: Oxford University Press, 2010.

Wilcox, Shelley. "The Open Borders Debate on Immigration." *Philosophy Compass* 4, no. 5 (2009): 813–21.

Williams, Randy. "Sorry, Get in Line." *Edmonton Journal*, September 14, 2010.

Wolanski, Paula. "Please Help Malgosia Get Stem Cell Therapy." GoFundMe, June 6, 2019. https://www.gofundme.com/f/please-help-malgosia-get-stem-cell-therapy.

World Medical Association. "World Medical Association International Code of Medical Ethics." World Medical Association, 2006. https://www.wma.net/policies-post/wma-international-code-of-medical-ethics/.

Yates, Connie. "Charlie Gard #charliesfight." GoFundMe, January 30, 2017. https://www.gofundme.com/f/please-help-to-save-charlies-life.

Young, Iris Marion. *Responsibility for Justice*. Oxford: Oxford University Press, 2010.

Zarzeczny, Amy, Timothy Caulfield, Ubaka Ogbogu, Peter Bell, Valorie A. Crooks, Kalina Kamenova, Zubin Master, Christen Rachul, Jeremy Snyder, and Maeghan Toews. "Professional Regulation: A Potentially Valuable Tool in Responding to 'Stem Cell Tourism.'" *Stem Cell Reports* 3, no. 3 (2014): 379–84.

Zettler, Patricia J., and Henry T. Greely. "The Strange Allure of State 'Right-to-Try' Laws." *JAMA Internal Medicine* 174, no. 12 (2014): 1885–86.

Zuckerman, Diana. "Right to Try National Law Would Exploit False Hope." *National Center for Health Research* (blog), March 16, 2017. http://www.center4research.org/right-to-try-exploit-false-hope/.

Zwolinski, Matt. "Structural Exploitation." *Social Philosophy and Policy* 29, no. 1 (2012): 154–79.

Zwolinski, Matt. "Sweatshops, Choice, and Exploitation." *Business Ethics Quarterly* 17, no. 4 (2007): 689–727.

Index